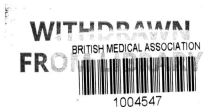

VASCULAR AND
ENDOVASCULAR SURGERY

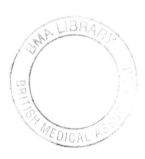

A Companion to Specialist Surgical Practice

Series Editors

O. James Garden
Simon Paterson-Brown

VASCULAR AND ENDOVASCULAR SURGERY

SIXTH EDITION

Edited by

Ian Loftus

MD FRCS

Professor of Vascular Surgery, St George's Vascular Institute,
St George's, University of London, UK

Robert J. Hinchliffe

MD FRCS

Professor of Vascular Surgery, Bristol Centre for Surgical Research,
Bristol NIHR Biomedical Research Centre, University of Bristol, UK

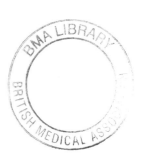

For additional online content visit ExpertConsult.com

ELSEVIER Edinburgh   London   New York   Oxford   Philadelphia   St Louis   Sydney   2019

ELSEVIER

First edition 1997
Second edition 2001
Third edition 2005
Fourth edition 2009
Fifth edition 2014
Sixth edition 2019

Notice

Practitioners and researchers must always rely on their own experience and knowledge in evaluating and using any information, methods, compounds or experiments described herein. Because of rapid advances in the medical sciences, in particular, independent verification of diagnoses and drug dosages should be made. To the fullest extent of the law, no responsibility is assumed by Elsevier, authors, editors or contributors for any injury and/or damage to persons or property as a matter of products liability, negligence or otherwise, or from any use or operation of any methods, products, instructions, or ideas contained in the material herein.

ISBN: 978-0-7020-7253-6

Printed in China
Last digit is the print number: 9 8 7 6 5 4 3 2 1

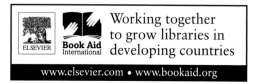

Working together
to grow libraries in
developing countries

www.elsevier.com • www.bookaid.org

Content Strategist: Laurence Hunter
Content Development Specialist: Lynn Watt
Project Manager: Umarani Natarajan
Design: Miles Hitchen
Illustration Manager: Nichole Beard
Illustrator: MPS North America LLC

Contents

Contents

Series Editors' preface

The *Companion to Specialist Surgical Practice* series has now come of age. This Sixth Edition takes the series to a different level since it was first published in 1997. The intention from the outset was to ensure that we could support the educational needs of those in the later years of specialist surgical training and of consultant surgeons in independent practice who wished for contemporary, evidence-based information on the subspecialist areas relevant to their general surgical practice. Although there still seems to be a role for larger reference surgical textbooks, and having contributed to many of these, we appreciate that it is difficult for them to keep pace with changing surgical practice.

This Sixth Edition continues to keep abreast of the increasing specialisation in general surgery. The rise of minimal access surgery and therapy, and the desire of some subspecialities, such as breast and vascular surgery, to separate away from 'general surgery' may have proved challenging in some countries. However, they also underline the importance for all surgeons of being aware of current developments in their surgical field. This series as a consequence continues to place emphasis on the need for surgeons to deliver a high-quality emergency surgical practice. The importance of evidence-based practice remains throughout, and authors have provided recommendations and highlighted key resources within each chapter. The ebook version of the textbook has also enabled improved access to the reference abstracts and links to video content relevant to many of the chapters.

We have recognised in this Sixth Edition that new blood is required to maintain the vitality of content. We are indebted to the volume editors, and contributors, who have stood down since the last edition and welcome the new leadership on several volumes. The contents have been comprehensively updated by our contributors and editorial team. We remain grateful for the support and encouragement of Laurence Hunter and Lynn Watt at Elsevier. We trust that our original vision of delivering an up-to-date affordable text has been met and that readers, whether in training or independent practice, will find this Sixth Edition an invaluable resource.

O. James Garden, CBE, BSc, MBChB, MD, FRCS (Glas), FRCS(Ed), FRCP(Ed), FRACS(Hon), FRCSC (Hon), FACS(Hon), FCSHK(Hon), FRCSI(Hon), FRCS(Engl)(Hon), FRSE
Regius Professor of Clinical Surgery, Clinical Surgery, The University of Edinburgh and Honorary Consultant Surgeon, Royal Infirmary of Edinburgh, Edinburgh, UK

Simon Paterson-Brown, MBBS, MPhil, MS, FRCS(Ed), FRCS(Engl), FCSHK, FFST(RCSEd)
Honorary Clinical Senior Lecturer, Clinical Surgery, The University of Edinburgh and Consultant General and Upper Gastrointestinal Surgeon, Royal Infirmary of Edinburgh, Edinburgh, UK

Editors' preface

This, the Sixth Edition of *Vascular and Endovascular Surgery*, continues the concept of previous editions, by providing the reader with an evidence-based contemporary approach to the recognition, assessment and management of vascular conditions.

In recent years, vascular surgery has gone through a period of evolution, perhaps more than many specialities. In some countries, such as the UK, vascular surgery has undergone a complete break from general surgery with the adoption of speciality status in its own right. This has required the creation of a vascular surgical curriculum and postgraduate examination independent of general surgery. With this, there continues to be a significant shift away from open surgery to endovascular interventions, throughout the vascular tree. These changes bring about multiple challenges to the vascular surgical practitioner in training and in established practice, not only in terms of providing a safe and effective clinical practice, but also to those with an interest in service provision. There also remain areas of vascular practice that are an essential core knowledge to other practitioners, including general surgeons, radiologists and cardiac surgeons.

We have embraced these changes and tried to balance the enthusiasm for modern techniques with available evidence, and provide key references within each chapter to guide surgical trainees and established consultants alike. Also in some chapters we have provided video links that we hope you will find interesting and complementary to the text.

We are indebted to the contributors for this and previous editions of the Companion Series. They have provided many hours of toil without compensation, other than the reward of continuing the tradition of teaching in vascular surgery, a tradition that we are proud to be a part of. It has been especially gratifying to work closely with new contributors who bring a fresh approach to many aspects of the text. Their enthusiasm has been matched by the editorial team who have worked especially hard to produce this Sixth Edition in such quick time, ensuring that the content is as contemporary as possible.

We hope you will continue to find this an invaluable resource, whether it be as part of surgical training, during preparation for an exam or complementing day-to-day clinical practice.

Acknowledgements

The editors would like to acknowledge and offer grateful thanks for the input of all previous editions' contributors, without whom this new edition would not have been possible. They would also like to thank the retiring volume editors of the previous editions, Jonathan Beard and Peter Gaines, who did a superb job in developing this volume to its current standard.

Ian Loftus
London
Robert J. Hinchliffe
Bristol

Evidence-based practice in surgery

Critical appraisal for developing evidence-based practice can be obtained from a number of sources, the most reliable being randomised controlled clinical trials, systematic literature reviews, meta-analyses and observational studies. For practical purposes three grades of evidence can be used, analogous to the levels of 'proof' required in a court of law:

1. **Beyond all reasonable doubt.** Such evidence is likely to have arisen from high-quality randomised controlled trials, systematic reviews or high-quality synthesised evidence such as decision analysis, cost-effectiveness analysis or large observational datasets. The studies need to be directly applicable to the population of concern and have clear results. The grade is analogous to burden of proof within a criminal court and may be thought of as corresponding to the usual standard of 'proof' within the medical literature (i.e. $P < 0.05$).

2. **On the balance of probabilities.** In many cases a high-quality review of literature may fail to reach firm conclusions due to conflicting or inconclusive results, trials of poor methodological quality or the lack of evidence in the population to which the guidelines apply. In such cases it may still be possible to make a statement as to the best treatment on the 'balance of probabilities'. This is analogous to the decision in a civil court where all the available evidence will be weighed up and the verdict will depend upon the balance of probabilities.

3. **Not proven.** Insufficient evidence upon which to base a decision, or contradictory evidence.

Depending on the information available, three grades of recommendation can be used:

a. Strong recommendation, which should be followed unless there are compelling reasons to act otherwise.
b. A recommendation based on evidence of effectiveness, but where there may be other factors to take into account in decision-making, for example the user of the guidelines may be expected to take into account patient preferences, local facilities, local audit results or available resources.
c. A recommendation made where there is no adequate evidence as to the most effective practice, although there may be reasons for making a recommendation in order to minimise cost or reduce the chance of error through a locally agreed protocol.

✓✓ Evidence where a conclusion can be reached **'beyond all reasonable doubt'** and therefore where a **strong recommendation** can be given. This will normally be based on evidence levels:
- Ia. Meta-analysis of randomised controlled trials
- Ib. Evidence from at least one randomised controlled trial
- IIa. Evidence from at least one controlled study without randomisation
- IIb. Evidence from at least one other type of quasi-experimental study.

✓ Evidence where a conclusion might be reached **'on the balance of probabilities'** and where there may be other factors involved which influence the recommendation given. This will normally be based on less conclusive evidence than that represented by the double tick icons:
- III. Evidence from non-experimental descriptive studies, such as comparative studies and case–control studies
- IV. Evidence from expert committee reports or opinions or clinical experience of respected authorities, or both.

Evidence that is associated with either a **strong recommendation** or **expert opinion** is highlighted in the text in panels such as those shown above, and is distinguished by either a double or single tick icon, respectively. The references associated with double-tick evidence are listed as Key References at the end of each chapter, along with a short summary of the paper's conclusions where applicable. The full reference list for each chapter is available in the ebook.

The reader is referred to Chapter 1, 'Evaluation of surgical evidence' in the volume *Core Topics in General and Emergency Surgery* of this series, for a more detailed description of this topic.

Contributors

Gillian Atkinson, MCSP
Clinical Specialist Physiotherapist (Amputees),
Mobility and Specialised Rehabilitation Centre,
Northern General Hospital, Sheffield, UK

Jill J.F. Belch, MBChB, MD(Hons), FRCP, FRS
Professor of Vascular Medicine, Division of Clinical
and Molecular Medicine, Ninewells Hospital and
Medical School, Dundee, UK

Romain Belmonte, MD
Department of Vascular Surgery, University Hospital
of Poitiers, Poitiers, France

Martin Björck, MD, PhD
Professor (Chair) of Vascular Surgery, Department
of Surgical Sciences, Vascular Surgery, Uppsala
University, Uppsala, Sweden

Stephen Black, MD, FRCS
Department of Vascular Surgery, St Thomas'
Hospital, London, UK

**Peter W.G. Brown, BSc, MBChB,
FRCS(Ed), FRCR**
Diagnostic Imaging, Sheffield Teaching Hospitals,
Sheffield, UK

Jan Brunkwall, MD, PhD, FEBVS
Professor and Chairman, Department of Vascular
Surgery, Heart Centre, University Hospital of
Cologne, Cologne, Germany

Patrick Coughlin, MBChB, MD, FRCS(Eng)
Consultant Vascular Surgeon, Vascular Surgery,
Addenbrooke's Hospital, Cambridge, UK

Robert Fitridge, MBBS, MS, FRACS
Professor of Vascular Surgery, The University of
Adelaide; Head of Unit, Vascular and Endovascular
Surgery, Royal Adelaide Hospital, Adelaide,
Australia

Lucinda Frank, MBChB, BSc
Clinical Fellow, Vascular Surgery, North Bristol NHS
Trust, Bristol, UK

Fran Game, MBBCh, FRCP
Consultant Diabetologist, Diabetes and
Endocrinology, Derby Teaching Hospitals NHS FT,
Derby, UK

Michael Gawenda, MD, PhD
Professor of Surgery, University of Cologne,
Cologne; Head of the Department of Vascular and
Endovascular Surgery, Euregio-Vascular-Centre,
St-Antonius-Hospital, Eschweiler, Germany

Manjit S. Gohel, MBChB, MD, FRCS, FEBVS
Consultant Vascular and Endovascular Surgeon,
Cambridge Vascular Unit, Addenbrooke's
Hospital; Honorary Senior Lecturer, Academic
Department of Vascular Surgery, Imperial College,
London, UK

Robert J. Hinchliffe, MD, FRCS
Professor of Vascular Surgery, Bristol Centre
for Surgical Research, Bristol NIHR Biomedical
Research Centre, University of Bristol, UK

Peter Holt, PhD, FRCS
Reader in Vascular Surgery, St George's Vascular
Institute, St George's Hospital, London, UK

Ian Loftus, MBChB, MD, FRCS
Professor of Vascular Surgery, St George's Vascular
Institute, St George's, University of London,
London, UK

**Jacobus van Marle, MBChB, MMed(Surg),
FCS(SA)**
Professor of Vascular Surgery, Department of
Surgery, Sefako Makgatho Health Sciences
University, Pretoria, South Africa

Ian McCafferty, BSc, MBBS, MRCP, FRCR
Consultant Diagnostic and Interventional
Radiologist, Imaging Department, Queen Elizabeth
Hospital, Birmingham, UK

Andrew R.I. Melville, MBBS, MA, MRCP
Core Medical Trainee, Northwick Park Hospital,
London, UK

Contributors

David C. Mitchell, MA, MBBS, MS, FRCS
Consultant Vascular and Renal Transplant Surgeon, Department of Surgery, Southmead Hospital, North Bristol NHS Trust, Bristol, UK

Ramesh Munjal, MS, FRCS
Consultant and Clinical Lead Neurological and Amputee, Rehabilitation, Mobility and Specialised Rehabilitation Centre, Sheffield Teaching Hospitals, Sheffield, UK

Kurian J. Mylankal, MBBS, MD, FRCS(Edin), FRACS
Consultant Vascular Surgeon, Vascular and Endovascular Surgery, Royal Adelaide Hospital, Adelaide, Australia

A. Ross Naylor, MBChB, MD, FRCS
Professor of Vascular Surgery, Vascular Surgery Group, Division of Cardiovascular Sciences, Leicester Royal Infirmary, Leicester, UK

Benjamin Patterson, PhD, MRCS
St George's NHS Foundation Trust, St George's Vascular Institute, London, UK

Jean-Baptiste Ricco, MD, PhD, FEBVS
Professor and Chief, Department of Vascular Surgery, University Hospital of Poitiers, Poitiers, France

Dirk A. le Roux, MBChB, FCS(SA), CVS(SA)
Consultant Vascular Surgeon, Department of Surgery, University of Witwatersrand, Johannesburg, South Africa

Prakash Saha, PhD, FRCS
Academic Department of Vascular Surgery, St. Thomas' Hospital, King's College London, London, UK

Marc L. Schermerhorn, MD
Chief, Division of Vascular and Endovascular Surgery, Beth Israel Deaconess Medical Center; Associate Professor of Surgery, Harvard Medical School, Boston, MA, USA

Indrani Sen, MS, MCh
Christian Medical College, Vellore, Tamil Nadu, India

Peter A. Soden, MD
Beth Israel Deaconess Medical Center, Boston, MA USA

Rob H.W. Strijkers, MD, PhD-candidate
Venous Surgery, Maastricht University Medical Centre and Cardiovascular Research Institute, Maastricht, The Netherlands

Andrew L. Tambyraja, MD, FRCSEd
Consultant Vascular Surgeon and Honorary Clinical Senior Lecturer, Royal Infirmary of Edinburgh and University of Edinburgh, UK

Ramesh K. Tripathi, MD, FRCS, FRACS(Vasc)
Professor of Vascular and Endovascular Surgery, University of The Sunshine Coast, Sippy Downs, Australia

Jos C. van den Berg, MD, PhD
Head of Service of Interventional Radiology, Centro Vascolare Ticino Ospedale Regionale di Lugano; Assistant Professor of Radiology, University Institute for Diagnostic, Interventional and Pediatric Radiology, Inselspital, University Hospital of Bern, Bern, Switzerland

Ramon L. Varcoe, MBBS, MS, FRACS, PhD
Associate Professor of Vascular Surgery, University of New South Wales, Consultant Vascular Surgeon, Prince of Wales Hospital; Director, the Vascular Institute, Prince of Wales Hospital, Sydney, Australia

Cees H.A. Wittens, MD, PhD
Professor of Venous Surgery, Head of Venous Surgery, Maastricht University Medical Centre, Maastricht, The Netherlands

1

Epidemiological risk factors for PAD, risk stratification and risk factor management

Patrick Coughlin

Introduction

Atherosclerotic peripheral artery disease (PAD) involving one or more major vessels of the lower limb is common.[1] Whilst previously a condition of high income countries (HIC), the global spread of abdominal adiposity and its associated metabolic disorders has led to a significant increase in PAD in lower and middle income countries (LMIC). Current estimates suggest that over 200 million people globally are affected by PAD, with a marked increase in those affected over the last decade (LMIC 29% increase, HIC 13% increase). PAD tends to affect older patients and likely occurs due to both genetic and environmental interactions that result in the development of atherosclerotic disease. The natural history of the lower limb in patients with symptomatic PAD (intermittent claudication) is somewhat benign, with up to 75% of patients noticing stabilisation or some improvement of their symptoms.[2] Patients with PAD, however, are at significant risk of major adverse cardiovascular events (MACE), noticeably due to concomitant atherosclerotic disease within the coronary, carotid and cerebral circulation. Disability and mortality associated with PAD have increased over the last 20 years, and this increase in burden has been greater among women than among men.[3] There are a number of studies that highlight this link between PAD and MACE, predominantly using the ankle–brachial pressure index (ABPI) as a marker of disease severity. Data from the Ankle Brachial Index Collaboration group showed that a low ABPI (<0.9) was associated with an increased risk of subsequent all-cause mortality (pooled RR 1.60, 95% CI 1.32–1.95), cardiovascular mortality (pooled RR 1.96,

95% CI 1.46–2.64), coronary heart disease (pooled RR 1.45, 95% CI 1.08–1.93) and stroke (pooled RR 1.35, 95% CI 1.10–1.65) after adjustment for age, sex, conventional cardiovascular risk factors and prevalent cardiovascular disease.[4] Furthermore, given the impending diabetes epidemic, this, alongside renal impairment, is associated with medial artery calcification leading to an inability to compress the arteries during ABPI measurement. An elevated ABPI (defined as >1.40) has also been identified with an increased risk of all-cause and cardiovascular (CV) disease mortality (adjusted risk estimates 1.77 all-cause mortality / 2.09 cardiovascular mortality).[5] This U-shaped relationship between ABPI and outcome is now well recognised (**Fig. 1.1**). The aims of this chapter are to undertake a contemporary review of the epidemiology of lower limb PAD; to analyse the role of reversible and irreversible risk factors on both disease progression and the incidence of MACE, and to determine the role of a number of disease-modifying therapies as part of 'best medical therapy' on reducing the risk of deleterious patient outcomes.

Epidemiology of PAD

Compared to coronary artery disease, there are few data available on the epidemiology of PAD. Incidence of PAD is defined as the rate of new (or newly diagnosed) cases of the disease (generally reported as the number of new cases occurring within a period of time). Prevalence is defined at the actual number of cases alive with the disease either during a period of time (period prevalence) or at a particular date in time (point prevalence).

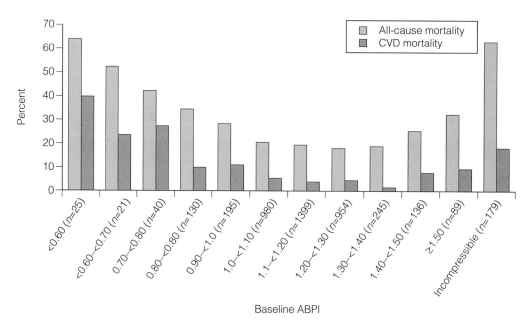

Figure 1.1 • Relationship between ABPI (ankle–brachial pressure index) and survival in patients in the Strong Heart Study.[5] There is a U-shaped relationship such that both low (<0.9) and high (>1.4) ABPI is associated with increased risk of CV and all-cause mortality.

The true incidence and prevalence of PAD is difficult to determine accurately, in part due to methodological issues related to the diagnosis of PAD but also due to continuing changes in cardiovascular risk factor prevalence and management. Differences are also encountered depending on sampling criteria and whether the diagnosis of PAD is based purely on symptomatic patients (intermittent claudication/critical limb ischaemia [CLI]) or whether one includes asymptomatic individuals. The population may be screened using a questionnaire-based approach (Rose questionnaire/Edinburgh Artery Questionnaire). These questionnaires tend to underestimate the diagnosis of claudication and a more objective analysis of limb perfusion (ABPI/reactive hyperaemia) may be more appropriate.

The ABPI has become an increasingly used diagnostic tool for PAD, with a value ≤0.9 signifying PAD. It is both a reproducible and reliable test. There are circumstances where a false-negative reading may be obtained and they include patients with medial artery calcification where arterial compression is difficult, the presence of mild arterial lesions (often seen in the iliac artery) and where significant collateralisation has occurred. In such circumstances, pre- and post-exercise ABPI measurement can help, but these are impractical to perform in population-based studies. A number of the initial validation studies of ABPI were performed prior to the advent of arterial duplex. As such, intra-arterial lower limb angiography was used as the gold standard against which the ABPI was compared. As this is an invasive test, not without risk, ABPI was only determined in selected patients with significant symptoms who were more likely to have severe arterial disease and this was compared against younger 'normal' controls. As such, the observed sensitivity and specificity values obtained were between 97% and 100%.[6,7] However, if one takes a more representative sample of patients seen in daily practice, then while the specificity of ABPI measurement is maintained at approximately 97%, the sensitivity falls to nearer 80%.[8]

There can be confusion in such epidemiological studies when determining whether solely symptomatic PAD or PAD as a whole (symptomatic *and* asymptomatic) are included. This gains some importance when discussing the merits of screening for PAD.

With regard to the epidemiology of PAD as a whole, nearly always determined by measurement of the ABPI, studies showed a prevalence of PAD of approximately 3–10% in the population as a whole, with this increasing to between 15 and 20% when focusing on older patients (>70 years of age).[9–11] More recent studies include the PARTNERS (PAD Awareness, Risk, and Treatment: New Resources for Survival) study, the National Health and Nutritional Examination Survey (NHANES) and the REGICOR study[12–14] (**Fig. 1.2**). The PARTNERS study screened 6979 subjects for PAD using ABPI (inclusion criteria – all subjects over 70 years OR age 50–69 years and at least one cardiovascular risk factor). PAD was detected in 29% of the population.

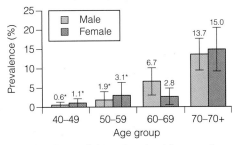

Figure 1.2 • Recent information about the prevalence of PAD from the US National Health and Nutrition Survey, confirming a steep age-related prevalence.

The NHANES recruited an unselected cohort of subjects over 40 years of age and found a prevalence of PAD of 2.5% in those aged 50–59 years, rising to 14.5% in those aged >70 years. The REGICOR study, studying a purely Mediterranean population, found the prevalence of PAD to be 4.5% (5.2% in 47 men and 3.9% in women). Other studies report prevalence of PAD from 3% to 20%, with variation depending upon methodology and the population examined. Interestingly, there appears to be little difference in prevalence between men and women, with ratios ranging from 0.8 to 1.2. The issue with regard to the method of assessment of PAD is borne out by the data from the British Regional Heart Study, where direct assessment of the femoral artery performed using ultrasound suggested that 64% of people aged 56–77 years have significant femoral atherosclerosis, of whom fewer than one-fifth were symptomatic.[15]

There are more limited data when one considers the incidence of PAD. The Limburg study, involving a cohort of 2327 patients selected from 18 primary care facilities in the Netherlands, found that after a follow-up period of 7.2 years the overall incidence rate for asymptomatic PAD was 9.9 (95% CI 7.3–18.8) per 1000 person-years at risk. The rate was 7.8 (95% CI 4.9–20.3) for men and 12.4 (95% CI 7.7–24.8) for women and more marked in those patients over the age of 65 years.[16] The REGICOR study collected data on 5434 individuals aged between 35 and 79 years.[17] In total, 118 new cases of confirmed PAD were identified, resulting in a cumulative population incidence rate of 377 cases per 100 000 person years, lower than that seen in other areas.

Intermittent claudication is a symptom of muscular lower limb pain brought on by exertion and relieved by rest, with CLI being at the more severe end of the symptom spectrum (night pain/rest pain/tissue loss). The prevalence of intermittent claudication varies, up to 3% at the age of 40 years rising to 6% at 60 years. While some of the data are historic, the largest studies performed over three decades ago are probably still the most reliable. These include the Edinburgh Artery Study, which screened large random samples of the general population using age/sex registers from general practices.[11] This study used both the WHO questionnaire and the ABPI to determine the prevalence of both symptomatic and asymptomatic lower limb PAD in a sample of 1592 participants (men and women) aged between 55 and 74 years. They found that the prevalence of intermittent claudication was 4.5% (95% CI 3.5–5.5) with major asymptomatic disease seen in 8.0% (95% CI 6.6–9.4).

The incidence also varies, in part depending on geography, with values as low as 0.2% in Iceland, 1.0% in Israel and 1.6% from the Edinburgh Artery Study.[11,18,19] More detailed data come from the Framingham dataset that showed an overall incidence of 7.1 per 1000 years in men and 3.6 per 1000 years in women, although the gender differences were not seen between the ages of 65 and 75 years.[20] Data from the REGICOR dataset suggest an incidence for symptomatic PAD of 102 per 100 000 person years.[14] This suggests that the incidence of PAD is lower in the Mediterranean area than reported from other areas and warrants more in-depth analysis.

The incidence of CLI has been estimated to be around 400 cases per million population per year, which equates to a prevalence of 1 in 2500 of the population annually.[21] For every 100 patients with intermittent claudication, approximately one new patient per year will develop critical ischaemia.[22]

What is clear is that the incidence of symptomatic PAD – namely intermittent claudication and CLI – increases steeply with age.[11,16]

When considering the effect of ethnicity, the most comprehensive data come from a study by Allison et al., who combined data from seven community-based studies within the USA.[23] The study showed that PAD was uncommon prior to the age of 50 years and yet was present in up to 20% of subjects over the age of 80 years. The rate of PAD in African Americans was double that seen in non-Hispanic Whites (NHW), with the rates for Hispanics, Asian Americans and Native Americans similar to those in NHW.

Natural history of PAD: limb-specific, cardiovascular morbidity and mortality

Limb-specific outcomes

There are a number of important methodological issues in determining the natural history of lower limb PAD. This relates to a higher chance that significant disease progression may result in either revascularisation or limb loss, or if associated with more aggressive atherosclerotic progression in other arterial beds, then a higher mortality risk. When considering symptom progression, then this is in part related to the degree of collateralisation, muscle adaptation, allied physical function/ability and adaptability so that there may be marked differences seen between pathological disease progress and symptom progression.

There is, however, a reasonable quantity of data on PAD progression using predominantly ABPI measurements as a marker of PAD.

The Cardiovascular Health Study, analysing a cohort of 5000 patients with normal ABPI, reported a 9.5% incidence of PAD over a 6-year follow-up period.[24] The Edinburgh Artery Study found between 7% and 15% of patients with initially asymptomatic PAD developed intermittent claudication over a 5-year follow-up period.[11] Nicoloff et al. reported a 37% deterioration in ABPI over a 5-year follow-up, which equated to clinical progression (defined as symptom change or need for revascularisation) in 22%.[25,26] A smaller study by Taute et al. from Germany found lower limb PAD progression occurred in 18.6% over a 5-year follow-up period and a study from San Diego, using a six-category scale of disease severity, found significant limb PAD progression in 30% of subjects over a follow-up period reaching nearly 5 years.[27,28]

When considering patients with intermittent claudication, the large population studies from Edinburgh and Basle suggest that only a quarter of patients will have significant deterioration in symptoms, with this being most frequent within the first year after diagnosis (7–9%) and after this occurring in only 2–3%.[2] Specifically, the risk of amputation is rare, occurring in only 1–3% of patients with intermittent claudication at 5 years.[2]

Association of PAD with atherosclerotic disease in other arterial beds

Atherosclerotic disease can be manifest in a number of arterial beds and as such PAD is associated with other vascular-related conditions, specifically within the coronary and cerebral circulations. The Cardiovascular Health Study, a cohort-based study from the USA of 5000 Medicare patients, showed that the diagnosis of PAD was associated with a 2.5 increased risk of a history of myocardial infarction, a twofold increased risk of angina and an approximately threefold increase in both congestive cardiac failure (×3.3) and a previous stroke (×3.1).[29] These findings are supported by the ARIC

study, a study of 15000 middle-aged subjects.[30] A diagnosis of PAD (ABPI <0.9) was associated with a twofold increase in coronary artery disease. The association is starker in older patients. A study of 1800 older patients (mean age 80 years) from New York showed that a diagnosis of PAD was associated with coronary disease in 68% of patients and with a history of ischaemic stroke in 42%.[31] These results are corroborated by the Reduction of Atherothrombosis for Continued Health (REACH) registry, a large multinational registry collating observational data about the spectrum of disease progression, cardiovascular (CV) outcomes and patterns of treatment in patients with atherosclerotic disease. The registry encompasses a total of 67888 patients, aged 45 years or more, from 44 countries with an inclusion criteria of either established CV disease or, if they were asymptomatic, with more than three risk CV risk factors (n = 12389). Among the symptomatic group, patients were enrolled on the basis of coronary artery disease (CAD; n = 40248), cerebrovascular disease (CVD; n = 18843) or PAD (n = 8273), with 16% of this group having polyvascular disease.[32]

Association of PAD with subsequent cardiovascular morbidity and mortality

Given this association of PAD with atherosclerotic disease in the coronary and cerebral circulation, it is unsurprising therefore that such patients have a higher subsequent cardiovascular event rate.[26] To determine the true effect of PAD specifically on cardiovascular event rates, appropriate logistic or proportional hazards regression models, with multivariable adjustment for conventional cardiovascular risk factors, are required.[26]

PAD acts as a marker for underlying atherosclerotic processes affecting other vascular beds. This is clinically important, to the extent that PAD has prognostic value independent of other known risk factors. A meta-analysis of 16 population-based cohort studies evaluated the association of ABPI with subsequent coronary events, CVD mortality and total mortality.[33] An ABPI of ≤0.90 was associated with approximately twice the 10-year event rates in each of these three categories. In addition, these results held across the full range of Framingham Risk Score categories.

Data from two decades ago suggested that PAD was associated with a ×2–3 increased risk of stroke, a fourfold increase in the risk of fatal myocardial infarction (MI) or cardiac-related death and a sixfold risk of death from any cardiovascular cause.[34,35] Coronary artery disease is the most common cause of death among patients with PAD (40–60%), with cerebral artery disease accounting for 10–20% of deaths. Other vascular events, mostly ruptured aortic aneurysm, cause approximately 10% of deaths.[2]

This relationship is also highlighted by the more recent REACH cohort.[32] Among patients within the whole cohort with established CV disease, CV death, MI or stroke rates were 23.0% for patients with CAD, 18.7% for patients with CVD and 33.6% for patients with PAD. Specifically, patients with a diagnosis of PAD were most likely to have subsequent vascular death (2.9 events per 100 person-years).

When considering intermittent claudication specifically, there remains a link with high cardiovascular event rates. The Whitehall study analysed a cohort of 18 403 patients aged between 40 and 64 years who were followed up over a 17-year period.[36] Within this cohort, 322 were felt likely to have a diagnosis of intermittent claudication, with an associated 40% mortality rate in this group during the study period. The study concluded that intermittent claudication was independently related to increased mortality rates. Such correlations are also seen in more recent studies by Kollerits et al. and the SHIP study ($n = 3995$, median follow-up 8.5 years), where a diagnosis of intermittent claudication was associated with an increased risk of all-cause mortality (Hazard Ratio 1.79).[37,38] Data from the GetABI study showed that there was an increased risk of a composite endpoint of all-cause mortality and severe vascular event in patients with symptomatic PAD compared to those with asymptomatic disease.[39]

CLI is associated with a higher burden of lower limb atherosclerotic disease. As such, mortality rates are notably higher in this specific cohort of patients. A recent meta-analysis of contemporary studies ($n = 50$ studies), showed that the estimated probability of all-cause mortality in patients with CLI was 3.7% at 30 days, 17.5% at 1 year, 35.1% at 3 years and 46.2% at 5 years. Men had a statistically significant survival benefit at 30 days and 3 years. The presence of ischaemic heart disease, tissue loss and older age resulted in a higher probability of death at 3 years.[40]

Epidemiological risk factors for PAD, risk stratification and risk factor management (Fig. 1.3)

Over the last 30 years there have been significant advances in the understanding and management of a number of risk factors associated with the

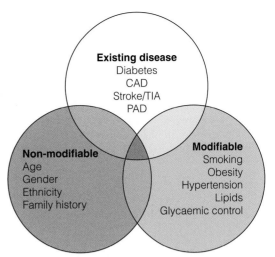

Figure 1.3 • Major CV risk factors can be grouped into: existing disease; non-modifiable risk factors; and modifiable risk factors, where placebo-controlled trials have shown the benefits of intervention.

development and progression of atherosclerotic disease. This includes a high quality of evidence from a number of well-conducted randomised controlled trials. Data from such studies have had a major influence on day-to-day clinical practice which has resulted in a decline in overall age-adjusted coronary mortality rates. Yet the onset of the 'diabetic epidemic' brings with it new challenges to maintain such reductions in cardiovascular morbidity and mortality.

Much of the data is from 'generic' cardiovascular studies, where patients with any form of atherosclerotic disease were recruited. Given both the significant association of PAD with coronary and cerebrovascular disease and the high MACE rate in PAD, extrapolation of such results into the PAD population is justified. As such, there is no overwhelming evidence that all patients with PAD should be receiving optimal secondary cardiovascular prevention strategies.

This is reflected in the most recent guidelines for the management of lower limb PAD issued by the National Institute for Health and Clinical Excellence (NICE) in the UK.[41] These guidelines delivered strategies for the management of recognised secondary cardiovascular risk factors. This guidance stated that all patients should be offered appropriate advice and treatment regarding these cardiovascular risk factors in line with the NICE guidance. This includes guidance regarding smoking cessation, diet, weight management and exercise, lipid modification/statin therapy, antiplatelet therapy and the prevention, diagnosis and management of diabetes and high blood pressure.

Age and gender

A number of studies have highlighted the effect of increasing age with PAD risk irrespective of gender.[11,42] The effect of gender is, however, less clear, with some studies, notably the Framingham Study, suggesting that the risk of PAD is doubled in men compared to women. Such a relationship was not evident in the Edinburgh Artery Study and indeed the reverse was seen in the Limburg study.[11,16]

Cigarette smoking

Smoking is associated with increased mortality rates from cardiorespiratory disease and numerous cancers. It has a detrimental effect on the vascular and platelet function and promoted the inflammatory cascades that are associated with development of atherosclerotic disease. True epidemiological assessment of its role can be somewhat problematic, specifically with regard to how one determines whether a subject is a smoker/ex-smoker (e.g. questionnaire-based/cotinine measurements) and an assessment of volume of smoking.

Smoking is, however, the strongest risk for PAD and all the largest epidemiological studies reported up to a fourfold increase in risk of PAD when compared to non-smokers.[26] There is also some evidence that suggests that even after having stopped smoking the risk of developing PAD is maintained for up to a further 20 years. However, the benefits of smoking cessation with regard to overall CV risk are evident within 5–7 years in men and 2–4 years in women.[43,44]

Once PAD has become evident, continued smoking is associated with up to a threefold increase in mortality risk and further risks of major amputation, the need for revascularisation and progression to CLI.[11]

As such, smoking is the modifiable risk factor for the prevention of unfavourable cardiovascular outcomes, with mechanistic evidence of short- and longer-term benefits.

Smoking and specifically nicotinine is addictive and, as such, smoking cessation is challenging. There are a number of strategies that are available to aid in smoking cessation:

- Nicotine replacement therapy (NRT). A meta-analysis of 117 studies analysing more than 50 000 participants compared any type of NRT with placebo/non-NRT control groups. The risk ratio (RR) of abstinence for any form of NRT relative to control was 1.60 (95% CI 1.53–1.68). The conclusions of this study were that all of the commercially available forms of NRT (gum, transdermal patch, nasal spray, inhaler and sublingual tablets/lozenges) can help people who make a quit attempt to increase their chances of successfully stopping smoking. NRTs increase the rate of quitting by 50–70%, regardless of setting. The effectiveness of NRT appears to be largely independent of the intensity of additional support provided to the individual.[45]

- Partial agonist of nicotinic acetylcholine receptors (nAChRs) (cytosine/varenicline). A recent Cochrane review concluded that cytistine increased the chance of quitting. Varenicline at standard doses had a two- to threefold increased chance of long-term smoking cessation when compared to non-pharmacological methods. More participants quit successfully with varenicline than with bupropion or with NRT.[46]

- Bupropion and other antiderpressants. The recent Cochrane review showed that Bupronion significantly improved long-term smoking cessation rates ($n = 13728$; RR 1.63 CI 1.49–1.76). The antidepressant nortriptyline also aids long-term smoking cessation. Evidence suggests that the mode of action of bupropion and nortriptyline is independent of their antidepressant effect and that they are of similar efficacy to nicotine replacement. Evidence also suggests that bupropion is less effective than varenicline.[47]

Diabetes mellitus

Increasing life expectancy allied to a global spread of obesity has resulted in a significant increase in the number of people with a diagnosis of diabetes mellitus (DM). The recent World Health Organisation (WHO) data state that there are approximately 422 million adults with diabetes worldwide. Approximately 85–905 of such cases are classified as type 2 diabetes mellitus and it is estimated that this overall figure will double by the year 2030. Given the associated risks of DM it is generally considered to be a coronary artery risk equivalent when it comes to determining those patients requiring intensive secondary risk factor management.

Apart from smoking, it is the most important risk factor for the development of PAD, with insulin resistance and hyperinsulinaemia also independent factors for PAD. Associated odds risk for developing PAD in patients with DM range from 1.89 to

4.05. In patients with DM, the distribution of atherosclerotic disease tends to be more distal, with a larger burden within the crural vessels, and this allied to the neuropathic complication seen results in a significantly increased lifetime risk of major amputation.[48]

There is strong evidence that glycaemic control is an independent predictor for macrovascular disease as well as microvascular disease. The UK Prospective Diabetes Study showed a strong association of PAD with HbA1c levels (a measure of glycaemic control), with a 1% increase equating to a 28% increase in risk of developing PAD.[49]

Once PAD is established there is less convincing evidence that strict glycaemic control reduces the risk of a subsequent cardiovascular event.[50] A meta-analysis of studies of glucose-lowering therapies suggested that intensive compared with standard glycaemic control reduces coronary events but did not affect cerebrovascular event rates or all-cause mortality. It is possible that both oral hypoglycaemics and insulin therapy may have differing effects on cardiovascular event rates. For example, the use of metformin in obese patients with diabetes has been shown to slow atherosclerotic progression and avert the development of DM in patients with insulin resistance.

What is evident is the benefit of modifying other cardiovascular risk factors in patients with DM. Specifically, statin therapy and blood pressure control have a greater effect in patients with diabetes than those without. Data from the UKPDS showed that for every 10 mmHg reduction in systolic blood pressure, there was a 12% reduction in overall cardiovascular risk as well as a 16% reduction in the risk of a major lower limb amputation or PAD-related mortality. This link between aggressive blood pressure control and reduction in cardiovascular events may be more relevant and effective clinically than tight glycaemic control.[51,52]

Blood pressure management (Fig. 1.4)

Hypertension is the most common cardiovascular risk factor worldwide. Recent guidance from NICE suggests prescribing antihypertensive drug treatment to people aged under 80 years with stage 1 hypertension (defined as having a clinic blood pressure of 140/90 mmHg or higher and subsequent ambulatory or home blood pressure monitoring (AHBPM) of 135/85 mmHg or higher) who have one or more of the following: (a) target organ damage, (b) established cardiovascular disease, (c) renal disease, (d) diabetes or (e) a 10-year cardiovascular risk equivalent to 20% or greater. If none of these criteria apply, then

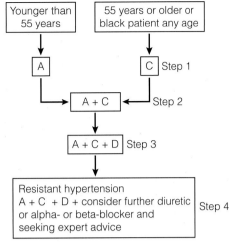

Figure 1.4 • Drug selection and drug sequencing for patients with hypertension. Algorithm published by the British Heart Foundation and endorsed by NICE. Beta-blockers are no longer recommended in step 1, but may be added at step 4. A, ACE inhibitor (consider angiotensin II-receptor antagonist if ACE-intolerant); C, calcium-channel blocker; D, thiazide-type diuretic. Black patients are those of African or Caribbean descent and not mixed-race, Asian or Chinese patients.

patients of any age (>/= 80 years) with stage 2 hypertension (defined as a clinic blood pressure of 160/110 mmHg or higher and subsequent AHBPM of 150/95 mmHg or higher) should be prescribed antihypertensive drug treatment.

There is overwhelming evidence of a direct relationship between levels of blood pressure control and associated cardiovascular event risk,[53] with more strict control of blood pressure associated with a greater reduction in risk. The aim is to achieve a target blood pressure of ≤140/90 or down to 130/80 in patients with diabetes mellitus or chronic renal failure. Yet even a small reduction in blood pressure can make large clinical differences. Current guidance is to prescribe as first line an angiotensin-converting enzyme (ACE) inhibitor for younger patients and a calcium antagonist for older patients, with beta-blockers, thiazides and other classes of antihypertensives reserved for second-line treatment. It is likely, however, that in most patients, monotherapy will not suffice and a combination of antihypertensives will be required to achieve optimal control. There are significant issues related to compliance, specifically as hypertension is not a 'visible' ailment. There is some evidence that even if the blood pressure is controlled within the defined normal range there is still some increased risk of subsequent cardiovascular events. This concept of 'pre-hypertension', with a systolic blood pressure between 120 and 139 mmHg requires further investigation.

A number of epidemiological studies point to the direct effect that hypertension has on the incidence of PAD, patients with PAD tending to have more problems related to systolic hypertension due to the degree of arterial calcification and subsequent lack of arterial elasticity associated with PAD.

Data from the Framingham Study showed that a blood pressure of >160/95 mmHg was associated with a 2.5 increased risk in men and a×4 increased risk of developing PAD in women over a follow-up period of 26 years. Furthermore, this is confirmed by a study which showed that a 10 mmHg increase in systolic BP was associated with an increase in risk of developing PAD (OR 1.3, 95% CI 1.2–1.5). This link of hypertension and PAD is also evident in the fact that 5% of patients diagnosed with hypertension have clinical evidence of PAD at the time of diagnosis.

There are many classes of antihypertensives and the vast majority of trials involving them have included PAD patients only as subgroups within larger studies on cardiovascular disease. As such, due to the issues associated with 'ad hoc' analyses there are few direct data available for PAD patients. One study that has reported on blood pressure control in patients with PAD is the Heart Outcomes Prevention Evaluation (HOPE) Study published back in 2000.[54] This randomised controlled trial determined the effect of the ACE inhibitor ramipril as an adjunct to other secondary risk factor interventions in patients with established cardiovascular disease or diabetes. The addition of ramipril significantly reduced overall major adverse cardiovascular events and this effect was also seen in the subgroup of patients recruited with a proven diagnosis of PAD (*n* >4000; **Fig. 1.5**). As part of the recruitment into this trial, patients were already receiving antihypertensive medication and as such blood pressure control was partially optimised. What was of great interest from the study was that despite only a small antihypertensive effect from ramipril (blood pressure reduction of approximately 3/2 mmHg), there was a marked reduction in cardiovascular event rate, suggesting that the protective effects were in part independent of the antihypertensive effect. This is supported by results from the PROGRESS study, which showed that stroke survivors with relatively normal blood pressure gained marked reduction in stroke recurrence and overall major cardiovascular event rates with ACE inhibitor therapy.[55] There is some evidence that drugs that block the RAAS (renin–angiotensin–aldosterone system) pathway do have effects above that of BP control, with established data available showing that ACE inhibitors and angiotensin-receptor blockers (ARBs) improve left ventricular function in heart failure and slow the progression of chronic kidney disease. Yet there is no doubt that the BP-independent benefits of ACE inhibitors and ARBs require further investigation, specifically with regard to possible positive effects that may occur at the vessel wall.

Dyslipidaemia

A link between cholesterol and the development of atherosclerotic disease has been evident for many years. There is now strong epidemiological evidence that a positive link exists between levels of total and low-density lipoprotein (LDL) cholesterol and the risk of major adverse cardiovascular events. Indeed, a reduction in LDL cholesterol levels of 1 mmol/L equates to a reduction in cardiovascular risk of 21%, irrespective of starting LDL cholesterol level.[56] Recently, there has been recognition that the total cholesterol to high-density lipoprotein cholesterol ratio is perhaps a better measure of CV risk but this is not in widespread use and is not reflected in current guidelines.

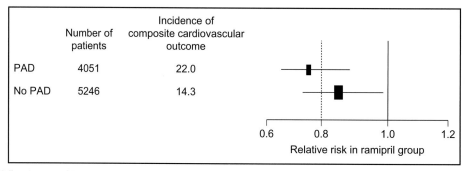

	Number of patients	Incidence of composite cardiovascular outcome
PAD	4051	22.0
No PAD	5246	14.3

Figure 1.5 • In the HOPE Study, analysis of subgroups according to baseline cardiovascular disease status shows that patients with PAD gain at least as much benefit from the ACE inhibitor ramipril as the study group overall.

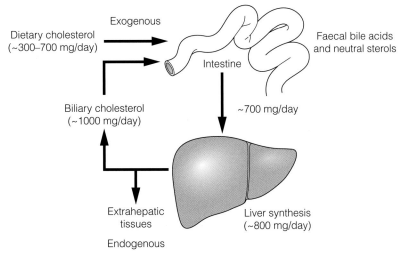

Figure 1.6 • Circulating cholesterol is derived from endogenous synthesis in the liver and exogenous sources (dietary intake and bile acids) absorbed through the gut. Statins block synthesis, ezetimibe blocks gut absorption. The drugs have additive effects on serum cholesterol.

Cholesterol is derived from two sources: (i) endogenous synthesis within the liver, which is in part secreted into the gastrointestinal tract via the biliary system, and (ii) gastrointestinal absorption of dietary cholesterol as well as reabsorption of that excreted within the biliary salts (**Fig. 1.6**).

As such, pharmacological manipulation has been targeted at these processes. The most commonly used therapies are HMG-CoA reductase inhibitors (statins), with this being the rate-limiting enzyme in cholesterol biosynthesis. Other pharmacological agents include ezetimibe, which inhibits cholesterol absorption, is not systemically absorbed and can be used as an adjunct to statin therapy.

Current guidance states that all individuals should have a LDL cholesterol level <3.2 mmol/L and in patients with any evidence of atherosclerotic disease or with a predicted 10-year cardiovascular risk of >20% a level of <2.6 mmol/L should be the aim. Those at highest risk should aim for a LDL cholesterol level of <1.8 mmol/L. Such guidelines are evolved from pooled analysis of a number of large studies and also evidence from the low- versus high-dose statin trials that showed that an increased dose resulted in a reduction in mortality risk.[57]

One of the difficulties of such guidance is achieving such reductions in LDL cholesterol levels using the first-generation statins (namely simvastatin); however, it may be more achievable to hit these targets using second-generation statins (atorvastatin/rosuvastatin). The role of statins in the management of cardiovascular disease is also developing, with recent evidence suggesting that early administration of statins may have a cardiovascular benefit in the setting of acute coronary syndromes. This may not be due to its primary effect on cholesterol synthesis but may actually occur due to other pleiotropic effects that are increasingly recognised with statin therapy. These include anti-inflammatory effects, plaque stabilisation and an increase in HDL cholesterol levels.

Specific to PAD, there is strong epidemiological evidence of elevated cholesterol levels conferring an independent risk of developing PAD. Specifically, data from the Framingham Study showed that a fasting cholesterol measure of >7 conferred a twofold increased risk of developing intermittent claudication. Secondly, low HDL cholesterol levels or an increased LDL:HDL cholesterol ratio also appear to be independent risk factors for PAD.[11]

When assessing the role of statins in secondary prevention in patients with PAD, a number of the studies are limited by inclusion of small numbers of patients with PAD, including the 4S and the CARE studies.[58] The Heart Protection Study did, however, have about 20% of its cohort of patients with PAD and showed that those patients with PAD treated with a statin had a reduction in cardiovascular event rate compared to those with PAD not treated with a statin (27.6% vs 34.3%)[59] (**Fig. 1.7**). The early statin studies (4S and CARE) focused on patients following an acute myocardial infarct with only 4% of patients recruited to the 4S study having a diagnosis of intermittent claudication at baseline. Statin treatment in the 4S study did result in a significant reduction in both the deterioration of claudication and the new onset of claudication in those patients not afflicted. There is some more recent evidence to suggest that statins may play a role in improving walking distances and QoL in

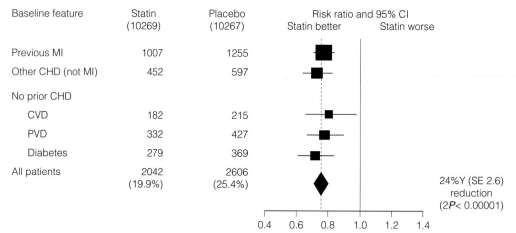

Baseline feature	Statin (10269)	Placebo (10267)	Risk ratio and 95% CI Statin better Statin worse
Previous MI	1007	1255	
Other CHD (not MI)	452	597	
No prior CHD			
CVD	182	215	
PVD	332	427	
Diabetes	279	369	
All patients	2042 (19.9%)	2606 (25.4%)	24%Y (SE 2.6) reduction (2*P* < 0.00001)

0.4   0.6   0.8   1.0   1.2   1.4

Figure 1.7 • In the Heart Protection Study, the benefits of simvastatin 40 mg were evident in those patients with peripheral vascular disease (PVD) at baseline and were independent of age, BP status and baseline cholesterol. Data from the Heart Protection Study Collaborative Group. MRC/BHF Heart Protection Study of cholesterol-lowering with simvastatin in 20,536 high-risk individuals. Lancet 2002;360:7–22.

patients with claudication, although the mechanism of action is unclear.[60,61]

Progress continues with regard to the availability of therapeutics to reduce cholesterol/LDL levels, with the development of pro-protein convertase subtilisin/kexin type 9 (PCSK9) inhibitors.[62] PCSK9 down-regulates expression of the LDL receptor within the liver and inhibition of this receptor with monoclonal antibodies has been shown to reduce the LDL-C level by over 50%, increase HDL-C levels and result in favourable changes generally in the lipid profile.

Antiplatelet therapy

There is some evidence that PAD is associated with a hypercoagulable state, with several studies confirming the association of high plasma fibrinogen levels with PAD. There is overwhelming evidence for the role of antiplatelet therapy in reducing MACE in patients with cardiovascular disease, with the seminal paper being the meta-analysis by the Antiplatelet Trialists' Collaboration which showed that antiplatelet therapy predominantly with a low-dose aspirin reduced the risk of non-fatal myocardial infarction, non-fatal stroke and vascular death in high-risk patients, including those with intermittent claudication.[63]

More recently, clopidogrel has become increasingly used as the first line monotherapy antiplatelet agent. This is based upon the results of the CAPRIE trial. The CAPRIE trial evaluated the efficacy and safety of clopidogrel compared to aspirin for secondary prevention in 19 185 patients with CV disease.[64] It showed a relative reduction in the risk of MI, ischaemic stroke and vascular death of 8.7% (*P* = 0.04) in favour of clopidogrel after a mean follow-up of 1.9 years, and an absolute risk reduction of 0.51% (NNT [number needed to treat] = 196 to avoid one ischaemic event during 1.9 years), although a subgroup analysis in PAD patients suggested that the clinical benefit of clopidogrel was greater than 8.7%. A recent cost-effectiveness analysis has reported that clopidogrel is more cost-effective than aspirin in patients with PAD.[65]

With regard to intermittent claudication, the most up to date Cochrane review (12 studies, 12 168 patients) of the role of antiplatelet agents in patients with intermittent claudication confirmed the benefit of antiplatelet agents with a reduction in all-cause and cardiovascular mortality. This benefit was, however, associated with a higher risk of adverse events, including gastrointestinal symptoms and events leading to cessation of therapy. Data on major bleeding was limited.

Current focus is now directed to the role of dual antiplatelet therapy as well as determining the role of the newer antiplatelet agents in current management protocols. Dual antiplatelet therapy has become widely used in patients with acute coronary syndromes and following percutaneous coronary intervention. The CHARISMA trial was performed to assess the effects of dual antiplatelet therapy (clopidogrel + aspirin) in patients with more stable atherosclerotic disease. Overall, there were some safety concerns with dual therapy yet in sub-group analysis there was some benefit in PAD patients compared with aspirin alone.[66]

Further data when looking at the role of dual antiplatelet therapy in patients with PAD are somewhat limited. A recent meta-analysis compared a number of different antiplatelet drugs in PAD patients with primary endpoints of a composite rate of major adverse cardiovascular events (MACE; including vascular deaths, non-fatal myocardial infarction and non-fatal stroke), and the rate of major leg amputations.[67] The primary safety endpoint was the rate of severe bleeding events. The authors analysed 49 RCTs comprising 34 518 patients with 88 358 person-years of follow-up with placebo as reference treatment. The take-home messages from this study were: (a) clopidogrel should be the indicated antiplatelet agent in PAD patients (RR 0.72, 95% CI 0.58–0.91, NNT = 80), (b) dual antiplatelet therapy with aspirin and clopidogrel can reduce the rate of major leg amputations following revascularisation (RR 0.68, 95% CI 0.46–0.99 compared to aspirin, NNT = 94), but carries a slightly higher risk of severe bleeding (RR 1.48, 95% CI 1.05–2.10, NNT = 215).

Newer antiplatelet agents are also becoming available. One such agent is ticagrelor, an antagonist of the $P2Y_{12}$ receptor. The results from the recent EUCLID study, a study investigating whether treatment with ticagrelor versus clopidogrel, given as antiplatelet monotherapy, will reduce the incidence of cardiovascular and limb-specific events in patients with symptomatic PAD, showed that there was no superiority of either therapy.[68]

Conclusions

Lower limb peripheral artery disease is becoming increasingly common and is now a global issue. While the natural history of the limb is somewhat benign it does present major impairment of day-to-day activities. What is of concern is the significant cardiovascular risk within this patient group, with PAD recognised as a coronary heart disease risk equivalent. Epidemiological studies have identified numerous risk factors that, in longitudinal follow-up studies in large populations, are associated with a higher incidence and more rapid progression of PAD. Due to the absence of suitably powered and conducted studies, there is a lack of level I evidence that interventions for such risk factors will improve clinical outcomes. As such, current recommendations are derived from studies of patients with other forms of cardiovascular disease.

Current guidance would suggest that all patients with PAD merit secondary prevention with disease-modifying therapies to lower BP and cholesterol levels, assist with smoking cessation, reduce platelet function and improve glycaemic control.

Key points

- There is a U-shaped relationship between ABPI and reduced life expectancy, with high ABPI measurements also associated with an increased risk of cardiovascular morbidity and mortality.
- The incidence of PAD increases steeply with increasing age and may be slightly more common in men.
- Although lower limb outcomes are relatively good in most patients with PAD, these patients are at very high risk of premature death from other cardiovascular events, as illustrated recently by the REACH registry.
- Risk factors for the development of PAD are similar to those for atherosclerotic disease in general, but smoking and diabetes may have a more significant impact in the lower limbs.
- Smoking cessation reduces the excess cardiovascular risk within a relatively short period, and treatments to alleviate nicotine withdrawal symptoms include NRT, varenicline or bupropion. NRT doubles quit rates at 1 year, relative to placebo, but the newer agent varenicline appears to be superior to NRT and bupropion.
- Glycaemic control for those with diabetes is important in the prevention of microvascular complications, but other factors in the diabetes syndrome, such as hypertension and dyslipidaemia, may be more important in the development of PAD.
- Lipid-lowering (statin) therapy increases walking distance and survival among patients with cardiovascular disease, and all PAD patients should be treated.
- Antiplatelet therapy is indicated in all patients with PAD.

Full references available at **http://expertconsult. inkling.com**

Key references

32. Bhatt DL, Steg PG, Ohman EM, et al. International prevalence, recognition and treatment of cardiovascular risk factors in outpatients with atherothrombosis. JAMA 2006;295:180–9. PMID: 16403930.
    The REACH registry is a large multinational observational study of >67 000 patients with cardiovascular disease, including patients with PAD.

42. Alberts MJ, Bhatt DL, Mas J-L, et al. Three-year follow-up and event rates in the international REduction of Atherothrombosis for Continued Health Registry. Eur Heart J 2009;30:2318–26. PMID: 19720633.
    The first outcomes from the REACH registry, which suggested that PAD patients had a high risk for MI and stroke.

44. Rosenberg L, Palmer JR, Shapiro S. Decline in the risk of myocardial infarction among women who stop smoking. N Engl J Med 1990;322:213–7. PMID: 2294448.
    Data identifying the benefits of smoking cessation.

46. Cahill K, Lindson-Hawley N, Thomas KH, et al. Nicotine receptor partial agonists for smoking cessation. Cochrane Database Syst Rev 2016;5:CD006103. PMID: 27158893.
    Up-to-date analysis of the evidence for a number of the treatments available with regard to smoking cessation.

49. Adler A. UKPDS 59: hyperglycaemia and other potentially modifiable risk factors for peripheral arterial disease in type 2 diabetes. Diabetes Care 2002;25:894–9. PMID: 11978687.
    A large study conducted in the UK that showed a strong association between glycaemic control and PAD.

65. Wong PF, Chong LY, Mikhailidis DP, et al. Antiplatelet agents for intermittent claudication. Cochrane Database Syst Rev 2011;11:CD001272. PMID: 22071801.
    Recent meta-analysis of antiplatelet therapy in patients with PAD.

2

Assessment of chronic lower limb ischaemia

Kurian J. Mylankal
Robert Fitridge

Introduction

Peripheral artery disease (PAD) refers to atherosclerotic stenosis or occlusion of the arteries outside of the heart and brain. It is a consequence of systemic atherosclerosis, which involves the arterial tree throughout the body and commonly affects the coronary, carotid, iliac, femoral and infra-inguinal arteries. For the purpose of this chapter, PAD will refer to its manifestations in the lower limb. PAD includes a wide range of symptomatology and disease severity. Although a proportion of individuals with PAD may be asymptomatic, others may experience exertional leg pain (intermittent claudication) which can subsequently progress to severe limb threatening ischaemia. Intermittent claudication (IC) is often the first symptom of PAD, most commonly located in calf muscles, and usually associated with atherosclerotic occlusion or stenosis involving the iliac or femoropopliteal segment. More severe limb ischaemia is usually associated with PAD affecting the lower limb vasculature at two or three anatomical levels. This results in significantly impaired tissue perfusion with rest pain, ulceration or gangrene involving the toes or forefoot. This is referred to as critical limb ischaemia (CLI). This chapter deals with the assessment of patients with chronic lower limb ischaemia and the principles of vascular imaging.

✔ Severity of PAD is commonly reported by two classification systems. The simplest is the Fontaine classification, which is based on clinical symptoms alone (Table 2.1). In contrast, the Rutherford classification is more detailed and takes into account clinical findings, Doppler assessment and ankle–brachial pressure index (ABPI) (Table 2.2). It is useful for reporting standards, but infrequently used in clinical practice.

Intermittent claudication

Intermittent claudication (IC) occurs as a result of reduced blood flow and tissue perfusion which is unable to meet the increased metabolic requirements of the exercising muscle groups. The classic feature of IC is of pain developing on walking in the muscle groups distal to the arterial obstruction, with relief of symptoms within 5–10 minutes of cessation of exercise. This pain reappears after walking a similar distance and is not felt at rest or within the first few steps taken. The symptoms have a chronic history and are described as an ache, cramp or tightening in the muscle that usually forces the patient to stop. Exercise tolerance is dependent on the balance between tissue perfusion and energy expenditure. In mild PAD, claudication may be felt only while walking uphill or walking quickly. Conversely, in individuals with restricted mobility from other comorbidities, PAD may not manifest with claudication symptoms. Claudication pain most commonly affects the calf muscles, which are extensively used whilst walking. However, in the presence of aorto-iliac disease, pain may be felt more proximally in the buttocks or thigh, as well as in the calf.

Osteoarthritis of the hip or knee, spinal stenosis and venous outflow obstruction should be considered in the differential diagnosis of IC. Other relevant

Table 2.1 • Fontaine classification of the severity of PAD

Fontaine stage		Description
I	Asymptomatic	PAD present but no symptoms
II	Intermittent claudication	Cramping pain in leg muscles precipitated by walking and rapidly relieved by rest
III	Rest pain	Constant pain in feet (often worse at night)
IV	Tissue loss	Ischaemic ulceration or gangrene

Table 2.2 • Rutherford classification of the severity of PAD

Grade	Category	Description
0	0	Asymptomatic
I	1	Mild claudication
I	2	Moderate claudication
I	3	Severe claudication
II	4	Ischaemic rest pain
II	5	Minor tissue loss
III	6	Major tissue loss

conditions to consider in the differential diagnosis of IC are described in Table 2.3.[1]

Patients with osteoarthritis of the hip with referred pain down the leg and a history similar to claudication usually experience some pain in the buttock or groin when turning their body and even in a sitting or supine position. Unlike the pain in IC, this is not relieved by standing still and requires easing the load off the arthritic joint. In addition, pain from osteoarthritis typically begins when walking and gets better after some exercise. Although the diagnosis can usually be established by history and examination alone, non-invasive investigations including an exercise test to exclude arterial disease will be reassuring.

Patients with spinal stenosis may have symptoms that are very similar to intermittent claudication although the history of pain may be inconsistent.[2] Sitting and leaning forward to straighten the lumbar lordosis relieves cord pressure although the pain symptoms may take 60 minutes or even longer to subside. A history of pain on standing as well as walking therefore suggests neurogenic claudication due to spinal stenosis.

Lumbar nerve route irritation may also cause aching in the calf or down the back of the leg from buttock to ankle. The sensation appears to be very similar to that of claudication, particularly when confined to the calf. Direct enquiry for these symptoms is helpful, but the key feature is again the need to sit or lie to obtain relief. Spinal flexion may release the involved nerve roots, whereas a straight leg raise will often precipitate the pain. When both sciatic nerve irritation or spinal stenosis and PAD coexist it can be extremely difficult to identify which is contributing most to the patient's symptoms.

In venous outflow obstruction, exercise-induced arterial flow augmentation is not matched by the venous outflow, resulting in high venous pressures within the lower limbs. Tense dilatation of the veins can mimic claudication-like symptoms. However, this is often described as a severe bursting pain and is relieved slowly with rest or leg elevation. A previous history of iliofemoral deep vein thrombosis and inspection findings of lower limb oedema and other stigmata of chronic venous insufficiency will often help with the diagnosis.

The cornerstones in the assessment of chronic lower limb ischaemia are a careful history, palpation of pulses and ABPI measurement. The important point is to verify that the clinical findings correlate well with the patient's symptoms. As the patients get older so does the arterial tree. The mere presence of PAD (i.e. reduced ABPI, atherosclerosis visible on ultrasound examination) does not mean that it is the cause of the symptoms. The history should include the duration of symptoms and the mode of onset. Most patients gradually become aware of pain on walking, which is typical in progressive PAD.

✔✔ The blood supply required by resting muscles is relatively small (130–150 mL/min) and may be increased five- to tenfold during exercise.[3]

Arterial occlusions can be well tolerated when collaterals are well developed, which may provide the same volume flow at rest compared to normal individuals.[4] Examples include the thigh muscles around the superficial femoral artery at the adductor canal, which is well collateralised by the profunda femoris artery. Similarly, in occlusions of the iliac arteries, where collaterals develop through the pelvis and buttock, this may result in normal resting ABPI and even a palpable foot pulse (**Fig. 2.1**). Significant PAD is usually associated with an ABPI of <0.9 (see later), but in such cases an exercise challenge will result in a fall in ankle pressures and disappearance of the distal pulses. If such patients undertake only limited physical activity they may be asymptomatic.

Ischaemic rest pain, ischaemic ulceration or gangrene of the feet requires urgent investigation and revascularisation in order to avoid limb loss from progressive tissue necrosis and/or infection. Unlike IC, in this situation the arterial perfusion is more severely compromised to the degree that it is unable to meet the basal metabolic requirements of the ischaemic tissues. Severely compromised tissue perfusion causes pain even at rest and the

Table 2.3 • Differential diagnosis of intermittent claudication

Condition	Location of pain or discomfort	Characteristic discomfort	Onset relative to exercise	Effect of rest	Effect of body position	Other characteristics
Intermittent claudication	Buttock, thigh, or calf muscles and rarely the foot	Cramping, aching, fatigue, weakness or frank pain	After same degree of exercise	Rapid relief with rest	None	Reproducible
Nerve root compression (e.g., herniated disc)	Radiates down leg, usually posteriorly	Sharp lancinating pain	Soon, if not immediately after onset	Not quickly relieved (also often present at rest)	Relief may be aided by adjusting back position	History of back problems
Spinal stenosis	Hip, thigh, buttocks (follows dermatome)	Motor weakness more prominent than pain	After walking or standing for variable lengths of time	Relieved by stopping only if position changed	Relief by lumbar spine flexion (sitting or stooping forward)	Frequent history of back problems, provoked by intra-abdominal pressure
Arthritic, inflammatory processes	Foot, arch	Aching pain	After variable degree of exercise	Not quickly relieved (and may be present at rest)	May be relieved by not bearing weight	Variable, may relate to activity level
Hip arthritis	Hip, thigh, buttocks	Aching discomfort, usually localized to hip and gluteal region	After variable degree of exercise	Not quickly relieved (and may be present at rest)	More comfortable sitting, weight taken off legs	Variable, may relate to activity level, weather changes
Symptomatic Baker's cyst	Behind knee, down calf	Swelling, soreness, tenderness	With exercise	Present at rest	None	Not intermittent
Venous claudication	Entire leg, but usually worse in thigh and groin	Tight, bursting pain	After walking	Subsides slowly	Relief speeded by elevation	Often history of iliofemoral deep vein thrombosis, signs of venous congestion, oedema
Chronic compartment syndrome	Calf muscles	Tight, bursting pain	After much exercise (e.g. jogging)	Subsides very slowly	Relief speeded by elevation	Typically occurs in heavy muscled athletes

15

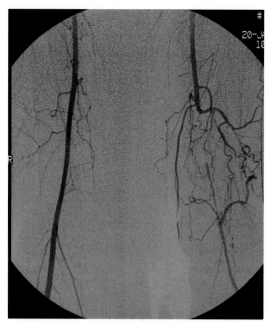

Figure 2.1 • Arteriogram showing well-collateralised occlusion of left superficial femoral artery. The patient had palpable foot pulses and almost normal resting ABPIs. These fell on the left side after exercise.

inability for cellular repair and regeneration results in ulceration and gangrene commonly over areas of minor trauma. Untreated, the prognosis is poor both for the patient and the leg and recognition of critical ischaemia is therefore vitally important. There have been several attempts at a consensus for the definition of critical limb ischaemia (CLI).

> ✓ The European Consensus defines critical limb ischaemia as rest pain for more than 2 weeks, and/or ulceration/gangrene, and an ankle pressure of <50 mmHg or a toe pressure of <30 mmHg.[5]

However, this definition has been criticised because the ankle pressures required for healing in the presence of ulceration or gangrene may be higher and are often falsely elevated, especially in patients with diabetes (see later).[6] The Trans-Atlantic Inter-Society Consensus (TASC) II suggests that an ankle pressure of <70 mmHg or a toe pressure of <50 mmHg is more realistic in the presence of ulceration or gangrene.

> ✓ The precise definition is more relevant for reporting standards than for clinical use and the TASC II document recommends that the term critical limb ischaemia should be used for all patients with chronic ischaemic rest pain, ulcers or gangrene attributable to objectively proven arterial occlusive disease.[1]

CLI may start with pain in the forefoot at night sufficient to disturb the patient's sleep when the patient is in supine position, cancelling the effect of gravity on blood flow to the lower limbs.[7] When the patient hangs the leg out of the bed or if they stand up and walk (thereby increasing the blood flow to the foot) the pain is relieved. If the patient constantly hangs their feet out of bed at night, or even sleeps sitting in a chair, the limb tends to swell due to dependent oedema. This oedema in turn increases the hydrostatic pressure of the peripheral tissue and compresses the already compromised capillaries and further interferes with tissue perfusion and nutrition. These patients may often require inpatient treatment with analgesics (usually including opiates) so that the limb can be kept in the supine position overnight to relieve the oedema prior to arterial reconstruction.

To the experienced eye the diagnosis of CLI seems obvious, but it is easy to miss a small ischaemic lesion on the heel or between the toes. When established necrosis or gangrene is present with absent limb pulses there is no doubt about the diagnosis. The stage of critical ischaemia without necrosis or gangrene (Rutherford II 4) is characterised by pallor when the leg is elevated above the heart and changing to a deep red colour when hanging down (Buerger's or Ratshow's test-positive). The red colour is caused by the dilated capillaries of the foot (**Fig. 2.2**). In critical limb ischaemia, the natural coping mechanisms for ischaemia including angiogenesis (new capillary formation) and arteriogenesis (enlargement of pre-existing capillaries) are exhausted and the capillaries are maximally vasodilated and hence unresponsive to pro-vasodilatory stimuli.[8,9] Therefore, it may take a while for pallor on elevation to occur but capillary refill will be abolished immediately.

Rare causes of ischaemia

The vast majority of cases of chronic lower limb ischaemia are caused by atherosclerotic PAD, but some rare conditions exist that tend to affect the younger age group. A good history of IC in a young patient should be taken seriously, as some of these conditions may progress rapidly to CLI. Resting ABPIs should be measured in all patients with leg pain on exercise, especially if foot pulses are absent. Those with a good history of IC and palpable foot pulses or normal ABPI should also undergo an exercise test and post-exercise ABPIs.

Persistent sciatic artery

In this congenital anomaly, the embryonic axial limb artery, the sciatic artery, does not obliterate and remains continuous with the popliteal artery, providing the major blood supply to the lower limb.

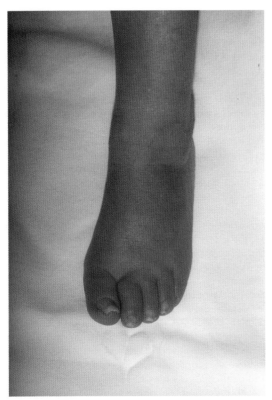

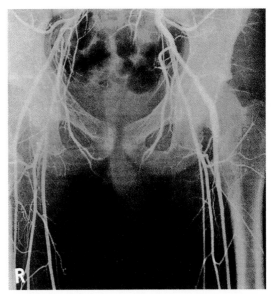

Figure 2.3 • Persistent bilateral sciatic arteries arising from the common iliac arteries with dilatation and intimal irregularity of the left sciatic artery at the level of the acetabulum.

Figure 2.2 • 'Sunset red foot due to dilated capillaries caused by critical (limb-threatening) ischaemia. Elevation of the foot will result in pallor (Buerger's or Ratshow's test-positive).

The anomaly is bilateral in 30% of cases and is commonly associated with failure of the iliofemoral vessels to develop normally. The presenting symptoms include pain and a pulsatile mass in the buttock due to aneurysmal degeneration of the artery as it emerges from the sciatic foramen. Thrombosis or distal embolism may lead to acute ischaemia. In a review of 159 patients with persistent sciatic artery, the mean patient age at the time of diagnosis was 59 years and 80% were symptomatic with IC, acute ischaemia, pulsatile mass or neurological symptoms from sciatic nerve compression.[10] Although pedal pulses may be present, the femoral pulse will be reduced or absent if the iliofemoral vessels are hypoplastic (Cowie's sign) and IC will result if neither system has developed properly (**Fig. 2.3**). Symptomatic patients can be treated by combined bypass grafting and endovascular exclusion of the aneurysm.[11] Asymptomatic patients should be monitored for aneurysm development.

Cystic adventitial disease (CAD)

CAD is caused by cyst formation in the adventitia of the artery due to implantation of mucin-secreting mesenchymal cells on the adventitial wall during development. It is a unilateral presentation and commonly affects the popliteal artery and less often the external iliac and femoral vessels. It predominantly affects males in the mid-30s who may present with IC. The contents of the cyst resemble that of a ganglion and the cysts may be connected to the synovium of the knee joint. IC may be severe and of rapid onset. The condition should be particularly suspected in young patients without significant risk factors for PAD. Pedal pulses sometimes disappear on knee flexion (Ishikawa's sign). Arteriography may show an unusually smooth 'hourglass' stenosis referred to as the 'scimitar' sign (**Fig. 2.4**). Ultrasound scanning will demonstrate the cystic abnormality with absence of flow within it and computed tomography (CT) may help delineate CAD from popliteal entrapment syndrome and aneurysm. The appearance of CAD on magnetic resonance imaging (MRI) is distinctive. CAD demonstrates homogenous low intensity signal on T1-weighted images and high signal intensity on T2-weighted images. On post-contrast T1-weighted images, the cyst does not enhance and can be seen compressing the arterial lumen.[12] The distinctive findings on MRI have resulted in this modality becoming the imaging technique of choice when the condition is suspected or diagnosed on ultrasound. Resection of the affected segment of artery and repair with an interposition vein graft via a posterior approach is the most widely practised technique and is mandatory in popliteal artery

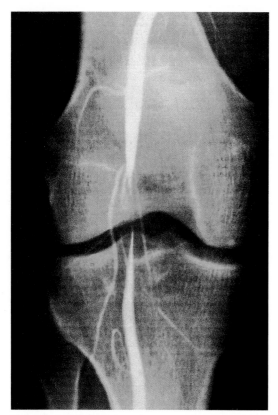

Figure 2.4 • Smooth 'hourglass' stenosis of popliteal artery due to cystic adventitial disease. A similar appearance may be seen in popliteal entrapment, especially during active plantar flexion.

thrombosis or in extensive arterial involvement.[13] Non-resectional techniques such as cyst excision or evacuation have been described with some success although a high incidence of recurrence has been observed with these techniques.

Popliteal artery entrapment

This condition should be suspected when a young patient, particularly an athlete, complains of claudication symptoms or classic critical limb ischaemia. Two-thirds of cases are bilateral and the popliteal vein is involved in 10%.[14] During the embryonic development, the medial head of the gastrocnemius muscle migrates from the posterior aspect of the fibula and lateral tibia across the popliteal fossa to its attachment to the posterior aspect of the medial femoral condyle. The popliteal artery simultaneously develops superficial to the popliteus muscle during this stage. These complex and dynamic changes associated with the fetal limb bud rotation and knee extension raise the chance for various anatomical variations to develop in the

relationship between the popliteal artery and the medial head of the gastrocnemius muscle. There are six variants of popliteal entrapment described. The popliteal artery is displaced medially by the migrating gastrocnemius muscle in Type I variant and the medial deviation is evident in radiological imaging. In Type II, the migration of the muscle is arrested by the already developed artery whereby the muscle has a more lateral insertion on the femoral condyle and hence the popliteal artery runs a straight course. In Type III, muscle slips or bands tether the artery to the medial or lateral femoral condyles as the artery develops within the muscle in the embryonic stage. Type IV variant is characterised by entrapment of the artery by the popliteus muscle and here a persisting axial artery replaces the popliteal artery. Type V refers to any of the above subtypes but with entrapment of both the popliteal artery and vein. In Type VI or '[functional variant', no anatomical abnormality is noted for the arterial compression and it may occur as a result of muscle hypertrophy (especially the medial head of gastrocnemius) from regular exercise. Continuous compression of the artery results in fibrotic change which progresses from the outer adventitial layer of the artery to the intima. As a consequence, aneurysmal degeneration and/or thrombosis may develop. Examination may reveal reduction or obliteration of pedal pulses during active plantar flexion. Duplex scanning or arteriography using this manoeuvre may also demonstrate kinking or compression of the popliteal artery. CT or MR scanning can also demonstrate the anatomical abnormality. Symptomatic patients should be treated by the division of the medial head of gastrocnemius and/or reconstruction of the popliteal artery. Surgery may be indicated for an asymptomatic contralateral limb whenever anatomical entrapment is detected.[15] In the functional variant of the condition, an anatomically normally positioned artery is compressed against a hypertrophied gastrocnemius or the soleal muscle ring. Functional entrapment, unlike the anatomical variant, should only be treated when symptomatic.[16]

Fibromuscular dysplasia (FMD)

FMD is a non-atherosclerotic and non-inflammatory arterial disease which is more commonly seen in women and usually affects the renal and carotid arteries. It can also affect the iliac, femoral or popliteal arteries although this is less common. In young people. FMD can cause IC or microembolisation and rarely critical limb ischaemia from arterial dissection. Depending on the layer of the arterial wall that is predominantly affected, three varieties of FMD are recognised – medial fibroplasia (most common type), intimal fibroplasia and adventitial fibroplasia.

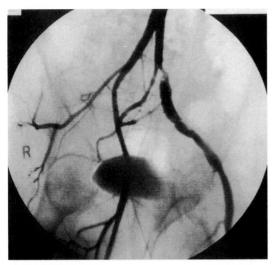

Figure 2.5 • Fibromuscular dysplasia affecting the left external iliac artery of a 12-year-old boy.

It is characterised by intra-arterial fibrotic webs that give rise to stenoses and post-stenotic dilatations giving the classic beaded appearance. The external iliac artery is the commonest site of involvement in the lower limb vasculature (**Fig. 2.5**). Patients with iliac FMD should be screened for renal and carotid involvement. Symptomatic stenoses usually respond well to angioplasty. Stenting should be reserved for cases with suboptimal angioplasty results or procedural complications following angioplasty.[17]

Endofibrosis of the iliac artery

This is a rare cause of arterial stenosis seen particularly in the external iliac artery among competitive cyclists. It is thought to develop as a result of repetitive trauma to the external iliac artery and the commonest presentation is intermittent claudication with maximal exertion. Clinical examination may be normal and occasionally a femoral bruit may be heard. Exercise testing with immediate post-exercise ABPIs and duplex ultrasound help confirm the lesion. Duplex ultrasound and contrast angiography may demonstrate concentric stenosis but the lesions may be very subtle at rest. Techniques widely reported for repair are endarterectomy and patch angioplasty and interposition graft.[18,19]

Buerger's disease

Buerger's disease (thromboangiitis obliterans) is a systemic vasculopathy associated with tobacco use that affects medium-sized arteries and veins in both the upper and lower limbs. It should be considered in any heavy-smoking young male claudicant, especially if they are of Middle or Far Eastern origin.[20] Vasospastic symptoms and superficial thrombophlebitis commonly occur and patients may progress rapidly to, or present with, CLI. The pathophysiology and management of this condition and other causes of vasculitis such as Takayasu's are covered in Chapter 12.

> ✔✔ The crural vessels are usually severely affected, with patent arteries to the knee joint and typical 'corkscrew' collaterals in the calf.[21]

History and examination

History

Duration of symptoms, relieving and exacerbating factors are central to the correct diagnosis of PAD and history taking should focus on eliciting this. Localising pain will help ascertain the anatomical level of atherosclerotic disease and subsequent clinical examination can further confirm this. Quantifying walking distance can help assess the limitations to mobility and progress or deterioration of symptoms over a period of time. Pain interrupting sleep, alleviated by dependency and sleeping in a chair are all features suggestive of CLI. It is also important to establish the impact of these symptoms on the patient's daily activities, ability to work and to remain independent.

> ✔✔ As all patients with PAD are at risk of myocardial infarction or stroke, a full history for other cardiovascular diseases and risk factors is essential (see Chapter 1).

In addition to direct enquiry for cardiovascular risk factors (smoking, diabetes mellitus, hypertension, dyslipidaemia, chronic kidney disease and a detailed drug and family history), the patient must be asked about a history of ischaemic heart disease, coronary stenting or bypass grafting and cerebrovascular disease, including transient ischaemic attacks and stroke. Although approximately 30% of patients with symptoms of limb ischaemia will have a history of myocardial infarction, it is not uncommon that angina or transient ischaemic attacks are diagnosed for the first time at initial vascular assessment. The investigation and treatment algorithm for these symptoms are usually based on a rational approach of prioritisation dependent on the severity of other comorbidities (see Chapter 3). Upper extremity exertional pain, postprandial abdominal pain and erectile dysfunction in men are other important potential clues to the presence of significant occlusive atherosclerotic disease in other vascular territories.

A systematic approach to history taking helps establish the correct diagnosis and institute optimal strategies/therapy to counter concomitant cardiac and cerebrovascular risks. In addition, it also helps develop a safe management strategy for PAD taking into consideration patient fitness to undergo interventions.

Examination

A thorough and systematic approach aims to establish the site and severity of PAD and elicit signs of atherosclerosis and its risk factors in any part of the cardiovascular system. General inspection for peripheral stigmata of cardiovascular disease such as cigarette staining of fingernails, scars from previous surgery, amputated limbs and toes, and xanthelasma should be sought. Measurement of blood pressure in both arms and the inter-arm difference, palpation of radial and brachial pulses (rhythm, rate and volume) and cardiac and pulmonary auscultation are mandatory to assess the extent of atherosclerotic involvement. Careful inspection of the feet for skin integrity including the interdigital web spaces and heel pressure points, skin colour and changes with elevation and dependency and temperature are noted. Abnormal femoral and foot pulses, lower extremity bruits, unilateral cool extremities, prolonged venous refill time and Buerger's test are findings highly suggestive of underlying PAD and capillary refill test, foot discolouration, atrophic skin and hairless extremities are unhelpful in the diagnosis of PAD.[22]

The body mass index (BMI) should be calculated by measuring height and weight. This is a good estimate of obesity, which may affect the patient's walking incapacity. Obesity may also affect anaesthetic risk as well as likelihood of surgical complications. In some cases, weight loss will reduce the patient's symptoms substantially.

Palpation of pulses is subjective, and is influenced by the sensitivity of the fingers, the experience of the examiner, the obesity of the patient and the warmth of the room. This should commence with a preliminary examination of the abdomen, assessing the aorta for the presence of an aneurysm and palpation for other abdominal masses. The femoral artery should be palpable in all subjects (**Fig. 2.6**). If it is occluded it can often be palpated as a hard cord due to atherosclerosis. If the pulse feels weak it is often because of proximal obstruction causing reduced femoral artery blood pressure. The popliteal pulse is more difficult to palpate, particularly in a well-muscled or obese subject, but should always

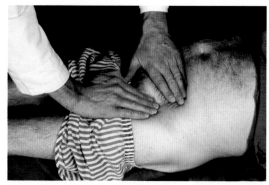

Figure 2.6 • Palpation of the femoral pulse may require both hands except in the thin patient. One hand pushes the lower abdomen out of the way and the other palpates the femoral artery/pulse.

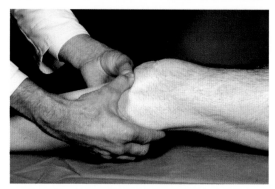

Figure 2.7 • A popliteal pulse is best felt using both hands with the leg relaxed in slight flexion.

be examined to exclude an aneurysm (**Fig. 2.7**). Palpation of the foot pulses should always be performed and described. It may be difficult when the foot is swollen or the room is cold. Presence or absence of foot pulses on physical examination is a 'weak' and subjective sign of PAD and should always be supplemented by objective measurements (ABPI). The absence of a single foot pulse may have little clinical significance and, although it should be recorded, it is not an indication for more detailed investigation. Auscultation of the neck, abdomen and groin should be performed to assess for bruits that may suggest stenoses of the carotid, renal/mesenteric and femoral arteries.

Exercise challenge

Patients present occasionally with a classic history of IC, but with palpable foot pulses. These patients may have been investigated previously for joint disease or lumbar nerve root irritation even though their history may be 'typical' of claudication. Most often, there is proximal aorto-iliac disease with collaterals through the pelvis, sufficient to produce adequate or even normal pulses at rest. In patients who complain of symptoms only on exercise, it is useful to examine the leg following an exercise challenge. This can be done quite simply by asking the patient to walk up and down the corridors of the outpatient clinic or on a treadmill if available. Exercising the calf muscle by repeated 'tiptoe' while leaning on the couch may be a practical alternative to this (**Fig. 2.8**). The patient returns to the couch so that the pulses can be examined immediately after exercising for 1 minute. More importantly, the post-exercise ABPI is measured and a drop in ABPI of >0.15 from baseline and/or drop in ankle pressure > 30 mmHg is significant.[23] In moderate to severe PAD, a sustained drop in post exercise ABPI

is noted which persists for the observation period of 10–15 minutes.

ABPI measurement using a hand-held Doppler device

The perfusion pressure at the ankle can be measured using a tourniquet and insonating the pedal arteries with Doppler ultrasound. The patient should be rested for more than 5 minutes, lying supine, and a standard blood pressure tourniquet applied just above the ankle, with the tourniquet being 50% wider than the limb diameter. The tourniquet cuff is inflated above the systolic pressure, when the pedal Doppler signal should disappear. On gradually lowering the cuff pressure, the Doppler signal reappears at the ankle systolic pressure (**Fig. 2.9**). The probe should be held at a 30–60° angle to the vessel in order to achieve the optimal signal. The systolic blood pressure is then taken from the brachial artery in the same way and the ABPI calculated as the ratio of the ankle to the brachial systolic pressures. Blood pressures should be assessed on both arms at the patient's first visit since 3–5% of PAD patients may have supra-aortic occlusive disease as well. The higher of the two brachial blood pressures should be used as the reference for calculating ABPI.

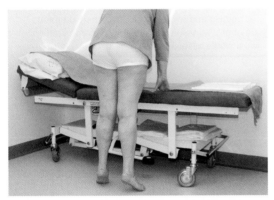

Figure 2.8 • Simple 'tiptoe' exercise of the calf muscle causes vasodilatation with disappearance of pulses and the emergence of bruits on examination immediately after the exercise.

✓ The systolic pressure at the ankle is normally higher, due to superimposed pulse waves down the arterial tree with an ABPI of 1.0–1.2. An ABPI of <0.9 suggests arterial disease and serves as the lower limit of normal. An ABPI of <0.5 is often associated with critical ischaemia.[1]

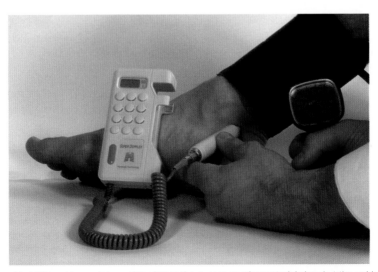

Figure 2.9 • A hand-held Doppler can be used to detect the presence of an arterial signal at the ankle. Assess the waveform – abnormal (monophasic/damped) or normal (biphasic/triphasic) – and measure the ABPI.

An ankle arterial pressure of 60 mmHg is required for ulcer healing in patients without diabetes and a higher pressure of 80 mmHg is generally required in the patient with diabetes. Falsely high ankle arterial pressures may be measured if the calf arteries are rigid due to calcification, as is often associated with diabetes and chronic kidney disease. The finding of very high or incompressible ankle pressures (systolic >200 mmHg or ABPI >1.3) should always raise suspicion of a false result. In such cases, measurement of toe pressures (see below) will reveal a true pressure as the small digital arteries infrequently become affected with medial calcification. Alternatively, if toe pressure measurement is not possible, the pedal Doppler signal should be assessed for normal triphasic or biphasic waveforms (see below, Waveform assessment and segmental pressures). When the Doppler signal in the foot is monophasic due to proximal disease, pressures above the brachial pressure suggest falsely high readings due to vascular calcification.

> ✔ ABPI assessment should be a routine part of a vascular examination.[1]

Assessment of ABPI is indicated for all patients with leg ulceration and foot ulcers. The technique is particularly important in diabetic 'neuropathic' ulcers or infection involving the toes or feet, where missed proximal arterial disease may lead to avoidable amputation due to rapidly progressing infection. The ABPI is also useful in elderly patients referred with foot symptoms that do not appear to be vascular and in these cases a normal measurement is reassuring.

Toe pressures

Toe pressure measurements may be useful when the calf arteries are incompressible or when severe distal arterial disease in the foot is suspected, i.e. in cases with high ABPI but non-healing ulcers at toe or forefoot level.

> ✔ A small toe cuff should be used and placed around the proximal phalanx of the great, second or third toe with a photoelectric cell on the toe distally.[24]

The toe pressure is most commonly measured using photo-plethysmography or continuous-wave Doppler techniques to detect the disappearance and reappearance of the pulse as the cuff is inflated and deflated. Laser Doppler, which utilises the Doppler shift phenomenon of reflected light from moving blood cells to measure microcirculatory blood perfusion, is an alternative technique for toe pressure assessment. A warm room is essential to avoid vasospasm and most often the feet need a 15- to 20-minute warm-up period. Toe pressures are expressed as an absolute value in mmHg and also as a ratio to brachial artery pressure, toe–brachial index (TBI). The absolute toe pressures are normally 20–40 mmHg less than the ankle pressures, which may be due to the sensitivity of the measurement technique. A normal TBI ranges from 0.8 to 0.9. An absolute toe pressure <30 mmHg is frequently associated with CLI and generally superficial foot ulcers heal with pressures greater than 40 mmHg (the higher the toe pressure, the more confident one can be that healing will occur).

> ✔ Critical ischaemia is unusual with toe–brachial pressure ratios >0.3 or absolute toe pressures >40 mmHg and two or more serial measurements are of greater value in predicting outcome than an initial single assessment.[25]

Risk factors

All patients should be investigated for risk factors for atherosclerosis as modification reduces both the risk of fatal and non-fatal cardiovascular events and the need for arterial reconstruction. The risk factors associated with PAD are essentially the same as those for ischaemic heart disease, and include smoking, lack of exercise, unhealthy dietary habits, dyslipidaemia, diabetes mellitus, hypertension, age and male sex (see Chapter 1).

All patients with PAD require a full blood count, erythrocyte sedimentation rate (ESR), urea and electrolytes, a random blood glucose and lipid levels. Anaemia can present with symptoms of leg ischaemia, as can polycythaemia. An elevated ESR (or viscosity) may indicate raised fibrinogen, which seems an important factor in the development of PAD and vascular thrombosis. Renal impairment is often associated with PAD and requires detection before contemplating both imaging and intervention. Arterial thromboembolism is relatively infrequent in patients under the age of 50 years. Young patients with PAD should have a thrombophilia screen as antiphospholipid antibodies or antithrombin III deficiency may lead to repeated rethrombosis following either angioplasty or reconstruction. Hyperhomocysteinaemia can cause accelerated atherosclerosis and should be excluded in young patients with PAD. Acute limb ischaemia in a younger patient with no history of PAD warrants thorough cardiac investigations work-up, including at least an electrocardiogram (ECG) and echocardiography.

Vascular laboratory

Waveform assessment and segmental pressures

The use of Doppler waveforms, originally implemented using hand-held continuous-wave Doppler devices, still has an important role in the investigation of PAD. The elasticity in normal arteries gives a characteristic triphasic waveform (see **Fig. 2.11c**). The blood pressure may be reduced distal to a stenosis and consequently the resistance in the peripheral vascular bed is reduced, changing the shape of this waveform. Distal to a moderate stenosis (50% diameter reduction) the waveform is usually biphasic, and with a >70% stenosis the waveform generally becomes monophasic (see **Fig. 2.11d**).[26] Waveform shape can be affected by distal disease, dilatation of

arteries, multisegment disease, complete occlusion of an artery and also ambient temperature. Waveform shape can only give an indication of disease and should be used in conjunction with segmental pressures to determine which segments in the leg are diseased, i.e. since percutaneous transluminal angioplasty (PTA) is minimally invasive and generally provides good results in the iliac arteries, knowing that a pressure-reducing lesion is located in this anatomical region may strengthen the indication for invasive treatment in a patient with severe IC.

Clinicians frequently see patients with multisegment disease. Segmental arterial pressures have some additional value in both determining the level of disease and predicting whether proximal arterial reconstruction will be adequate to treat critical ischaemia (**Fig. 2.10**). However, duplex ultrasound, CT or MR arteriography are more useful in this respect.

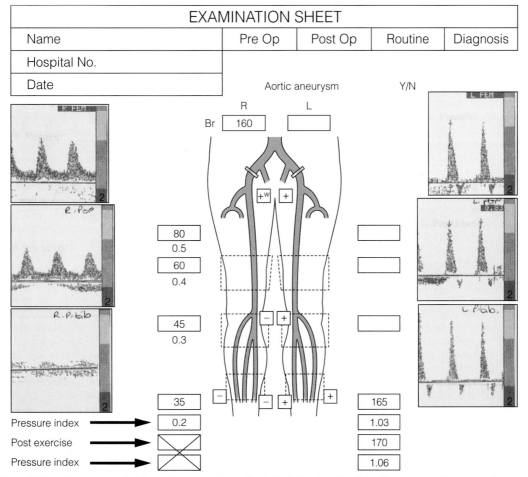

Figure 2.10 • Segmental arterial waveforms may help discriminate the functional significance of multisegment disease, such as the right iliac and superficial femoral occlusions in this patient. Theoretically, normalising the low thigh pressure will approximately double the ankle arterial pressure to a level that should relieve ischaemic rest pain.

Transcutaneous oximetry

This technique can be used to measure the partial pressure of oxygen diffusing through the surface of the skin as an indirect measure for oxygen tension in the underlying tissue. It was hoped that $tcPO_2$ measurements of calf skin might be used to determine whether healing would occur following below-knee amputation.[27] Unfortunately, $tcPO_2$ is unreliable for this purpose as the changes in the proximal skin perfusion after amputation of the limb cannot be predicted. However, a recent systematic review suggests that $tcPO_2 \geq 25$ mmHg is a favourable indicator for ulcer healing. Along with a toe pressure ≥ 45 mmHg, this may be reassuring for the treating clinician and a predictor of a positive outcome.[28]

Duplex ultrasound (DUS)

DUS has emerged as the most important non-invasive imaging modality to confirm and assess severity of PAD. DUS allows the visualisation of arteries in real time using grey-scale (B-mode) imaging and detailed haemodynamic evaluation of blood flow by colour-flow Doppler mapping, power Doppler and spectral Doppler. DUS is non-invasive and cost-effective which has also resulted in its widespread use in serial imaging to assess disease progression and surveillance following intervention. It is an operator-dependent examination and reliability of DUS is dependent on the experience and knowledge of the operator and interpreting clinician.

✓✓ DUS of the extremities has been given a class 1 recommendation (supported by multiple randomised controlled trials or meta-analyses) for the diagnosis, the anatomical location and determining the degree of stenosis of PAD, as well as for routine surveillance after lower limb bypass with a venous conduit.[29]

Lower extremity scanning requires a variety of transducers. Lower frequency transducers (2 MHz or 3 MHz) are suitable for deeper structures, such as the abdominal aorta and iliac arteries and a higher frequency (5 MHz or 7 MHz) is required for the infrainguinal segments. In general terms, the higher the probe frequency, the greater will be the resolution and hence the highest frequency transducer that provides satisfactory depth of view should be used for the examination.

DUS of lower limb arterial disease is dependent on high quality B-mode which visualises echogenic plaques and the anatomy of the artery/disease. Colour-flow Doppler and spectral Doppler are two types of ultrasound displays which are often used simultaneously during arterial imaging. Colour flow Doppler depicts both direction of blood flow and mean velocity and is used to visualise blood flow by colour encoding Doppler information and displaying the colour through the colour box positioned within the grey-scale image. The colour box is subdivided into small sample regions or colour pixels and represents the mean velocity within that region. By convention, flow towards the transducer is depicted in red and flow away from the transducer in blue. The display of blood flow includes different shades of blue and red to represent the flow velocity and this colour allocation is dependent on the colour map provided by the manufacturer. Colour filling will only occur where blood is moving and can therefore be used to enhance the grey-scale image by identifying 'soft' echolucent atheroma or thrombus as an area of absent colour filling. Colour flow allows identification of increased blood velocity by a change in colour within the lumen of the artery. Severe stenosis can be seen as grey echoes reducing the diameter of the colour filling and a 'mosaic' of colours indicates increased velocity and turbulence. However, colour flow Doppler does not provide a quantitative means of determining the severity of a stenosis other than by direct luminal diameter or area loss measurement (**Fig. 2.11a, b**).

Accurate quantification of the severity of the stenosis requires the use of spectral Doppler. In this form of ultrasound image display, flow velocities are graphically represented on the Y axis against time on the X axis. Continuous wave Doppler and pulse wave Doppler are two types of spectral Doppler with some differences. As the name implies, in continuous wave Doppler the transducer is emitting and receiving ultrasound waves continuously and hence can measure velocities along an entire line of interrogation. For the same reason, it can detect very high velocity flow although it cannot pinpoint where along the line this arises from. In contrast, in pulse wave Doppler the transducer emits a pulsed ultrasound signal which is pinpointed to a specific depth by the sampling box. The change of frequency (Doppler shift) in the reflected signal is determined by the transmitted frequency, angle of insonation and the velocity of blood flow. Modern DUS machines allow automated calculation of blood velocity but the accuracy of this relies heavily on the correct determination of the position of the pulsed-wave Doppler box and angling of the central cursor to the axis of blood flow. The peak systolic velocity is measured in the normal artery proximal to a stenosis and then in the stenosis identified by colour flow. The shape of the Doppler waveform (triphasic, biphasic or monophasic), degree of spectral broadening (range of velocity profiles within the wave spectra secondary to turbulence) and change in peak systolic velocity relative to the upstream

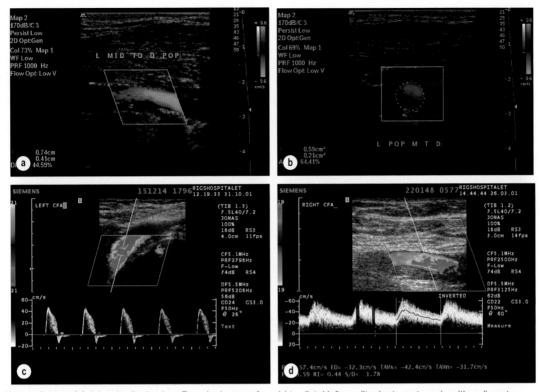

Figure 2.11 • (a) A longitudinal colour Doppler image of a mid to distal left popliteal artery stenosis with a diameter reduction of approximately 50%. **(b)** The area reduction of the same lesion on transaxial imaging is 60–70%. **(c, d)** Doppler waveforms from common femoral artery, just proximal to stenosis **(c)** and distal to stenosis **(d)**. Notice how the waveform is triphasic with steep acceleration phase signalling high resistance **(c)**, and monophasic and dampened distal to the stenosis, where the stenosis has caused a pressure drop with reduction in resistance as a result **(d)**.

Table 2.4 • Diagnostic criteria for peripheral artery diameter reduction

Degree of stenosis	PSV(cm/s)	Velocity ratio (Vr)	Spectral waveform of distal artery.
Normal	<150	<1.5	Triphasic, normal PSV
30–49%	150–200	1.5–2	Triphasic, normal PSV
50–75%	200–400	2–4	Monophasic, reduced PSV
>75%	>400	>4	Damped, monophasic reduced PSV
Occlusion	No flow, proximal and distal collaterals help estimate occlusion length		Damped, monophasic reduced PSV

PSV, peak systolic velocity; Vr, PSV ratio across a stenosis

normal artery all help to determine the severity of a given stenosis (Table 2.4).[30] In the peripheral arteries, a twofold increase in the peak systolic velocity generally indicates a 50% narrowing of the artery, while a fourfold increase in velocity ratio with monophasic waveform indicates a high grade stenosis. Distal to a stenosis, the Doppler waveform changes shape due to damping with reduction in peak systolic velocity and a slower acceleration time (time from end diastole to peak systole; **Fig. 2.11c**).

Certainty of the diagnosis of a complete occlusion as opposed to high-grade stenosis with trickle flow within an artery may be difficult and depends heavily on the experience of the sonographer. The shape of the Doppler waveform proximally and distally, colour-flow images and the presence of collaterals all contribute to differentiating these lesions. Difficulties can arise with deep or tortuous arteries, where signal return is reduced and optimum angles of insonation are difficult to obtain. Multiple stenoses along the length of an artery reduce the accuracy of flow velocity measurements in the assessment of more distal stenoses. Power Doppler imaging, which is dependent on the amplitude of Doppler signals and independent of flow velocity and direction, is a sensitive imaging technique that can help in such situations to differentiate arterial occlusion from high-grade stenosis. The sonographer must thus use valuable years of experience and knowledge of more subtle changes in blood velocity to determine the severity of a given stenosis when there are tandem or multiple stenoses.

Assessment of suprainguinal arteries

This can be achieved by direct assessment of the iliac arteries although this poses challenges due to respiratory movements, the depth of arteries, arterial tortuosity, overlying bowel gas and arterial wall calcification obscuring the vessel lumen. Changing the plane of insonation may often help find an acoustic window through obscuring and distracting anatomy and pathology. It is critical that sonographers communicate difficulties encountered during scanning to the referring physician.

> ✔ Aorto-iliac DUS arterial assessment using a peak systolic velocity ratio >2 has been shown to match catheter angiography in detecting a >50% stenosis with a sensitivity of 82% and specificity of 92%.[31]

Changes in the Doppler waveform proximal and distal to an inadequately viewed segment often give an indication of the extent of disease and the need for further investigation. Evaluation of the Doppler waveform in the common femoral artery is an indirect method for assessing the iliac arteries. If it is triphasic, the likelihood of a severe obstructive lesion in the aorto-iliac segment is very low.[32]

> ✔ In experienced hands, DUS is accurate at identifying disease from the common femoral to the distal popliteal artery, with a sensitivity of 84–87% and specificity of 92–98% compared to catheter angiography.[30,33]

Assessment of femoro-popliteal segment

DUS assessment of the superficial femoral artery can give accurate information regarding flow and stenoses although insonation at the level of the adductor canal may pose technical challenges. The crural arteries can be more difficult, especially when there is severe proximal disease.[34,35] In large calves, the depth of insonation attenuates the signal return, making it difficult to visualise the proximal crural arteries.[35] Accuracy can be improved by using a low frequency transducer such as a curved-array abdominal probe, which allows for deeper penetration albeit at the cost of reduced image quality. Alternatively, power Doppler, which is more sensitive to slow flow, can help detect the optimum tibial artery for revascularisation.

Radiological investigations

The choice of imaging modality for the investigation of chronic lower limb ischaemia was reviewed as part of the August 2012 UK National Institute for Clinical Excellence (NICE) Clinical Guideline 147, 'Lower limb peripheral artery disease: diagnosis and management'.[36] The question as to the most clinical and cost-effective method for assessment of PAD revealed eight relevant publications from which the following broad recommendations were made.

> ✔✔ 1. Offer duplex ultrasound as first-line imaging to all people with peripheral artery disease for whom revascularisation is being considered.
> 2. Offer contrast-enhanced magnetic resonance angiography (CE-MRA) to people with peripheral artery disease who need further imaging (after duplex ultrasound) before considering revascularisation.
> 3. Offer computed tomography angiography (CTA) to people with peripheral artery disease who need further imaging (after duplex ultrasound) if CE-MRA is contraindicated or not tolerated.[36]

Most vascular centres use DUS as the first-line imaging modality to investigate PAD due to its greater availability, lower cost and limited access to MR scanner time. However, relying solely on DUS prior to lower limb revascularisation risks underestimation of the severity and number of sites of vascular disease, particularly at challenging-to-reach anatomical areas such as the iliac and proximal infragenicular crural arteries. CE-MRA, on the other hand, provides better overall diagnostic accuracy and may also serve as a first-line imaging modality.[37] CE-MRA with images processed by maximum intensity projection (MIP) provides angiogram quality images that can be viewed from any projection. DUS can then be utilised in a complementary role, focused on problem-solving, to address specific equivocal haemodynamic questions that may affect the treatment strategy. This optimises the sonographer's time and eliminates redundant duplication of imaging normal arterial segments twice.

Magnetic resonance angiography (MRA)

The basic principles of MRI rely on a large external magnetic field which magnetises the subject protons to align parallel to the field, a magnetic field gradient which helps alter the direction of the external magnetic field and a radiofrequency field provided by resonant coils placed in close proximity to the area of interest. The resonant frequency of the protons is tapped into by the receivers to process the final image by a complex mathematical algorithm. The contrast seen in MRI depends on the characteristics of the imaging object. It is referred to as T1-weighted and T2-weighted images. MR angiography (MRA) and MR venography (MRV) are dependent on T1-weighted images and here fat, methaemoglobin, flow and contrast agents will appear bright. T2-weighted images display fluids as bright and are not used for MRA. There are several MR techniques for the assessment of vessels and vessel patency, all of which continue to evolve at a rapid pace. Modern MR scanners provide high-quality angiographic images without exposing the patient to radiation. In addition, MRA avoids the need for image manipulation to remove overlying bone and calcification from the arterial wall. MRA can be performed by contrast-enhanced techniques (CE-MRA) and non-contrast techniques such as time of flight (TOF) MRA and phase contrast MRI. The non-contrast techniques utilise the ability to differentiate signal characteristics of flowing blood from static tissues for image acquisition. TOF MRA poses significant challenges with inadequate signals from deeper vessels with poor image resolution, flow-related artefacts especially in areas of stenosis, and prolonged scan time. Phase contrast MRI, although has >90% sensitivity and specificity for detection of stenosis compared to digital subtraction angiography, once again is limited by prolonged image acquisition time.[38] In recent years, these two techniques have been supplanted by 3-dimensional contrast-enhanced MRA (CE-MRA). However, safety concerns related to gadolinium-based CE MRA and nephrogenic systemic fibrosis (see below) over the last decade have led to a revival of interest in non-contrast MRA. ECG-gated partial Fourier fast spin echo (FSE), balanced SSFP with arterial spin labelling and quiescent-interval single-shot MRA are some of the newer techniques being developed. Early studies with single-shot MRA have shown over 85% sensitivity and 95% specificity for detecting significant stenosis when comparing with CE-MRA.[39]

CE-MRA employs subtraction, bolus chase and stepping-table movements for image acquisition. It provides a non-invasive, 3-dimensional luminal assessment of vessels without the risk of iodine-based contrast agents and ionising radiation. It has now become the preferred first-line imaging technique for the investigation of PAD in many centres. This is advocated in international guidelines, as well as by the TASC II document and the NICE Clinical Guideline 147 on the diagnosis and management of PAD.[1,36]

✔✔ In a meta-analysis of 32 studies including 1022 patients, CE-MRA was concluded to have high accuracy for identifying or excluding clinically relevant arterial steno-occlusions in adults with PAD symptoms.[40]

Technique

There are a wide variety of techniques for performing peripheral lower limb MRA that depend on the MR hardware, software sequences, moving or continuous-table capability, peripheral and surface coils, preferred contrast agent and injection protocol. As crural (tibial) vessel venous contamination has been the Achilles heel of consistently high-quality peripheral MRA, techniques have been developed to overcome this by obtaining this imaging station either faster using parallel imaging (acceleration techniques) or by first using dynamic time-resolved MRA, followed by the more usual three- or four-station stepping-table 'bolus chase' technique (**Fig. 2.12a**). More recent developments have included greater efforts at imaging the distal calf and foot vessels as distal intervention has become of increasing importance (**Fig. 2.12b**).

Contraindications

Contraindications to MRA include the presence of a pacemaker or certain types of metallic prosthetic cardiac valve implants, intracranial aneurysm clips, cochlear implants or metallic intraocular foreign bodies. Up to 5% of patients may be claustrophobic in the MR bore, which may be overcome using open bore systems or by using psychotherapy relaxation techniques. Occasionally, sedation or rarely a general anaesthetic may be required.

Nephrogenic systemic fibrosis (NSF) is a phenomenon of skin, muscle and organ fibrosis that occurs in a setting of severe chronic or acute renal failure following exposure to gadolinium-based contrast agents (GBCA), which are widely used in MRI. Clinical features include skin manifestations such as skin plaques, joint contractures, cobblestone skin appearance, marked induration or peau d'orange of the skin, skin puckering, superficial skin plaques and dermal papules to multi-organ involvement, which is associated with an increased mortality.

Impaired gadolinium clearance by the kidney leads to tissue accumulation of gadolinium and the toxicity is primarily attributed to the dissociation of gadolinium ion (Gd^{3+}) which competitively binds with components of the extracellular matrix and also with readily available phosphates, carbonates and citrates to form insoluble molecules. Non-complexed Gd^{3+} deposits have been documented in skin, kidney, liver and brain.

The worldwide incidence of NSF has significantly reduced since the United States Food and Drug Administration (FDA) and European Medicine Agency (EMA) alert in 2007. The European Medicines Agency has classified GBCAs based on their risk for NSF into Class 1, 2 and 3. The incidence of NSF is significantly high in Class 1 GBCA, ranging from 3 to 7% in patients with reduced renal function.[41] Class 3, which includes macrocyclic non-ionic GBCAs such as gadobutrol (Gadovist) and gadoteridol (Prohance) have a low incidence of NSF.

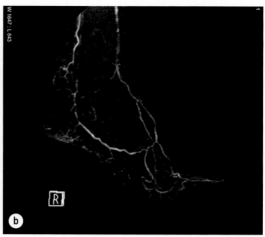

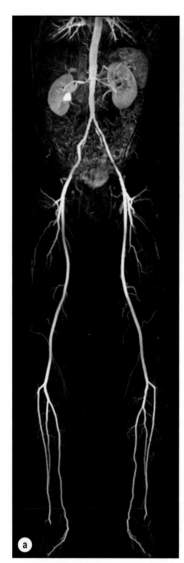

Figure 2.12 • **(a)** Coronal MIP of contrast-enhanced aorta and lower limb MRA at 3 T using a stepping, bolus chase technique and image fusion. **(b)** Sagittal MIP of optimal arterial filling during dynamic contrast-enhanced MRA of the foot.
Images provided by Dr A. Holden, Auckland City Hospital.

Although several therapies have been attempted with variable results, only restoration of renal function by renal transplantation and recovery of acute renal failure has been shown to slow or arrest the progression of NSF.[42,43] Hence there is a greater emphasis on preventative measures.

General recommendations for avoidance of NSF are to use the lowest possible dose of GBCA and avoid re-administration of GBCA for several days to a week.

Computed tomographic angiography

Initial CT imaging had a rotating emitter producing the X-ray beams and a series of image detectors placed opposite to register the axial slice images.

In conventional CT, the table moved to a new position to acquire the next cross-sectional slice. In spiral CT, the table moves continuously through the gantry whilst the X-ray emitter and detector are rotated 360°. This allows for acquiring continuous volume data rather than discontinuous data from separate cross-sectional slices with the added benefit of quicker scan time and lower radiation exposure. Multislice (multidetector) CT, as the name suggests has multiple rows of detectors which enable scanning a larger volume with multiple separate slices simultaneously. This reduces the scan time dramatically and also eliminates many artefacts seen in single-row scanners. Because a volume of tissue has been scanned, these slices can be reconstructed in any plane (multiplanar and curved planar reconstructions) and it allows acquisition of high-resolution images of less than 0.6 mm³ voxel (volume element) size. Multidetector CT scanners with 256 slice capabilities are currently in routine use.

> ✓✓ The UK National Clinical Guideline 'Lower limb peripheral artery disease: diagnosis and management' (NICE Clinical Guideline 147, August 2012), recommends CT angiography to people with peripheral arteryl disease who need further imaging prior to revascularisation (after Duplex ultrasound) if CE-MRA is contraindicated or not tolerated.[36]

Computed tomographic angiography (CTA) enables visualisation of vessels by administration of intravenous contrast and the acquisition speed of spiral CT helps chase the bolus of contrast as it passes through the tissue imaged. Multislice CT enables capture of inflow and outflow images simultaneously by using a single acquisition and contrast media injection. CTA today is invaluable in the acute setting for the diagnosis of acute bleeding and vessel injuries and has a high sensitivity (92%) and specificity (93%) for detecting a stenosis of >50% in the lower limb arteries.[44]

Complex reconstructions can be performed, with the subtraction of bone or other detail that may obscure the arteries. As arterial wall calcification is close to the Hounsfield unit of arterially opacified blood, care must be taken to ensure that no normal part of the vessel has been subtracted when using automated subtraction algorithms. This also applies to vessels that lie in close proximity to bone, for example the tibial arteries, which may be subtracted if the bones are automatically removed. The radiologist must therefore review the source data in the plane of greatest spatial resolution as well as the reconstructions. Heavy calcification within the lower limb arterial tree has greatly limited its use for the assessment of chronic lower limb ischaemia, particularly in the calf of patients with diabetes.

Maximum intensity projection (MIP) images can be constructed, selecting the highest-density voxel along a given plane or planes (**Fig. 2.13c**). This produces a 2-dimensional angiographic-like image that can be rotated to allow multiple viewing angles. A variety of 3-dimensional volume-rendered reconstructions can also be displayed in colour, with preset colour maps determined to best display the anatomy required (**Fig. 2.13a,b**). These images are useful for surgical and endovascular planning, producing accurate vessel diameters, permitting consideration of catheter selection to take place ahead of interventions, or allowing planning of optimal angulation of fluoroscopic and digital subtraction angiographic tube positions.

Contrast media

Iodinated intravascular contrast media, whether for use in catheter angiographic procedures or for vascular or tissue enhancement in CT examinations, continues to pose risks for the development of contrast-induced nephrotoxicity (CIN). This is most commonly defined as an increase in serum creatinine (SCr) by more than 25% of the baseline value or a 44 μmol/L (0.5 mg/dL) absolute increase of SCr occurring within 72 hours, following the intravascular administration of a contrast medium in the absence of an alternative aetiology.[45]

In a multivariable analysis several risk factors have been identified for CIN (Box 2.1).[46] Methods to reduce the incidence of CIN have been highly contentious and have included using alternative imaging techniques, varying the choice of contrast, minimising contrast volume, pharmacological manipulation by stopping nephrotoxic drugs, and intravenous volume expansion.[47] Prehydration remains a cornerstone in our management strategy for prevention of CIN although evidence to support a particular hydration strategy, fluid composition (sodium bicarbonate vs sodium chloride) or pharmacological agent (N-acetyl cysteine) is lacking.[48–50] Most clinicians consider an eGFR <45 mL/min as a trigger for pre-hydration before contrast imaging.

> ✓✓ The CIN Consensus Working Panel agreed that for an estimated glomerular filtration rate (eGFR) of 30–59 mL/min, intravenous volume expansion reduces the risk for CIN and that patients should receive adequate intravenous volume expansion with isotonic crystalloid (1.0–1.5 mL/kg per hour) for 3–12 hours before the procedure and for 6–24 hours afterwards. If the eGFR is <30 mL/min, a nephrology consultation is recommended with dialysis planning should CIN occur.[51]

Much debate has surrounded which contrast agent might have an advantage in reducing the incidence of CIN, with much support for the use of iso-osmolar, non-ionic contrast media over low-osmolar, non-ionic agents. In addition, there is emerging evidence that both intra-arterial and intravenous administration of contrast media pose similar risk of CIN and volume of contrast media administered may be a greater determinant of CIN.[52,53]

> ✓✓ In the PREDICT study, a randomised double-blind comparison of CIN after low- or iso-osmolar contrast agent exposure, 248 patients with moderate to severe chronic kidney disease and diabetes mellitus were randomised to receive at least 65 mL of iopamidol 370 (low-osmolar) or iodixanol 320 (iso-osmolar) for a CT procedure. There was no significant difference in the incidence of CIN at 48–72 hours after contrast administration.[54]

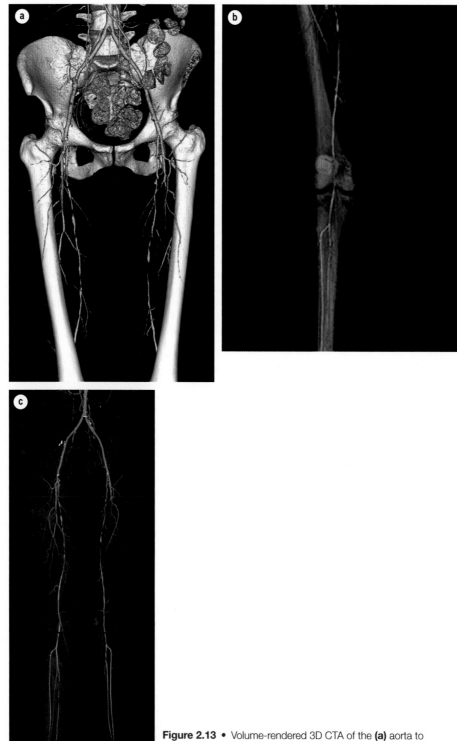

Figure 2.13 • Volume-rendered 3D CTA of the **(a)** aorta to femoral and **(b)** femoro-popliteal segment in a young patient with diabetes and renal failure presenting with chronic bilateral lower limb ischaemia. Bilateral multifocal high-grade stenosis of both the superficial femoral arteries is noted. **(c)** Composite stitched coronal MIP of bilateral lower limb CTA from aorta to ankle.

Box 2.1 • Risk factors for contrast-induced nephropathy (CIN) identified in multivariable analysis

- Chronic kidney disease (stage 3 or greater: eGFR <60 mL/min/1.73 m^2)
- Diabetes mellitus (type 1 or 2)
- Volume depletion
- Nephrotoxic drug use (NSAIDs, ciclosporin, aminoglycosides)
- Preprocedural haemodynamic instability
- Other comorbidities:
  - Anaemia
  - Congestive heart failure
  - Hypoalbuminaemia

eGFR, estimated glomerular filtration rate; NSAIDs, non-steroidal anti-inflammatory drugs.

Metformin is excreted unchanged in the urine. In the presence of renal failure, either pre-existing or induced by iodinated contrast medium, metformin may accumulate in sufficient amounts to cause the serious complication of lactic acidosis. Metformin does not cause renal failure.[45] Contrast agents should therefore be administered with caution, particularly those with known renal impairment, and it is essential that the renal function is checked in these patients prior to the examination. If >100 mL of intravenous iodinated contrast is to be administered for intra-arterial contrast, metformin should be withheld for 48 hours after the procedure.

✔ If there is biochemical evidence of renal impairment, i.e. serum creatinine >120 µmol/L, metformin should also be withheld for 2 days before and after contrast administration. Serum creatinine should be rechecked 48 hours post procedure and the metformin reinstituted only if renal function remains stable (less than 25% increase compared to baseline).

Patients with a baseline serum creatinine of >150 µmol/L should not be taking metformin. If patients are referred on metformin despite this level of chronic kidney disease, the metformin should be discontinued indefinitely and the patient referred back for alternative hypoglycaemic therapy prior to the procedure.

Catheter angiography

Digital subtraction angiography (DSA) is often referred to as the gold standard in the investigation of PAD due to superior image resolution and also the ability to perform both diagnostic and interventional procedures at the same sitting. However, as an invasive procedure placing patients at some risk of harm this has now given way to non-invasive imaging modalities and is no longer recommended for diagnostic imaging of PAD. Diagnostic angiography is also expensive, requires a day-case bed, ties up numerous members of angiography suite staff and negatively impacts on time available for planned therapeutic interventions.[55] Modern practice has thus changed and use of DSA is reserved for situations where there is an intention to proceed to endovascular intervention.

Technique

An initial standard X-ray exposure is captured and digitised and this is referred to as the mask image. This mask image is subsequently subtracted from subsequent images known as the live images. This allows for the display of contrast opacifying the arterial lumen without the visual distraction of adjoining anatomy. There are some applications of DSA that facilitate optimal visualisation and improve procedural success.

Roadmapping is a technique where an unsubtracted fluoroscopic image is superimposed over a live fluoroscopic image. This enables the observation and manipulation of guide wires and catheters in real time through a virtual image of the vessel. Image overlay or fade is superimposition of a live fluoroscopic image on a reference image and this again provides a virtual image of the vessel during intervention.

Single injection multi-linear arteriography or bolus chase angiography permits visualisation of entire lower limb arteries in sequence from a single injection of contrast agent. Image acquisition occurs during a continuous longitudinal movement of the image intensifier. As this technique takes a considerably longer time, patient movement can affect the image quality. In addition, asymmetrical disease severity in the lower limbs can limit its use.

Cone-beam CT is an advanced application that has multiple uses. Using this technique, a 3D image data set is created by rotating the C-arm around the patient and this allows for CT images during interventions, 3D angiography and 3D road mapping.

Pre-procedural planning is critical to the outcome of any intervention. Access vessel and puncture site is chosen based on a likely low risk of complications and reasonable proximity to site of intervention (frequently the common femoral artery). Standard angiographic access is by the modified Seldinger technique.[56] Arterial puncture under ultrasound guidance is widely accepted as safe practice and an 18-gauge puncture needle is used. Once pulsatile backbleeding is confirmed through the needle, a floppy tip guidewire, usually a J-tip, is advanced via the central lumen of the needle into the artery lumen under fluoroscopic guidance. A sheath is advanced over this wire or alternatively a catheter may be used bareback. A flush catheter with multiple side holes allows for even distribution of contrast in diagnostic studies. Injection of contrast can be performed by power injector or by manual injection and both have distinct advantages. Large high flow arteries such as the aorto-iliac segments may require a higher pressure to dispense the contrast for satisfactory images. A micropuncture set with a 21-gauge needle may be used in scarred groins, pulseless arteries, calcified arteries or for antegrade access to the femoral artery. With care, diagnostic angiography is safe with 4-Fr catheters in most patients. Adequate analgesia is essential to ensure a pain-free and cooperative patient who will comply with the instructions to avoid movement artefacts, especially during imaging of the crural (tibial) arteries and plantar arch.

Carbon dioxide (CO_2) angiography

CO_2 creates a radiographic contrast image due to its reduced radio-density. With modern advances in digital subtraction technology, it is now possible to achieve good quality angiographic images. The use of CO_2 is not associated with nephrotoxicity and allergic reactions and hence valuable in patients with renal impairment requiring endovascular intervention and patients with contrast allergy. Complications related to CO_2 angiography are extremely rare during investigations of the lower limb arteries.[57] However, caution needs to be exercised in the use of CO_2 in situations where there is a risk of gas trapping and ischaemia as in mesenteric and carotid angiography.

Risks and limitations

The risks of conventional catheter angiography are related to contrast media or technique.

Contrast related
Risks and limitations
The risks of conventional catheter angiography are related to contrast media or technique.

Contrast related
- Allergic: Allergic reactions are not dose related and probably result from mast cell degranulation. The incidence of severe anaphylactic reactions due to ionic contrast media is 0.01–0.02%, but non-ionic low-osmolar iodinated contrast agents

are 5–10 times safer than their predecessors. Patients with severe asthma or hay fever are at increased risk of an allergic reaction, which may be severe. Steroid prophylaxis should be considered. Patients with known contrast allergy should be imaged using alternative techniques.
- Toxic: These are dose related and manifest themselves as a metallic taste in the mouth, feelings of warmth, nausea or vomiting, cardiac arrhythmias and pulmonary oedema. They are more likely to occur in patients with severe vascular disease.
- Renal (CIN – see above).

Technique related
- Pseudoaneurysm/haematoma: Haematoma around the puncture site is common. This can be reduced by using smaller catheters and a good manual haemostasis arterial compression technique for at least 10 minutes. Arterial closure devices are rarely indicated for diagnostic angiography although this may allow faster ambulation of patients and be useful with uncorrected clotting profiles.
- Dissection: A dissection flap is usually caused by poor technique using undue force or hydrophilic guidewires or from closure devices, which may disrupt the integrity of plaques. Although small flaps are rarely a problem, larger or antegrade flaps may significantly slow blood flow or occlude the artery.
- Infection is rare with good aseptic technique.
- Arteriovenous fistula: As the femoral artery and vein are contained within the femoral sheath they may both be punctured during arterial access when a blind puncture is performed. Where ultrasound is available, this should be used to avoid anterior wall plaques and accurately identify the common femoral artery.
- Embolisation: If atheroma lining the artery is inadvertently dislodged, it will embolise distally. This may be retrieved using suction aspiration but may need surgical embolectomy or bypass surgery.

Radiation safety
Clinicians should have a clear understanding of the risks involved with radiation exposure to the patient and staff, as well as the measures to reduce radiation dose. The main source of radiation to the operator is scatter and scatter decreases as the

inverse square of the distance from the source. In addition, fluoroscopic field size significantly affects scatter radiation. Image intensifier positioning close to the patient, beam collimation, minimising fluoroscopic screening time and angiographic run, and protective personal equipment including lead shields, lead aprons, thyroid shields and eye protection, are important strategies to limit radiation exposure.

Classification of aorto-iliac, femoral popliteal and infrapopliteal disease

Atherosclerotic arterial lesions in PAD may be focal or extensive and involve multiple segments of the lower limb arteries. Hence, it is important to have a universally acceptable classification system that clearly defines the extent and complexity of these lesions for the purpose of standardised reporting and also planning intervention.

The Trans-Atlantic Inter-Society Consensus for the management of peripheral artery disease (TASC II) document derived a simplified nomenclature to classify lesions in the aorto-iliac, femoropopliteal and, more recently, the infrapopliteal arterial regions[1,58] (Tables 2.5–2.7). The TASC classification reflects the location and extent of the arterial

lesions and also gives recommendations for the revascularisation options most suited, taking into consideration the risks of a specific intervention and its durability. TASC A lesions are best treated by endovascular techniques, which yield excellent results and D lesions are best treated by open techniques, as endovascular techniques yield suboptimal results. Endovascular methods yield good results and hence are favoured for TASC B lesions unless an open revascularisation procedure is required for a lesion in close proximity. Type C lesions should be treated by open techniques and endovascular means are reserved for patients considered to be at high risk for open procedures. However, with the advances in endovascular technology and skillsets of interventionists, the subsequent TASC II supplementary document recommends an endovascular first strategy as acceptable when considering revascularisation of even complex arterial lesions. The risks and benefits of endovascular and open surgery have to be carefully considered along with the experience of the interventionalist and institution when making this decision.

Acknowledgement

This text is based on the earlier chapter by Henrik Sillesen and John R. Bottomley in the 5th edition of this volume.

Table 2.5 • TASC classification of aorto-iliac lesions

TASC A lesions	Unilateral or bilateral CIA stenoses Unilateral or bilateral single short (≤3 cm) EIA stenosis
TASC B lesions	Short (≤ cm) stenosis of infrarenal aorta Unilateral CIA occlusion Single or multiple stenosis totalling 3–10 cm involving the EIA not extending into the CFA Unilateral EIA occlusion not involving the origins of internal iliac or CFA
TASC C lesions	Bilateral CIA occlusions Bilateral EIA stenosis 3–10 cm long not extending into the CFA Unilateral EIA stenosis extending into the CFA Unilateral EIA occlusion involving the origins of internal iliac and/or CFA Heavily calcified unilateral EIA occlusion with or without involvement of the origins of the internal iliac and/or CFA
TASC D lesions	Infrarenal aortoiliac occlusion Diffuse disease involving the aorta and both iliac arteries Diffuse multiple stenoses involving the unilateral CIA, EIA and CFA Unilateral occlusions of both CIA and EIA Bilateral EIA occlusions Iliac stenoses in patients with AAA not amenable to endograft placement

CIA, common iliac artery; EIA, external iliac artery; CFA, common femoral artery; AAA, abdominal aortic aneurysm.

Table 2.6 • TASC classification of femoropopliteal lesions

TASC A lesions	Single stenosis ≤10 cm in length
	Single occlusion ≤5 cm in length
TASC B lesions	Multiple lesions (stenoses or occlusions), each ≤5 cm
	Single stenosis or occlusion ≤15 cm not involving the infrageniculate popliteal artery
	Heavily calcified occlusion ≤5 cm in length
	Single popliteal stenosis
TASC C lesions	Multiple stenoses or occlusions totalling >15 cm with or without heavy calcification
	Recurrent stenoses or occlusions after failing treatment
TASC D lesions	Chronic total occlusions of CFA or SFA (≥20 cm, involving the popliteal artery)
	Chronic total occlusion of popliteal artery and proximal trifurcation vessels

CFA, common femoral artery; SFA, superficial femoral artery.

Table 2.7 • TASC classification of infrapopliteal lesions

TASC A lesions	Single focal stenosis, ≤5 cm in length, in the target tibial artery with occlusion or stenosis of similar or worse severity in the other tibial arteries
TASC B lesions	Multiple stenoses, each ≤5 cm in length, or total length ≤10 cm or single occlusion ≤3 cm in length, in the target tibial artery with occlusion or stenosis of similar or worse severity in the other tibial arteries
TASC C lesions	Mutliple stenoses in the target tibial artery and/or single occlusion with total lesion length >10 cm with occlusion or stenosis of similar or worse severity in the other tibial arteries
TASC D lesions	Multiple occlusions involving the target tibial artery with total lesion length >10 cm or dense lesion calcification or non-visualisation of collaterals. The other tibial arteries occluded or densely calcified

Key points

- The Fontaine classification for the severity of PAD has the benefit of simplicity and is clinically useful.
- Risk factors must be identified and treated in all patients with PAD.
- A careful history is essential, especially in patients with coexisting spinal problems.
- Patients with a good history of claudication and palpable pulses should be examined after exercise and/or an exercise ABPI test performed.
- Rare causes of ischaemia should not be forgotten, especially in younger patients.
- Documentation of the severity of ischaemia by Doppler pressures/waveforms is mandatory in all patients with absent or weak pulses who are complaining of leg pain, weakness or numbness.
- Further investigation is not warranted unless revascularisation is being considered.
- Critical limb ischaemia requires urgent investigation and revascularisation in order to avoid limb loss due to progressive tissue necrosis and/or infection.
- Offer Duplex ultrasound as first-line imaging to all people with peripheral artery disease for whom revascularisation is being considered. Offer CE-MRA or CTA to people with peripheral artery disease who need further imaging (after Duplex ultrasound) before considering revascularisation.
- Contrast-induced nephrotoxicity remains a serious concern for all procedures requiring iodinated contrast medium. Serum creatinine or eGFR must be known and provided on all patients at risk for developing this complication and must also be checked at 48 hours post contrast injection.
- Nephrogenic systemic fibrosis is a rare but potentially serious condition occurring in chronic kidney disease patients receiving gadolinium-based contrast agents. Serum creatinine levels or eGFR must be known and provided on all patients referred for CE-MRA who are at risk of developing this condition (stage 3, 4 and 5 chronic kidney disease).

- CTA provides detailed angiographic imaging in peripheral artery disease but is limited in severely calcified arteries. It is particularly useful in the acute assessment of limb ischaemia where potentially embolising sources may be identified.
- Catheter angiography is invasive and is no longer recommended as a first-line imaging modality in the diagnosis of PAD. It should be limited to patients in whom therapeutic intervention is planned at the same time and when inadequate information is obtained from non-invasive investigations.
- TASC II classification of aorto-iliac, femoropopliteal and infrapopliteal arterial disease reflects the location and extent of the arterial lesions.

🌐 Full references available at **http://expertconsult. inkling.com**

Key references

1. Norgren L, Hiatt WR, Dormandy JA, et al. Inter-Society Consensus for the Management of Peripheral Arterial Disease (TASC II). Eur J Vasc Endovasc Surg 2007;33(Suppl 1):S1–75. PMID: 17140820.
A working group comprised of members from sixteen societies from around the world collaborated in producing this abbreviated document which focuses on diagnosis and management of PAD based on current evidence.

36. NICE Lower limb peripheral arterial disease: diagnosis and management. National Institute for Health and Clinical Excellence: Clinical guideline [CG147]. August 2012. https://www.nice.org.uk/ guidance/cg147/chapter/1-guidance.
(1) Offer duplex ultrasound as first-line imaging to all people with peripheral arterial disease for whom revascularisation is being considered.

(2) Offer CE-MRA to people with peripheral arterial disease who need further imaging (after duplex ultrasound) before considering revascularisation.

(3) Offer computed tomography angiography to people with peripheral arterial disease who need further imaging (after duplex ultrasound) if CE-MRA is contraindicated or not tolerated.

37. Collins R, Burch J, Cranny G, et al. Duplex ultrasonography, magnetic resonance angiography, and computed tomography angiography for diagnosis and assessment of symptomatic, lower limb peripheral arterial disease: systematic review. BMJ 2007;334(7606):1257. PMID: 17548364.
A systematic review that compared the diagnostic accuracy of DUS, CE-MRA and CTA for assessment of PAD. CE-MRA had the highest diagnostic accuracy for detection of stenosis of 50% or more.

44. Heijenbrok-Kal MH, Kock MC, Hunink MG. Lower extremity arterial disease: multidetector CT angiography meta-analysis. Radiology 2007;245(2):433–9. PMID: 17848679.
A meta-analysis comparing CTA and DSA showed that CTA is an accurate imaging modality for assessment of >50% stenosis in PAD.

49. Brar SS, Hiremath S, Dangas G, et al. Sodium bicarbonate for the prevention of contrast induced-acute kidney injury: a systematic review and meta-analysis. Clin J Am Soc Nephrol 2009;4(10):1584–92. PMID: 19713291.
A meta-analysis that included 2290 patients showed no benefit for hydration with sodium bicarbonate compared to sodium chloride for prevention of CIN in the large randomised trials.

50. Investigators ACT. Acetylcysteine for prevention of renal outcomes in patients undergoing coronary and peripheral vascular angiography: main results from the randomized Acetylcysteine for Contrast-induced nephropathy Trial (ACT). Circulation 2011;124(11):1250–9. PMID: 21859972.
A large randomised trial with 2308 patients failed to demonstrate a protective effect from acetylcysteine use in preventing CIN in the at-risk patient.

52. McDonald JS, Leake CB, McDonald RJ, et al. Acute kidney injury after intravenous versus intra-arterial contrast material administration in a paired cohort. Invest Radiol 2016;51(12):804–9. PMID: 27299579.
In a cohort of 1969 patients from this retrospective study, the risk of CIN from intra-arterial and intravenous administration of contrast agent was similar.

54. Kuhn MJ, Chen N, Sahani DV, et al. The PREDICT study: a randomized double-blind comparison of contrast-induced nephropathy after low- or isoosmolar contrast agent exposure. AJR Am J Roentgenol 2008;191(1):151–7. PMID: 18562739.
An RCT of 263 patients with moderate to severe renal failure and diabetes showed that the incidence of CIN was not significantly different following exposure to low or iso-osmolar contrast agent.

3

Medical treatment of chronic lower limb ischaemia

Peter A. Soden
Marc L. Schermerhorn

Introduction

Peripheral artery disease (PAD) is a common condition. A recent meta-analysis of 34 studies estimated that over 202 million people worldwide suffer from PAD and the prevalence is increasing.[1] In the Edinburgh Artery Study of men and women aged 55–74 years of age, 4.5% had symptomatic PAD.[2] However, a further 8% had evidence of major asymptomatic disease and 17% had abnormal hemodynamic parameters suggesting minor PAD. Five years later all new cases of intermittent claudication in the study group were in patients who were previously found to have asymptomatic disease.[3] It is believed that the current ratio of symptomatic to asymptomatic PAD is approximately 1:3.[4,5]

PAD is also a strong risk factor for cardiovascular disease, which has been estimated to be at least as great as for patients with a history of previous myocardial infarction.[6] In a survey of 1886 patients with PAD, 58% had coronary artery disease and 34% had suffered a cerebrovascular event.[7]

In the Reduction of Atherothrombosis for Continued Health (REACH) registry of patients with either known cardiovascular disease or who were at increased cardiovascular risk, the highest cardiovascular event rate was in the 5986 patients with PAD.[8] At 1-year follow-up 18.2% of PAD patients had suffered a cardiovascular death, myocardial infarction (MI), stroke, or had been hospitalised for a cardiovascular event compared with 13.3% of the coronary artery disease group and 10% of the cerebrovascular disease group.

Risk factors associated with PAD are similar to those that have also been identified in coronary artery disease. These include both demographic and comorbid conditions (**Fig. 3.1**).[4,9–12] Patients older than 64 years appear to be at highest risk for having PAD (**Fig. 3.2**).

The cost associated with PAD is significant. In 2001 the US Medicare programme spent an estimated $4.3 billion on PAD-related treatment.[13] As invasive treatment of PAD continues to increase, the costs associated with PAD are likely to increase in the future as well.

The key aims for treatment of PAD should include reduction of cardiovascular risk, improvement of symptoms, and disruption of disease progression. This chapter will address the diagnosis and detection of PAD; as well as medical management to affect cardiovascular risk, symptoms related to PAD, and prevention of PAD progression.

PAD diagnosis and screening

Knowing the associated risk factors for PAD combined with a thorough history and physical examination are the first steps to effectively diagnosing PAD. However, there are numerous additional aetiologies that can mimic symptomatic PAD, which include venous claudication, nerve root compression, symptomatic Baker cyst, chronic compartment syndrome, spinal stenosis and arthritis. Physical examination findings that support a PAD diagnosis include absent or weak pulses, distal hair loss, non-healing wounds, or dry skin related to apocrine gland dysfunction. Supplementing the

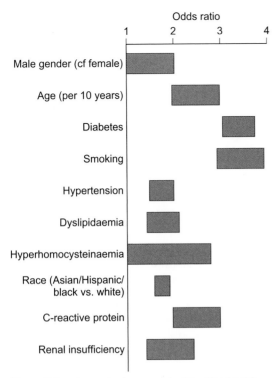

Odds ratio

Figure 3.1 • Approximate range of odds ratios for risk factors for symptomatic peripheral artery disease.[4]

often spared from calcification, with a TBI of <0.7 indicating PAD.[15] Additionally, further non-invasive testing using pulse volume recordings and segmental pressures can be helpful in localising significant lesions and quantifying the magnitude of the deficit. In the setting of a normal ABPI but a compelling story for PAD, exercise ABPIs can be measured using a treadmill, climbing stairs, or walking a hallway in patients able to undergo such testing. A drop in ABPI of 15–20% after the specified exercise would be considered consistent with PAD. Pedal plantar flexion testing (toe raises) has been used in patients who are unable to perform exercise testing. Further imaging modalities are available to better characterise a patient's PAD after the diagnosis is made, and include arterial duplex, computed tomographic angiography (CTA), magnetic resonance angiography (MRA) and contrast arteriography.

Given the associated cardiovascular risk with PAD it is not surprising that ABPI alone can be used as a marker for future cardiovascular risk (**Fig. 3.3**).[15] The Atherosclerotic Risk in Communities Study found that the lower the ABPI the greater the risk of cardiac and cerebrovascular disease.[16] Despite this, however, general screening for PAD has not been endorsed by any professional society at this time.[17] Some professional societies believe there are 'high-risk' populations who should be screened for PAD in the absence of symptoms, while others believe there is still not enough evidence to support this practice as there is potential harm in identifying and over-treating asymptomatic PAD (Table 3.1).[4,17–21]

Once the diagnosis of PAD has been made patients can be categorised based on clinical presentation as being asymptomatic, having intermittent claudication (IC), or chronic limb-threatening ischaemia (CLI), which includes both rest pain and tissue loss related to gangrene. For purposes of our discussion on medical management we will focus on symptomatic PAD (which includes IC and CLI), except when asymptomatic disease is specifically noted.

clinical history with measurement of an ankle-brachial pressure index (ABPI) using an ABPI <0.90, has been shown to be a reasonable alternative to the gold standard of invasive arteriography for the diagnosis of PAD.[4,14] The non-invasive nature, low cost and reproducibility of ABPI makes it an ideal tool for diagnosis of PAD in primary and secondary care settings. In the setting of ABPI measurements, >1.4, secondary to non-compressibility of the arteries from calcification, a toe–brachial index (TBI) is a useful alternative as the digital arteries are

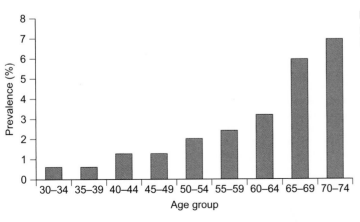

Figure 3.2 • Weighted mean prevalence of intermittent claudication in large population-based studies.[4]

Figure 3.3 • Adjusted odds of a cardiovascular event by ankle–brachial index. MI, myocardial infarction; CV, cardiovascular. [4]

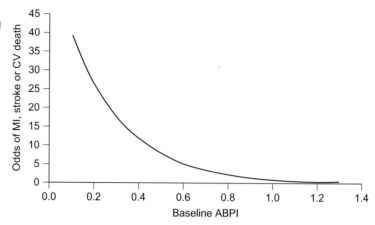

Table 3.1 • Recommendations for screening for PAD in asymptomatic patients

Society for Vascular Surgery (2015)

Insufficient data on benefit or harm in patient-important outcomes

US Preventative Services Task Force (2013)

Insufficient evidence to determine the balance of benefits and harms of screening for PAD with ABPI to prevent future cardiovascular disease outcomes

TASC II (2007)

Screen all patients ages 50–69 who have a cardiovascular risk factor, all patients >69 years regardless of risk factors, and all patients with a Framingham risk score of 10-20%

American College of Cardiology/American Heart Association (2011)

Screen all patients >65 years and all patients >50 years with a history of smoking or diabetes

European Society for Cardiology (2015)

Screening with ABPI is recommended in select populations considered at high risk for cerebrovascular disease

Modifying cardiovascular risk

There is strong evidence that patients with symptomatic PAD have increased cardiovascular risk and therefore benefit from risk reduction strategies, which include exercise, smoking cessation, curbing obesity and medications to control comorbid risk factors. Non-invasive options should always be the first line intervention provided to patients with claudication and at least a supplement to interventions performed in those with CLI. The National Health and Nutrition Examination Survey (NHANES) between 1999 and 2004 demonstrated that in those older than 39 years with PAD, the proportion of patients on statins was only 30% and on aspirin was only 36%.[22] Furthermore, this study

also reported that use of these therapies resulted in a 65% lower all-cause mortality in patients with PAD who did not have known cardiovascular disease at the time. Clearly, risk factor control plays a big role in improved survival for patients with PAD. The REACH registry of patients at increased cardiovascular risk, most being treated in the primary care setting, also showed that patients with PAD were receiving suboptimal medical treatment and few were controlled within target ranges for blood pressure, cholesterol and blood sugar, regardless of geographic region.[23] Furthermore, in patients referred to specialists, only 70% were on antiplatelet therapy and 44% were taking a statin.[24] As awareness around the importance of cardiovascular risk reduction increases, the proportion of at-risk patients on appropriate medical therapy has increased but there is more work to be done.[25]

It should be noted that many of the current recommendations for risk-factor modification in PAD have been extrapolated from studies on secondary prevention in coronary artery disease. Thus there is a gap in the evidence regarding treatment of PAD patients specifically, but most practitioners believe that the strength of the association between PAD and coronary disease makes such extrapolations credible.

Smoking cessation

Smoking is associated with worsening atherosclerosis, increased cardiovascular death, and accelerated graft failure.[26,27] For PAD patients smoking cessation has been shown to reduce death from coronary disease, and decrease lower extremity interventions and amputations.[28] Advising and assisting patients to quit smoking is one of the most modifiable and beneficial interventions a practitioner can perform in the population with PAD. Supplementing counselling on smoking cessation with nicotine replacement and the antidepressant bupropion has been shown to be most effective in 12-month abstinence from smoking rates compared to each alone.[29] This has led some societies to recommend prescribing pharmacologic interventions such as varenicline, bupropion and nicotine replacement to assist in smoking cessation.[30]

Treatment of diabetes

Diabetes mellitus is thought to worsen atherosclerosis as a consequence of arterial wall degeneration in addition to increases in platelet aggregation, blood viscosity and fibrinogen levels.[31] Tight glucose control, with a haemoglobin A1C level below 7% is recommended.[32] In addition, tighter control of diabetes has been shown to reduce the development of microvascular complications such as neuropathy.

Additional lifestyle modifications

Other potentially modifiable behaviours include dietary indiscretion and inactivity as they relate to cardiovascular health. Diet can have a profound effect on lipid metabolism and atherogenesis, as well as its effect on weight and diabetes mellitus. Exercise also plays an important role in cardiovascular health and will be discussed further below.

Management of dyslipidaemia

The treatment of dyslipidaemia with statins reduces the risk of a cardiovascular event in patients with atherosclerosis.[33] It appears that the benefits of statins are independent of their lipid-lowering properties and have more to do with their ability to decrease oxidative stress and vascular inflammation, as well as their protection against thrombosis through platelet influence.[34] The 2013 American College of Cardiology/American Heart Association (ACC/AHA) guidelines recommend consideration of statin therapy for primary prevention in all patients with a 10-year risk of atherosclerotic vascular disease of >7.4% and no longer recommends treating to a particular lipid target level.[35] The UK National Institute for Health and Care Excellence (NICE) offer similar recommendations for statin therapy in at-risk populations without treatment to a particular lipid level target.[36] High-dose statin therapy (e.g. atorvastatin 40–80 mg daily or rosuvastatin 20 mg daily) should be considered for all patients with symptomatic vascular disease who are <75 years old and not on haemodialysis. Moderate statin

doses should be considered for all other patients with symptomatic PAD or with >7.4% 10-year risk of atherosclerotic vascular disease.

Antiplatelet and antithrombotic medications

Antiplatelet therapy is recommended in all patients with PAD if not contraindicated. The Antiplatelet Trialists' Collaboration, which included 102 459 patients with cardiovascular disease, reported a 2.4% reduction in cardiovascular events for those treated with an antiplatelet agent.[37] When patients with claudication were evaluated in subgroup analysis, an 18–23% reduction in cardiovascular events was found. This result has been replicated for both aspirin and clopidogrel in lowering the risk of myocardial infarction and stroke in patients with symptomatic PAD.[37–39] More recently there has been a suggestion that certain patients with symptomatic PAD may benefit from dual antiplatelet therapy.[40,41] The risk of bleeding should be factored into the decision to start a patient on dual antiplatelet therapy. The ACC/AHA recommends that a single antiplatelet agent should be prescribed in all patients with symptomatic PAD to reduce the risk of stroke, myocardial infarction and vascular death and that clopidogrel is a safe alternative to aspirin.[30]

For patients with asymptomatic PAD the benefits of antiplatelet agents are unknown at this point. The Aspirin for Asymptomatic Atherosclerosis Trial randomised 3350 patients to aspirin versus placebo and found no difference in vascular events through 8 years, although there were criticisms regarding the measurement of ABPI used to stratify patients.[42] Currently there is no evidence to suggest that warfarin decreases the rate of adverse cardiovascular events in patients with PAD and it has been associated with increased bleeding complications in other patient populations. Therefore, unless indicated for other reasons, warfarin should not be prescribed for the treatment of PAD to reduce cardiovascular risk.

Blood pressure medication

Hypertension is a risk factor for PAD, stroke, coronary artery disease, congestive heart failure and chronic renal insufficiency.[43] In the Heart Outcomes Prevention study, 4051 patients with PAD treated with ramipril had a 25% reduction in cardiac events compared to controls.[44] TASC II guidelines consider angiotensin-converting enzyme inhibitors and thiazide diuretics to be first-line medications for control of hypertension in patients with PAD.[4] Beta-adrenergic blockers are also an acceptable choice for control of hypertension in patients with

PAD and there is no evidence that this medication reduces walking distance or worsens claudication pain, as was previously suspected.[45] The ACC/AHA guidelines for treatment of PAD state that angiotensin-converting enzyme inhibitors (ACE-I) are also reasonable in patients with asymptomatic PAD to reduce the risk of cardiovascular events, although there is no strong evidence.[30]

Homocysteine-lowering medications

Roughly 30% of patients with PAD have elevated homocysteine levels compared with only 1% of the general population.[4] Elevated homocysteine levels are thought to be associated with endothelial dysfunction and injury. In addition, people with PAD also exhibit increased production of hydrogen peroxide, increases in Factor XII and V, and decreases in Protein C, thrombomodulin and heparin sulfate activity.[46] This led some to believe that folic acid and cobalamin (Vitamin B12) may help reduce the risk of cardiovascular events in those with hyperhomocysteinemia. However no data to date have proved this and currently there are no level 1 recommendations to prescribe these medications in the setting of PAD.[4,47,48]

Medical treatment for symptomatic PAD

It is important that all patients receive clear and appropriate advice about their condition and how they can improve their prognosis.

Exercise

Exercise therapy is thought to be the best initial therapy for claudication.[49] It has been clearly demonstrated to improve pain-free ambulation and walking performance.[4,50] There is good evidence that exercise leads to improvement in muscle and vascular endothelial cell function and increases collateral vessel growth.[50] Beyond improving the symptoms of claudication, exercise also reduces cardiovascular risk.[51] This benefit is lost when a sedentary lifestyle is resumed and therefore sustained exercise regimens are key to achieving long-term results. There is also a correlation between ABPI and a patient's exercise routine, suggesting that a sustained active lifestyle could help prevent PAD.[52] This has led multiple professional societies to recommend formal exercise therapy in patients with claudication.[4,30,53]

Walking, compared to other forms of lower extremity exercise (e.g. cycling, stair climbing, tip-toe raises, dancing, and static and dynamic leg exercises), has been shown to be superior.[54] In fact, independent predictors of increased walking distance with an exercise programme from a meta-analysis of 21 rehabilitation studies included the type of claudication pain endpoint used (meaning walking distance until maximum pain instead of onset of pain), mode of exercise (walking vs other), and duration of the exercise programme.[49] Current recommendations are for supervised walking exercise programmes 3×/week for >30 minutes each session for more than 6 months. Neither lower extremity strength training nor upper extremity aerobic exercise appear to augment the benefits of walking exercise programmes.[55]

Intervention (angioplasty and stenting) has been studied as both a supplement and an alternative to exercise therapy for claudication. Multiple studies have shown that after both endovascular lower extremity intervention and bypass, supplementing with a structured exercise regimen improves long-term maximal claudication and walking distance.[56,57] The CLEVER trial randomised 111 patients with claudication to optimal medical care, optimal medical care with supervised exercise, or optimal medical care with stent revascularisation and found that at 6 months peak walking time was greatest in the supervised exercise group, whereas improvements in quality of life were greatest in the stent revascularisation group.[58] However, at 18 months there was no difference in quality of life metrics between the supervised exercise and stent revascularisation groups.[59] Markov models on a 5-year time horizon have found structured exercise therapy to be more cost-effective than endovascular revascularisation.[60]

The data supporting benefits of exercise are mostly from structured and supervised programmes; however, reimbursement for such therapy ranges widely across the USA and Europe and is rarely fully covered. Given this, for those patients placed on home-based walking regimens frequent assessment of progress by patient and provider is needed to ensure adherence.

Patients with CLI may have more physical restrictions on their ability to walk but low-intensity exercise should be encouraged in those patients who are able. This would likely involve close attention to footwear and foot care as well as involvement of physical therapy services to assist in establishing a suitable regimen tailored to the individual patient with CLI.

Pharmacologic interventions

Pharmacologic management of PAD is aimed at symptom control and slowing the progression of atherosclerotic disease. In addition to cardiovascular risk reduction, primary pharmacologic intervention is utilised most often in patients with claudication whereas it is often used as a supplement to revascularisation or after failed intervention in those with CLI.

Naftidrofuryl oxalate

This vasoactive drug works by enhancing aerobic glycolysis and oxygen consumption in ischaemic tissues. A meta-analysis based on individual patient data reported that individuals with PAD receiving naftidrofuryl walked 37% further than those getting placebo at 6 months.[61] This benefit in claudication was further verified in a subsequent Cochrane review.[62] The National Institute for Health and Care Excellence (NICE) evaluated the evidence of four vasoactive drugs used in the treatment of intermittent claudication – cilostazol (Pletal), naftidrofuryl oxalate (Praxilene), pentoxifylline (Trental) and inositol nicotinate (Hexopal) – and found that there was no conclusive evidence of an advantage of one agent over the other; however naftidrofuryl oxalate was more cost-effective.[63] As a result, naftidrofuryl was recommended by this group as the only vasoactive agent to be used out of this group of medications for treatment of symptoms related to claudication.

Cilostazol

This vasoactive drug is more commonly used in the USA. It is a phosphodiesterase inhibitor that suppresses platelet aggregation and promotes vasodilatation. Randomised controlled trials have shown its benefit in 6-month maximum and pain-free walking distance compared to pentoxifylline (mean change from baseline: cilostazol 107 metres vs pentoxifylline 64 metres, $P <0.001$ and cilostazol 94 m vs pentoxifylline 74 m, $P <0.001$, respectively) and placebo (cilostazol 107 m vs placebo 65 m, $P <0.001$ and cilostazol 94 m vs placebo 57 m, $P <0.001$, respectively).[64,65]

Levocarnitine

This is a carrier molecule involved in the transport of long-chain fatty acids. Supplementation with levocarnitine results in an increase in the availability of energy substrate for skeletal muscle metabolism. It has been shown to improve pain-free and maximum walking distance compared to placebo but not to exercise alone.[66,67] Currently there are no strong recommendations for its use.

HMG-CoA reductase inhibitors (Statin)

In addition to the cardiovascular protection there is some evidence that statins may alter vasomotor tone and stimulate angiogenesis and have been shown to improve pain-free walking time in patients with claudication.[68] However, the CLEVER trial, which had a medication-only arm, did not show statins to significantly improve claudication symptoms.[58] PAD patients should be on a statin for cardiovascular protection regardless, but further study is warranted to investigate the potential limb-based benefits of statins to both better understand the mechanism and to determine what dose of statin is best.

Pentoxifylline

This was one of the first medications used to treat symptoms related to PAD and works through reducing blood viscosity and interrupting platelet aggregation, which results in improved oxygenation to compromised areas in PAD. Port et al. in 1982 demonstrated that it improved both pain-free and maximal walking distance versus placebo.[69] However, later placebo controlled and comparative studies have not shown improvement in PAD symptoms from pentoxifylline and therefore it is currently not commonly used in either Europe or the USA.[65,70]

Ramipril

Ramipril is already considered a first-line therapy for hypertension in patients with PAD for protection against cardiovascular events. In a recent double-blinded randomised controlled trial ramipril was also associated with improvements in pain-free and maximal walking distances.[71] Further investigation is needed before ramipril can be recommended for this use.

Other medications

Prostaglandins are thought to work in PAD through vasodilatation and inhibition of platelet aggregation. In recent trials this group of medications showed mixed results, especially in patients with claudication.[72,73] Buflomedil, an alpha-1 and -2 antagonist resulting in vasodilatation, has shown positive effects on treadmill performance in PAD patients; however, these findings were from small studies and need further confirmation before conclusions about its use in PAD can be made.[74,75] L-Arginine, an amino acid precursor of endothelial-derived nitric oxide, which acts through vasodilatation of vascular smooth muscle cells has also been studied, with inconsistent results, and is also currently not recommended for PAD.[76]

Intermittent Pneumatic Compression

Intermittent pneumatic compression of the calf and foot has been shown to increase popliteal artery blood flow. It is thought to accomplish this through increases in the arteriovenous pressure gradient, reversal of vasomotor paralysis and enhanced release of nitric oxide. The role of this therapy is not clearly defined yet but studies have shown its benefit in patients with both claudication and CLI who do not have good revascularisation options.[77,78] An additional benefit is that this therapy can be used by patients in the comfort of their own homes. Further research is needed to establish where this therapy is most effectively utilised.

Angiogenesis

There is much hope for pro-angiogenic factors to help in symptomatic PAD but this research is still in its infancy. In early human trials the use of growth factors, including vascular endothelial growth factor, fibroblast growth factor and platelet-derived growth factor, has been associated with increased vascularity and limb blood flow. However, these trials were small and without controls.[79] There are also potential risks with such a therapy, such as new vessel growth at other sites including the eye and malignant lesions.

In addition to injecting growth factors to encourage angiogenesis, stem cell therapy is also being studied: autologous stem cell therapies aspirated from bone marrow mononuclear cells or endothelial progenitor cells and directly injected concentrated solutions of these cells back into the individual patient's ischaemic tissue. Early trials using this method have shown promise but much work remains before this can become recommended therapy.[80,81] Allogenic stem cell therapies are being studied for this purpose as well. Further understanding of the human genome will likely lead to numerous additional areas to target intervention.

Advancements in wound care are not the focus of this chapter but are also an integral component of caring for patients with more advanced PAD. There are multiple medical interventions that can assist revascularisation procedures and expedite wound healing leading to improved preservation of limbs for these patients.

Conclusions

PAD remains under-diagnosed and under-treated. There are numerous risk factors for PAD which should be used to raise a clinician's awareness for the potential of PAD in a patient with lower extremity pain. History, clinical exam and measurement of ABPI, which can all be performed efficiently in an office visit, are enough to diagnose PAD. A diagnosis of PAD is also an indicator of increased cardiovascular risk and risk factor modification can have a profound impact, for both the extremity and the cardiovascular system. Smoking cessation and exercise therapy, in addition to control of other risk factors, should be initial steps to the treatment of all patients with claudication and should be a supplemental to revascularisation procedures for patients with CLI. Medical therapies focused on improving limb-based symptoms have been less efficacious. The key to improving the treatment of PAD seems to be in raising awareness of the condition and organising effective risk factor and lifestyle interventions.

Key Points

- PAD can be diagnosed on history, examination and a reduced ABPI.
- Low ABPI is a marker of cardiovascular risk.
- Patients with leg pain on walking should have ABPI measured.
- Further evidence is needed to recommend screening of the adult population for reduced ABPI.
- Supervised exercise should be available and offered to patients with intermittent claudication.
- Smoking cessation should be recommended and monitored at each clinical visit.
- There are effective behavioural and pharmacologic interventions to assist in smoking cessation, which should be utilised for all patients with PAD.
- Naftidrofuryl or cilostazol may be of value in patients who cannot undertake (or in addition to) exercise programmes and do not wish interventional treatment.
- All patients with symptomatic PAD should be on a statin and antiplatelet agent, unless they have a strong contraindication for one of these medications.
- The role of dual antiplatelet therapy in patients with symptomatic PAD for secondary prevention of cardiovascular events is unclear and requires further investigation.
- Angiogenesis is an exciting concept but at present needs considerable further evaluation before it can be put into practice.

🌐 Full references available at **http://expertconsult. inkling.com**

Key references

4. Norgren L, Hiatt WR, Dormandy JA, et al. Inter-Society Consensus for the Management of Peripheral Arterial Disease (TASC II). J Vasc Surg 2007;45(Suppl S):S5–67. PMID: 17223489.

The majority of patients with PAD are thought to be asymptomatic. Out of those with symptoms, few with claudication go on to develop CLI but risk factors for this include increased age, diabetes, smoking, and lipid abnormalities. Exercise therapy in addition to control of risk factors has been proven to help improve symptomatic PAD.

8. Steg PG, Bhatt DL, Wilson PW, et al. One-year cardiovascular event rates in outpatients with atherothrombosis. JAMA 2007;297(11):1197–206. PMID: 17374814.

Patients with PAD have a higher rate of cardiovascular events compared to similar patients with coronary artery disease or cerebrovascular disease. Furthermore, the risk of a cardiovascular event increased with each additional arterial lesion.

9. Selvin E, Erlinger TP. Prevalence of and risk factors for peripheral arterial disease in the United States: results from the National Health and Nutrition Examination Survey, 1999–2000. Circulation 2004;110(6):738–43. PMID: 15262830.

Risk factors for PAD include increasing age, black race, current smoking, diabetes, hypercholesterolaemia, and kidney disease.

14. Caruana MF, Bradbury AW, Adam DJ. The validity, reliability, reproducibility and extended utility of ankle to brachial pressure index in current vascular surgical practice. Eur J Vasc Endovasc Surg 2005;29(5):443–51. PMID: 15966081.

Ankle to brachial pressure index has a key role in the assessment of symptomatic PAD.

20. Rooke TW, Hirsch AT, Misra S, et al. 2011 ACCF/ AHA Focused Update of the Guideline for the Management of Patients With Peripheral Artery Disease (updating the 2005 guideline): a report of the American College of Cardiology Foundation/ American Heart Association Task Force on Practice Guidelines. J Am Coll Cardiol 2011;58(19):2020– 45. PMID: 21963765.

Ankle to brachial pressure index is an important diagnostic tool in high risk populations and in those identified as having PAD every effort should be made to reduce risk factors for progression of disease, especially smoking cessation.

21. European Stroke Organization, Tendera M, Aboyans V, Bartelink ML, et al. ESC Guidelines on the diagnosis and treatment of peripheral artery diseases: Document covering atherosclerotic disease of extracranial carotid and vertebral, mesenteric, renal, upper and lower extremity arteries: the Task Force on the Diagnosis and Treatment of Peripheral Artery Diseases of the European Society of Cardiology (ESC). Eur Heart J 2011;32(22):2851– 906. PMID: 21873417.

ABI is an excellent tool for identifying PAD and the treadmill test is a good secondary test for those with borderline ABIs but a consistent clinical story for PAD.

30. Anderson JL, Halperin JL, Albert NM, et al. Management of patients with peripheral artery disease (compilation of 2005 and 2011 ACCF/ AHA guideline recommendations): a report of the American College of Cardiology Foundation/ American Heart Association Task Force on Practice Guidelines. Circulation 2013;127(13):1425–43. PMID: 23457117.

Pharmacologic interventions should be considered, alongside counselling, to assist in smoking cessation. Exercise therapy should be recommended for patients with PAD.

50. Stewart KJ, Hiatt WR, Regensteiner JG, et al. Exercise training for claudication. N Engl J Med 2002;347(24):1941–51. PMID: 12477945.

Exercise therapy has proven efficacy in treating claudication and is best done through formal supervised exercise programmes if possible.

53. Society for Vascular Surgery Lower Extremity Guidelines Writing Group, Conte MS, Pomposelli FB, Clair DG, et al. Society for Vascular Surgery practice guidelines for atherosclerotic occlusive disease of the lower extremities: management of asymptomatic disease and claudication. J Vasc Surg 2015;61(3 Suppl):2S–41S. PMID: 25638515.

Risk factor modification as well as additional medical management are the first line interventions for claudication in PAD. Currently the Society for Vascular Surgery does not recommend screening asymptomatic patients for PAD with ABI measurements.

4

Intervention for chronic lower limb ischaemia

Ramon L. Varcoe

Introduction

Peripheral artery disease (PAD) is a process characterised by the formation of atheromatous plaque within the arteries of the lower extremity. Typically, this leads to luminal stenosis or occlusions of those major blood vessels. Patients who suffer from the condition may either be asymptomatic, or complain of a broad variety of clinical symptoms ranging from calf claudication to ischaemic tissue loss. Interventional therapy for PAD has traditionally been reliant upon open vascular surgery, such as endarterectomy and bypass to achieve definitive revascularisation. However, since the advent of peripheral angioplasty in the mid-1960s there has been a large increase in its use, driven in large part by technological advances in what we now know as the field of endovascular surgery. Herein we seek to outline the contemporary literature and recommend an evidence-based approach to revascularisation of patients with chronic lower extremity ischaemia.

Presenting symptoms

The spectrum of symptoms that may occur when lower extremity PAD becomes symptomatic range from intermittent claudication (IC), through to ischaemic rest pain, ulceration and gangrene.

Intermittent claudication is muscular discomfort that occurs reproducibly upon exercise and is relieved after a short period of rest. It occurs when muscular oxygen demand increases above its limited metabolic supply. It most often affects the calf muscles but can also affect more proximal muscle groups such as the thigh, hip and buttock. It is typically described as cramp, ache, fatigue or a combination of the three,

and is graded according to severity (Table 4.1). The decision to intervene is based upon an individualised patient assessment that considers severity of symptoms, quality of life (QoL), risk of intervention and predicted durability of treatment.

Critical limb ischaemia (CLI) is the chronic manifestation of an ischaemic process (>2 weeks) with symptoms that include rest pain, ulceration or gangrene. Whilst ulceration may be triggered by a non-ischaemic process such as trauma or neuropathy, a non-healing ulcer perpetuated by ischaemia is also considered CLI. Ischaemic rest pain may be constant or nocturnal. It is typically present in the distal portion of the foot and often relieved by hanging the leg dependent. It should not be confused with neuropathic symptoms, which are common in diabetes mellitus. When gangrene occurs it typically affects digits and pressure areas such as the heel. Often forming an eschar, it may remain dry or develop an underlying suppurative infection.

Exercise therapy

✔✔ There is a body of evidence to support the effectiveness of supervised exercise therapy (SET) for the resolution of intermittent claudication symptoms[1] and multiple guidelines recommend its use as first-line therapy for IC.[2–4]

Such a programme must be supervised walking,[3–5] 30–60-minute treadmill walks per day and be associated with risk factor modification and best medical therapy (BMT) to be most effective. The patient is instructed to walk until they experience moderate claudication, stop until symptoms resolve, then repeat until the predetermined time period

Table 4.1 • Classification of peripheral artery disease

Fontaine's Classification		Rutherford-Becker Classification	
Stage	Symptom	Category	Symptom
I	Asymptomatic	0	Asymptomatic
II	Intermittent claudication	1	Mild claudication
		2	Moderate claudication
		3	Severe claudication
III	Ischaemic rest pain	4	Ischaemic rest pain
IV	Ulceration or gangrene	5	Minor tissue loss
		6	Major tissue loss

has elapsed. The speed, inclination and treadmill walking time is incrementally increased throughout the programme.

The CLEVER (Claudication: Exercise Versus Endoluminal Revascularization) study was a randomised, multicentre, clinical trial.[5] One-hundred and eleven participants with aorto-iliac occlusive disease were randomised to SET with BMT, endovascular revascularisation (ER) with BMT or general advice to exercise and BMT. SET consisted of a 26-week programme of 60-minute treadmill walking followed by telephone counselling to encourage ongoing exercise participation. After 18 months of follow-up functional walking improvement and QoL were persistently improved in both the SET + BMT and ER + BMT groups. Those two groups could not be separated in their effectiveness, attesting to the value of each; and both of those strategies were superior to BMT with general advice to exercise.

In the CETAC study, 151 patients were randomised to either SET or ER for PAD of the aorto-iliac or femoropopliteal arterial segments and both groups received BMT.[6] SET consisted of a 24-week programme whereby participants walked for 30 minutes on a treadmill twice a week, were encouraged to walk for an additional 30 minutes three times per week at home and continue walking for at least 1 hour per day after the programme was complete. After a mean follow-up period of 7 years both groups had significantly improved maximum walking distance, pain-free walking distance and QoL. There was no difference between the two groups in any of those outcome measures. This trial demonstrated the long-term effectiveness of SET as an alternative therapy, equivalent to ER.

Despite this compelling evidence to support the use of SET, ER has become the first-line treatment of choice in most advanced healthcare regions. The reasons for this are multifactorial. First, ER offers a fast treatment with almost instant relief of symptoms. It is less labour-intensive than SET, which requires effort and persistence. Moreover, SET is frequently unavailable or not reimbursed in countries with insurance-based healthcare, a fact that is disappointing given the additional benefits of exercise in obesity reduction, blood pressure control, lipid lowering and glucose control, over-and-above that of claudication treatment.

Medical therapy

All patients with macroscopic arterial disease benefit from risk factor management. Optimal medical therapy should be instigated in conjunction with interventional therapy and continued long term to prevent secondary cardiovascular morbidity. Medical treatment for PAD, and risk factor modification have been comprehensively described in Chapter 3.

Global trends toward revascularisation treatment

There are more than 200 million people living with PAD around the world and the incidence is increasing.[7,8] In high-income countries there has been an increase in the proportion of patients undergoing endovascular revascularisation procedures, with decreasing open-surgical revascularisation procedures, in-hospital mortality and major amputation.[8] Factors that may be driving this trend include the association of endovascular procedures with reduced in-hospital mortality, length-of-stay and cost when compared to surgical revascularisation.[8,9] However, a causal relationship linking the endovascular approach to reduced amputation and improved outcomes remains to be demonstrated.

A regional approach to intervention

Aorto-iliac occlusive disease

The aorto-iliac segment is a frequently diseased vascular territory, which may be found both in isolation (claudication) and in conjunction with multilevel, occlusive disease in CLI. Isolated aorto-iliac revascularisation may be sufficient to address symptoms in patients who also have concomitant infrainguinal disease, and it is often necessary to maximise inflow in order to maintain infrainguinal revascularisation strategies. It is therefore recommended that all vascular specialists have a thorough knowledge of treatment options for aorto-iliac occlusive disease.

The open-surgery, gold-standard for the treatment of aorto-iliac occlusive disease is aorto-(bi)-femoral (ABF) or bi-iliac bypass, which has durable patency that remains unchallenged by all other peripheral bypass operations.[10] However, whilst those patency rates are excellent one must also consider the risk of major complications, which may occur in up to a quarter of patients, sexual dysfunction in up to 40% and perioperative mortality rates as high as 5%.[10,11] It is this burden of risk which has led some to question whether a first-line, endovascular approach is more appropriate for most patients with aorto-iliac disease.

Revascularisation of aorto-iliac disease

Percutaneous interventions have gained increasing popularity, driven by patient preference, enhanced safety and the increasingly complex patient comorbidities encountered in an ageing population. Moreover, minimally invasive procedures have demonstrated reduced length-of-stay requirements and intensive care utilisation, making them extremely attractive.

Whilst in the past it was common for endovascular therapies to face insurmountable technical challenges to wire passage and stent delivery during the treatment of extensive aorto-iliac disease, dedicated chronic-total-occlusion (CTO) wires and catheters, bi-directional techniques and re-entry devices have contributed to very high technical success in contemporary experience.[4,12] This has made possible the percutaneous treatment of even the most extensive aorto-iliac occlusion for the skilled interventionist.

Surgical treatment for aorto-iliac disease

Several open surgical options exist to revascularise the lower limbs in the presence of aorto-iliac occlusive disease. They include extra-anatomical bypass (femoro-femoral crossover and axillo-(bi)-femoral bypass), aortic endarterectomy and ABF bypass.

ABF has been performed since the advent of the synthetic aortic graft in the early1950s. The aorta may be approached from a trans- or retro-peritoneal route, and the bypass may be configured with either a proximal anastomosis that is end-to-end, or end-to-side. The latter configuration has the advantage of preserving flow to the distal inferior mesenteric, aberrant renal or internal iliac arteries; however, no patency advantage has been demonstrated with either technique and the decision as to which method is best remains contentious amongst vascular

surgeons. An individual patient approach appears reasonable, dependent upon patient anatomy and disease morphology.

Patency rates with ABF are considered the gold standard for the treatment of aorto-iliac occlusive disease. A meta-analysis by De Vries et al. analysed 23 studies published between 1970 and 1996. Primary patency at 5 and 10 years was 91% and 86.8%, respectively, in those with claudication.[10] For those with critical limb ischaemia the rates were slightly lower at 86.8% and 81.8%. However, despite those excellent surgical results, current practice in most units is to favour an endovascular-first approach for the majority of patients, morphology permitting, due to the relatively high perioperative risk. De Vries et al. found a combined 30-day mortality rate of 4.4% which was higher in the older series (4.6% in studies published prior to 1975; 3.3% 1975–1996; $P = 0.01$). Furthermore, major morbidity rates were 19.7% (12.1% systemic complications; 7.6% local) and in series that looked specifically at sexual dysfunction morbidity was noted in as many as 40%, with a combination of retrograde ejaculation and iatrogenic impotency.[11,13]

Extra-anatomic bypass is a less morbid operation than ABF, but it suffers from lower 5-year primary patency rates of 51% (range 44–79%) for axillo-uni-femoral, 71% (range 50–76%) for axillo-bi-femoral and 75% (range 55–92%) for femoro-femoral bypass.[4] For that reason, most vascular surgeons are likely to reserve those options for patients with severe comorbidities or a hostile abdomen where transperitoneal surgery is best avoided.

It should be noted that many of the studies included in the meta-analyses which have evaluated open-surgical techniques for aorto-iliac occlusive disease are from an era when open surgery was used in the majority. Although outcomes from vascular surgery have generally improved over the years, care must be taken in their interpretation to consider that they are likely to have included patients with relatively minor disease who would be treated with angioplasty or stenting using current standards of practice. The inclusion of those relatively simple cases means that the patency and morbidity results from these studies may be skewed towards longevity and safety relative to the real-world application of ABF using present-day treatment algorithms.

Percutaneous treatment for aorto-iliac disease

Patients often prefer minimally invasive therapeutic options, as they experience less pain, less operative risk and a faster return to normal activities.

The TASC II document pooled results of 2222 iliac artery angioplasty procedures for both claudication (76%) and critical ischaemia (24%). They found a high technical success rate of 96% (range 90–99), as well as 1-, 3- and 5-year primary patency rates of 86% (range 81–94%), 82% (range 72–90%) and 71% (range 64–75%), respectively, demonstrating both the technical feasibility and durability of percutaneous transluminal angioplasty (PTA) for aorto-iliac occlusive disease.[4] In other contemporary findings from a large, single-centre study describing an experience with 505 aorto-iliac lesions treated with angioplasty ± stenting over a 9-year period, the authours found a technical success rate of 98%.[14] Eight-year primary and primary-assisted patency rates were 74% and 81%, respectively, illustrating the durability of the procedure, and safety was demonstrated with a 30-day mortality of 0.5%, comparing favourably to open surgery.

New techniques and technology have allowed us to treat ever more extensive patterns of disease, including long infrarenal aortic occlusions that extend into the iliac arteries (**Fig. 4.1**). These have traditionally been considered only suitable for open surgery. The most important technical aspect of treating advanced aorto-iliac occlusive disease proximal to the aortic bifurcation is the reliable passage of guidewire into the aortic true lumen from below. When the occlusion approaches the renal arteries then accurate localisation of the true lumen entry point becomes particularly critical in order that stents can be deployed in the true lumen but as far distal to the renal arteries as possible. These two aspects of treatment are reliably achieved utilising a bidirectional approach (combined antegrade from an upper limb access and retrograde from a femoral access) and by using re-entry devices with fine, retractable needles that can accurately facilitate a point of re-entry.

Percutaneous vs open surgery for aorto-iliac occlusive disease revascularisation

Whilst it is generally accepted that an endovascular-first approach should be the treatment of choice for those with less extensive disease (TASC A and B; for details of TASC classification see Table 2.7, p. 34), there are few robust data with which to compare the two methods of revascularisation for more complex and extensive disease patterns. Current evidence is largely based on single-centre, retrospective studies with no large-scale, contemporary, randomised clinical trials to compare endovascular and open surgery for the treatment of TASC C and D aorto-iliac lesions. However, a contemporary meta-analysis has identified all studies that included TASC C and D disease between 1989 and 2010. Data were extracted for 1625 patients from all 28 studies that evaluated endovascular revascularisation (ER) and 3733 patients from the 29 studies which evaluated open bypass surgery. ER was found to be safer (complication rate 13.4% vs 18.0%, $P < 0.001$; 30-day mortality 0.7% vs 2.6%, $P < 0.001$) and incur a shorter length-of-stay (4 days vs 13 days, $P < 0.001$). The complications observed in the ER studies were more likely to be minor and self-limiting, such as

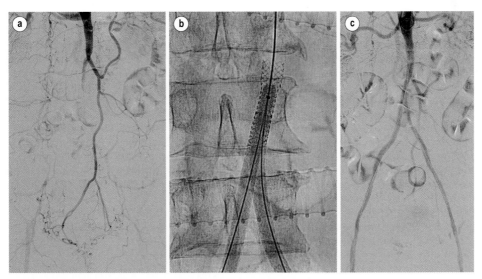

Figure 4.1 • **(a)** Complete occlusion of the aorta (distal to the inferior mesenteric artery), common and external iliac arteries. **(b)** Post-dilatation after implantation of two self-expanding iliac stents within a single large balloon-expandable stent for the aorta. **(c)** Completion subtraction angiogram demonstrating unimpeded flow and complete revascularisation.

haematoma and fever; whereas cardiac complications were frequent after bypass surgery, as were wound and graft infections. Findings favouring the more invasive procedure were that bypass surgery had increased primary patency rates at 1, 3 and 5 years of 94.8% vs 86.0%, 86.0% vs 80.0% and 82.7% vs 71.4%, respectively (all P <0.001), with a similar difference seen in secondary patency. It is apparent that ER is safer and less invasive, whilst surgery remains more durable. The published data reinforce the fact that both approaches are reasonable and should be considered a standard part of the armamentarium in the everyday clinical practice of patients with aorto-iliac disease. A reasonable approach is to apply the most appropriate form of treatment, matched to the individual patient's needs, disease morphology and risk factors. That may favour the durability of OS for the young, fit patient with claudication or a minimally invasive strategy for the elderly patient with tissue loss. Some argue that an endovascular-first approach to all patients remains reasonable as long as that procedure does not impact future surgical options.

Angioplasty vs stent vs covered stent

The Dutch Iliac Stent Trial randomised 279 patients with mostly stenotic disease to undergo either primary stent placement (n = 143) or PTA (n = 136) between 1993 and 1997.[15] At a mean follow-up of 6.3 and 5.7 years for the two groups respectively, there was no difference between the group who ultimately received stents versus those who underwent uncomplicated PTA. The group that fared best were those that underwent PTA and had bailout stenting. Those patients had superior preservation of symptomatic relief and long-term quality of life. No difference was observed between ankle-brachial pressure index (ABPI) or patency between any of the groups. The authors concluded that PTA with selective stenting strategy was the preferred method of iliac revascularisation.

The STAG trial was a contemporary, British, multicentre randomised controlled trial (RCT) which recruited 118 patients with iliac artery occlusions to undergo either PTA (n = 55) or primary iliac stenting (n = 57) (6 were excluded due to protocol violations).[16] Primary stent placement resulted in increased technical success rates (98% vs 84%; P = 0.007) and reduced major complication rates (5% vs 20%; P = 0.010) compared with simple PTA. There was no difference in primary patency after a median follow-up period of 721 days and the authors concluded that primary stent placement was preferable to improve technical success and reduce complications.

Whilst there is no randomised trial that has compared self-expanding and balloon-expandable stents for the iliac artery there are 24-month follow-up data from the BRAVISSIMO European prospective, multicentre registry.[17] That study enrolled 325 patients with aorto-iliac occlusive disease (n = 190, TASC A and B; n = 135 TASC C and D) and followed them with duplex ultrasound. They found similar primary patency rates of 88.0%, 88.5%, 91.9% and 84.8% for TASC A, B, C and D groups, respectively. There was a trend toward better patency for self-expanding stents (92.1%), compared with balloon expandable (85.2%) or a combination of both stent types (75.3%) (P = 0.06). These results suggest that more advanced disease may also be treated with endovascular intervention and that both stent types are reasonable to use in the aorto-iliac segment. However, when stenting the iliac arteries, it is worthwhile to consider the common and external iliac segments as separate regions with individual characteristics that favour different stent types. The common iliac artery is well suited to a balloon-expandable stent, which has placement accuracy and increased radial strength to overcome the calcification that is common in this region. Typically, disease involving the aortic bifurcation will be treated with bilateral stents placed in a 'kissing' configuration to reduce the risk of plaque-shift compromising the contralateral flow lumen. The external iliac artery is exposed to increased range of movement and mechanical strain upon hip flexion which may benefit from a more flexible, self-expanding stent. The external iliac is also prone to rupture during dilatation which may lead to sudden, catastrophic blood loss. This should always be considered and a range of covered stents kept available to expeditiously deal with such events.

Covered stents may also be used as primary therapy in the iliac arteries due to their known property of in-stent restenosis reduction. COBEST (Covered versus Balloon Expandable Stent Trial) was an Australian, multicentre trial which enrolled 125 patients with iliac occlusive disease (TASC B–D) and randomised them to treatment with a PTFE-covered (Advanta V12; Atrium) or a bare-metal stent (both self-expanding and balloon-expandable varieties were used) chosen at the operator's discretion.[18] Subgroup analysis after 18 months found better patency of the TASC C and D lesions treated with covered stents (HR 0.136; 95% CI 0.042–0.442; P = 0.0056). There was no such patency difference observed in the TASC B subgroup.

✔ The COBEST trial results suggested that covered stents may confer protection from restenosis and should be considered in more severe patterns of aorto-iliac occlusive disease.

Common femoral artery disease

Common femoral artery (CFA) disease has continued to be treated almost exclusively by open surgery. This is partly due to the nature of the disease as well as the technical difficulties with using stents in this region.

The CFA is prone to the development of eccentric and calcified atheromatous plaque with a predilection for the posterior artery wall (**Fig. 4.2**). Upon handling, the plaque is often friable and it frequently involves the bifurcation, proximal superficial femoral (SFA) and profunda femoris arteries. Whilst PTA can be effective in treating CFA disease, there is a risk of embolisation and if stents are required there is not a good solution for dealing with the bifurcation. Furthermore, it is a commonly held belief that the CFA is a flexion point that puts stents at risk of fracture, and that following implantation the blood vessel cannot be used as an access site for future arterial access. Whilst neither of these points are entirely true, with the majority of vessel flexion taking place through the distal external iliac artery[19] and sheath insertion through well-incorporated self-expanding stents, a simple, safe manoeuvre, it helps explain the general reluctance to use endovascular techniques in this short arterial segment.

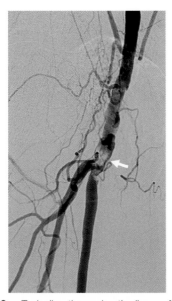

Figure 4.2 • Typically, atherosclerotic disease found in the common femoral artery is calcified and eccentric (*arrow*). It frequently involves the origins of both superficial femoral and profunda femoris arteries, making femoral endarterectomy preferable to percutaneous transluminal angioplasty and stent implantation.

Common femoral endarterectomy

The CFA is located superficially within the femoral triangle and is easily accessed through surgical exposure under either local or general anaesthesia. Common femoral endarterectomy (CFE) can be extended proximally into the distal external iliac artery or distally into the profunda femoris and SFA. The longitudinal arteriotomy is commonly patched using the adjacent great saphenous vein, synthetic material (polytetrafluoroethylene [PTFE] or polyethylene terephthalate [Dacron]) or even an occluded segment of SFA which can be resected, endarterectomised and used as patch material. Whilst that manoeuvre may be used to avoid the risk of infection associated with synthetic material, it prevents the option of future endovascular recanalisation of the occluded SFA and is therefore not recommended.

CFE is generally considered a safe surgical procedure; however, most published literature is based on single-centre case series of fewer than 100 patients. One exception is a large North American study that retrospectively reviewed admission and 30-day outcomes data of 1843 patients which was recorded prospectively in the American College of Surgeons National Surgical Quality Improvement Program (ACS-NSQIP) database.[20] That study found 30-day mortality to be 3.4%, wound complications 8.4% (86% were after discharge) and return to the operating theatre in 10%, indicating that CFE may not be as benign as previously thought. There remains little doubt that the procedure has excellent durability. In one single-centre study 121 CFEs were performed over 8 years. They obtained complete follow-up (mean 4.2 years) in 111 patients (115 limbs). The 7-year primary patency, assisted primary patency and limb salvage rates were 96%, 100% and 100%, respectively; whilst freedom from further revascularisation and survival rates were 79% and 80%, respectively.[21] Another contemporary study, again from a single centre, demonstrated 1- and 5-year primary patency of 93% and 91%, respectively, in 65 CFE in 58 patients.[22]

In contemporary practice CFE is often combined with an endovascular procedure to revascularise occlusive disease of the inflow or outflow arteries (**Fig. 4.3**). These so-called 'hybrid' procedures offer a durable solution for the CFA with fewer incisions to avoid long wounds, lymphatic disruption and the need to find long lengths of venous conduit.

Profundaplasty

Endarterectomy and patch repair of the profunda femoris artery (profundaplasty) may be performed in isolation to improve lower extremity perfusion, or as an adjunct during an inflow (aortofemoral) or outflow (femoropopliteal/tibial) bypass procedure. Under those circumstances, it may be convenient

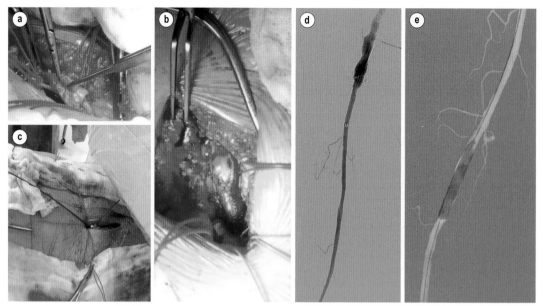

Figure 4.3 • A hybrid procedure may involve common femoral endarterectomy followed by an endovascular intervention through that exposed artery or its patch repair. **(a)** Posterior wall plaque being removed during common femoral endarterectomy. **(b)** Arterial repair with a saphenous vein patch. **(c)** A sheath is introduced after direct patch puncture under fluoroscopic guidance. **(d)** Subtraction angiography with injection of contrast through the sheath. **(e)** Percutaneous transluminal angioplasty of an atherosclerotic lesion at the adductor canal.

to use the profunda femoris as the location of the proximal/distal anastomosis or extend the hood of the graft from the common femoral artery into the profunda artery. Profundaplasty, in isolation, has value in improving direct perfusion to the thigh and indirect to the calf/foot via geniculate collaterals. It may reduce the severity of claudication and ischaemic rest pain but is unlikely to result in wound healing in cases of ulceration or gangrene.

Percutaneous treatment for the common femoral artery

There are only very few reports in the literature of endovascular treatment for isolated common femoral disease, with most reporting good outcomes in small patient cohorts. However, there is one large, prospective multicentre study with published experience using PTA alone, provisional stenting and atherectomy with PTA in 167 patients.[23] Over a 7-year period they treated 114, 15 and 38 patients in each of those groups, respectively. The entire cohort underwent a mean follow-up period of 42.5 months. Twelve-month primary patencies were reported as 78.4% for PTA alone, 100% for provisional stenting and 94.5% for atherectomy with PTA; with only 3% suffering major complications and 0.6% perioperative death. They concluded that percutaneous CFA interventions are safe and effective in selected patients.

The Endovascular Versus Open Repair of the Common Femoral Artery trial (NCT01353651) was a 117-subject, French, multicentre RCT designed to compare CFE with direct stenting for the CFA. Results published in 2017 found that stenting was safer, with a 1-month combine endpoint of mortality and/ or major morbidity rate of 12.5% vs 26% ($P=0.05$) and a shorter length of hospital stay (3.2 vs 6.3 days; $P<0.0001$). At 2-years of follow up primary patency, freedom from TLR and overall survival rates were statistically indistinguishable between the two groups. Suggesting that there is a role for the less invasive treatment, particularly in the medically comorbid.[23a]

Superficial femoral artery disease

The SFA extends from the CFA bifurcation to the adductor hiatus. It runs through the muscular borders of the adductor canal and comes under a great deal of mechanical strain during hip and knee flexion.[24] This results in the development of dense atherosclerosis, particularly in smokers, with stenosis and heavy calcification a common feature. It also poses a mechanical challenge to the implantation of permanent metallic devices, such as stents.

Surgical bypass

Surgical bypass can be performed using synthetic material (PTFE or Dacron) or autogenous vein. To maximise patency, proximal anastomosis at a site with adequate inflow should be undertaken. This would typically be the CFA, but may be the SFA or profunda femoris artery depending on the pattern of disease and length of available conduit. The distal anastomosis would be to the most proximal vessel sufficiently free of disease to suture which can provide at least one in-line blood vessel to the foot, although bypass to a blind segment of popliteal artery ('isolated popliteal segment') is well described. The most common distal anastomotic sites are the above- and below-knee popliteal arteries. Anastomosis to the above-knee popliteal artery is now infrequent given that these patients are usually claudicants (rather than having more extensive disease and CLI) and are usually treatable by angioplasty if necessary. The crural vessels may also be used for the distal anastomosis. They are accessible throughout their lengths with varying approaches and degrees of technical difficulty. The choice of crural vessel to use is based on that which is least diseased and which provides continuous run-off to the foot. The quality of the outflow system is an important determinant of graft patency.

✔✔ The great saphenous vein is the preferred conduit and may be used in situ after valvotomy, or be reversed. There is no difference in patency between in situ and reversed grafts,[25] but in situ grafts provide an appropriately small distal segment for use in tibial bypass and therefore may be preferred at the ankle. Vein may be harvested in one single incision or by leaving skin bridges to better approximate the wound and relieve tension. It may then be tunnelled in an anatomical or subcutaneous plane to facilitate future surgical access for patch graft repair. No patency advantage has been demonstrated for any of these techniques over another. If ipsilateral great saphenous is not available then contralateral great saphenous, spliced small saphenous, arm vein or synthetic material should be used in that order.[26] Conduit should preferably be a single graft but splicing and/or repair of varicose segments is sometimes required. Synthetic graft should be used as a last option, and has very poor patency rates below the knee. If a tibial anastomosis is to be performed with synthetic material a vein cuff configured as a Miller cuff, Taylor patch or St Mary's boot is generally recommended to improve patency through minimising compliance mismatch, reducing mechanical injury and expanding the distal anastomosis to lessen the impact of perianastomotic intimal hyperplasia.[26] There is no short-term difference in patency rates between PTFE and Dacron,[25] but long-term patency may be superior with the latter.[26,27]

The patency of surgical bypass has traditionally been evaluated using a combination of ankle–brachial index (to compare with the preoperative value), history of symptom return, clinical examination and occasionally duplex ultrasound to check for flow within the graft.

✔✔ The PREVENT III trial is the largest prospective, randomised, double-blind, multicentre trial to have performed an objective evaluation of patency rates for venous bypass surgery in patients with critical limb ischaemia (CLI).[28] Some 1404 subjects were enrolled to determine whether a novel molecular therapy agent (edifoglide) was useful in the prevention of vein graft failure. Whilst no difference was detected as a result of the drug the dataset serves as a useful cohort to determine the patency rates of vein bypass. Binary restenosis was defined as >70% on angiography, >50% with recurrent symptoms, ABPI <0.4, toe pressure <30 mmHg or duplex ultrasound stenosis with a peak systolic velocity ratio of >3.0 or velocity >300 cm/s; insensitive standards compared with those used to evaluate endovascular therapy patency in contemporary trials (>50% on angiography or peak systolic ratio >2.0–2.5). Twelve-month graft primary patency, limb salvage and patient survival rates were 61%, 88% and 84%, respectively. There was no difference in patency when vein bypass was performed at a distal anastomotic site above or below the knee. This trial gives us a well-defined and rigorously adjudicated measure of patency with which to compare other methods of SFA revascularisation in patients with CLI.

✔ Bypass graft surveillance programmes with duplex ultrasound have been used to detect patency-threatening lesions before complete thrombosis. This is thought to be worthwhile as these lesions are common and may often be asymptomatic prior to complete graft occlusion. Several studies have demonstrated a patency advantage with intense duplex surveillance over the first 2 years, the period where significant intimal proliferation is most common.[29,30] However, there is conflicting evidence, with a large RCT showing that duplex surveillance after venous femoral distal bypass grafts leads to no significant clinical benefit or quality of life improvement at 18 months.[31] Most guidelines recommend at least 2 years of formal, structured, combined clinical and ultrasound surveillance for vein bypass grafts.[4,32] This is not true for synthetic bypass, where patency failure is less likely to be preceded by a detectable stenotic lesion.

Percutaneous treatment for the superficial femoral artery

Since the first percutaneous transluminal angioplasty in 1964 there has been an ever-expanding number of endovascular options developed to treat occlusive disease of the SFA. Angioplasty itself has become more sophisticated and its technique has matured. There has been extensive development in the field of stents, stent grafts, atherectomy and drug-coating technology. However, evidence of effectiveness has often lagged behind the rapid pace of technological evolution. When comparative trials have been performed, they have usually included a high proportion of claudicants with short to moderate length, single-level disease, and most have compared the investigational technology to conventional balloon angioplasty. These trials have largely focused on angiographic outcomes and not patient-centred measures.

Nitinol self-expanding stents

☑☑ Nitinol self-expanding stents have superior effectiveness to PTA. A contemporary meta-analysis accumulated results from 17 randomised clinical trials (627 subjects) which used either primary nitinol stenting or PTA for symptomatic femoropopliteal occlusive disease (mean length 74.6 mm nitinol stent group, 66.7 mm PTA group).[33] They found that the nitinol stent group had higher rates of technical success (95.8% vs 64.2%, P <0.001), and at 12-month follow-up lower rates of both target lesion revascularisation (TLR) (OR 2.47, 95%CI 0.72–8.49, P =0.065), a subjective endpoint that can be susceptible to bias, and binary restenosis (OR 3.02, 95% CI 1.3–6.71, P <0.001), with similar safety outcomes. Whilst lower rates of restenosis have been demonstrated, the neointimal proliferation that does form within these permanent metallic implants is a bulky lesion that poses a particular challenge to future attempts at endovascular intervention which may be difficult to cross and frequently recoil after angioplasty. It is for this reason that many interventional specialists have explored alternative technologies.

Stent grafts

Stent grafts covered in PTFE offer a theoretical advantage over uncovered stents. The PTFE acts as a barrier to neointimal migration and proliferation which can then only compromise the lumen at the proximal and distal edges of the stent (edge-restenosis). The VIBRANT trial randomised 148 subjects with symptomatic and complex (TASC C and D) SFA disease to a bare-metal, nitinol stent or Viabahn stent graft at 19 US centres.[34] Although this differing pattern of edge-restenosis was observed, there was no difference in primary patency rates over a follow-up period of 3 years. Given that stent grafts are costly and cover collaterals, which may be important if future patency is lost, their use is difficult to justify as part of routine practice.

Atherectomy

Atherectomy is another technology that has theoretical advantages over stenting. It debulks the atheromatous plaque and leaves behind no permanent implant. However, it may pose a risk of distal embolisation and there are concerns about its potential to stimulate restenosis through aggressive vessel wall injury. Whilst no randomised, comparative data exist, the DEFINITIVE LE study was a large, prospective, multicentre, single arm trial which demonstrated the effectiveness of directional atherectomy through satisfactory 12-month primary-patency rates with a low incidence of perforation and distal embolisation.[35]

Drug-coated balloon angioplasty

☑☑ Angioplasty balloons coated with the antiproliferative drug paclitaxel (DCB) offer a novel method of revascularisation and drug delivery which also leaves behind no permanent metallic implant and has the potential to be combined with other therapies, such as atherectomy and stenting. A 2016 meta-analysis examined data from eight multicentre RCTs which each compared DCB to PTA for stenotic femoropopliteal lesions.[36] These studies each assessed short-to-moderate-length lesions, ranging in length between 4.3 cm and 8.9 cm, with proportion of total occlusions ranging from 26% to 100%. The meta-analysis found that paclitaxel-coated balloons were superior to PTA in reducing TLR at 12 months, an effect which persisted during longer follow-up. However, there was some evidence of differential efficacy, with not all paclitaxel-coated balloons having as pronounced an anti-restenotic effect. It is likely that this relates to the differing excipient (spacer) molecule, which plays a major role in determining efficiency of drug transfer and the deposition of drug reservoirs into the arterial wall. It may also be related to the different formulation (crystalline or amorphous) or concentration of paclitaxel, which ranges between 2.0 and 3.5 µg/mm[6] in commercially available balloon catheters, as well as the stability of the drug coating as it traverses the haemostatic sheath and target arteries.

Drug-eluting stents

☑☑ Nitinol, paclitaxel-eluting, self-expanding stents (DES) have demonstrated efficacy in the SFA, superior to both PTA and bare-metal stents (BMS). The ZILVER PTX trial randomised subjects with symptomatic femoropopliteal disease (91% claudicants) to DES (n=236) or PTA (n=238).[37] Of those in the PTA arm who required a bailout stent, a secondary randomisation took place to DES (n=61) or BMS (n=59). After 5 years the drug-eluting stent was superior to PTA in freedom from persistent or worsening symptoms of ischaemia (79.8% vs 59.3%, P <0.01), primary patency (66.4% vs 43.4%, P <0.01), and freedom from TLR (83.1% vs 67.6%, P <0.01). Similarly, clinical benefit (81.8% vs 63.8%, P=0.02), patency (72.4% vs 53.0%, $P=0.03$), and freedom from TLR (84.9% vs 71.6%, $P=0.06$) with provisional DES were improved over provisional BMS. A smaller multicentre, single-arm study evaluated a newer generation of paclitaxel and polymer-coated DES in 57 participants from Europe, Australia and New Zealand. The MAJESTIC study found a 12-month primary patency rate of 96.4% in relatively complex, moderate-length lesions which included a high proportion of diabetes, severe calcification and chronic total occlusions.[38] These results are the best of any interventional study in the SFA to date, underscoring the value of combining antiproliferative drug with biomechanical scaffolding. Results at 24 months have been presented but not yet published. They show a drop-off in the primary patency to 78.2%, but excellent maintenance of clinical effectiveness with freedom from clinically driven TLR rate of 91.3%.

The femoropopliteal area is becoming increasingly crowded with new technology; however, studies comparing the latest devices are lagging well behind the expanding therapeutic arsenal. The IMPERIAL trial (NCT02574481) is currently recruiting 465 subjects from 75 global centres to make a 2:1 randomised comparison between those two paclitaxel-coated stents for the treatment of SFA disease. BASIL (Bypass vs Angioplasty in Severe Ischaemia of the Leg)-3 is a randomised, pragmatic, multicentre, three-arm, open-label trial of alternative revascularisation strategies, designed to evaluate the clinical benefit and cost-effectiveness of drug-coated balloons, drug-eluting stents, and plain balloon angioplasty with bailout bare-metal stent revascularisation for severe limb ischaemia secondary to femoropopliteal disease. It is aiming to recruit 861 subjects from approximately 60 vascular centres in England, Wales, Scotland and other European Union states over a 36-month period. More comparative trials such as these are expected to follow.

Surgical bypass vs percutaneous intervention

Direct comparisons of surgical bypass and endovascular revascularisation methods are very much needed; however, they are limited due to variations in vascular anatomy, extent of disease and indications for treatment.

The BASIL trial was a randomised controlled trial designed to compare infrainguinal vein bypass with PTA for patients with severe limb ischaemia and was published in 2005.[9] They found broadly similar amputation-free survival and overall survival rates during the first 2 years of follow-up. A subsequent analysis showed that there was an increase in overall survival for the bypass group beyond 2 years

of follow-up. Conversely, endovascular therapy was found to be safer with equivalent QoL outcomes and was significantly less costly. In that trial the endovascular therapy arm did not use stents, drug-eluting devices or atherectomy; adjunctive procedures that are now commonplace and known to improve patency rates and add cost compared with PTA alone.

✅ In a meta-analysis which included 23 unique studies (12 779 patients) that evaluated the comparative effectiveness of endovascular and surgical revascularisation between 1995 and 2012 the authors commented on the dearth of high-quality evidence.[39] There was only one directly comparative RCT. Their analysis of these mostly observational studies found no difference in all-cause mortality, lower extremity amputation or amputation-free survival between the two forms of treatment. Rates of primary patency favoured endovascular revascularisation at 1 year (OR 0.63, 0.46–0.86), and secondary patency at both 1 year (OR 0.57, 0.40–0.82) and 2–3 years (OR 0.49, 0.28–0.85).

The Best Endovascular versus Best Surgical Therapy in Patients with Critical Limb Ischemia (BEST-CLI) trial (NCT02060630) expects to enrol 2100 participants over 120 North American centres, with the intent to randomise 1:1 to open surgery with venous conduit or best contemporary endovascular treatment. Enrolment is ongoing, having just surpassed 700 enrolled subjects in late 2016. The ZILVERPASS study (NCT01952457) is currently recruiting 220 subjects with extensive symptomatic SFA disease to compare between a paclitaxel DES and prosthetic bypass. The outcomes of these comparative trials are eagerly awaited.

Popliteal artery disease

The popliteal artery is one of the most challenging infrainguinal vessels to treat with endovascular means and warrants individual consideration beyond that of the SFA. Coursing between the adductor hiatus and the origin of the anterior tibial artery it suffers repeated biomechanical stresses during knee flexion and has a tapering diameter which provides sizing challenges for most current generation implantable devices.[40] Management may be challenging, and with few randomised trials dedicated to answering questions of technical success and durability the correct approach remains contentious. The popliteal artery is also the location for several non-atherosclerotic disease processes such as aneurysm, cystic adventitia disease and popliteal entrapment, which may occasionally make accurate diagnosis a challenge and should be considered in younger patients with few vascular risk factors.

Percutaneous treatment for the popliteal artery

Due to the repetitive and extreme physical forces that exist on devices implanted into the popliteal artery it has been attractive for interventionists to consider options that leave behind no permanent implant. In the past PTA has played a primary strategic role with early generation stents thought to be at high risk of fracture and technical failure.

The TASC II guidelines recommended PTA for patients with stenoses or occlusions up to 15 cm in length of both the superficial femoral and popliteal arteries, if the infrageniculate popliteal artery or trifurcation are not involved.[4] Despite these recommendations there are few studies dedicated to assessing the performance of PTA in the popliteal artery. What scientific reports are available reveal generally disappointing patency rates, inferior to that seen in the superficial femoral artery and as low as 30–45% at 12 months.[41] This has led many interventional specialists to seek more durable solutions for PAD of the popliteal artery.

Atherectomy

Directional atherectomy may be used for debulking atheroma from the popliteal artery, but it has been rarely assessed in clinical studies. In a subset analysis of the DEFINITIVE LE study, 162 target lesions in 158 subjects with short popliteal artery lesions (mean length 5.8 cm) were assessed after 1 year. They found a promising 80.3% core-lab-adjudicated, duplex and angiography-assessed primary patency with a low 3.7% bailout stenting rate.[42] It may be that atherectomy has a role in the popliteal artery, particularly in debulking heavily calcified atheroma which may be otherwise resistant to angioplasty or stenting.

Nitinol, self-expanding stents

✅ The ETAP (Endovascular Treatment of Atherosclerotic Popliteal Artery Lesion-Balloon Angioplasty Versus Primary Stenting) trial is the only RCT to have addressed endovascular treatment for the popliteal artery specifically.[41] It was a prospective, multicentre trial conducted on single, de novo, popliteal artery lesions throughout nine European centres. Lesions were not included if they involved the SFA or extended to the crural arteries. Two hundred and forty-six subjects were randomised to either nitinol stent placement ($n = 127$) or PTA ($n = 119$), and evaluated with colour duplex ultrasound at 6 and 12 months. Twelve-month primary patency was significantly higher in the nitinol stent group compared to PTA (67.4% vs 44.9%; $P = 0.002$) and clinically driven TLR was significantly lower (14.7% vs 44.1%;

$P = 0.0001$). This difference was solely accounted for by a 25.2% acute failure rate in the PTA group due to either residual stenosis >30% or a flow-limiting dissection that did not resolve after prolonged balloon dilatation. In a secondary analysis where provisional bailout stenting was not considered loss of patency and TLR, no difference was observed between the groups at 12 months. The authors concluded that primary PTA with provisional bailout stenting for short lesions of the popliteal artery is a reasonable strategy. However, 12-month primary patency under 70% for such short popliteal lesions is not particularly impressive for either strategy and leads one to wonder whether surgery or newer generation devices may offer improved durability in that regard.

Novel devices for the popliteal artery

There are several new devices with early, observational data to support their use in the popliteal artery. These include drug-coated balloons, the hybrid Tigris stent (W.L. Gore, Flagstaff, USA), a dual component design made of a single nitinol wire interconnected by an expanded-PTFE lattice structure with a heparin-bonded surface, the BioMimics 3D (Veryan, West Sussex, UK), a nitinol stent with unique three-dimensional helical geometry and swirling flow properties and the Supera stent (Abbott Vascular, Santa Clara, CA, USA) made from six nitinol wires interwoven around a duly-sized mandrill. The latter stent is extremely flexible, fracture- and kink-resistant with high-resistive radial strength properties which make it ideal for use in the popliteal artery. The largest of these observational, single-centre studies was a retrospective review of 101 patients who had Supera stents placed in the popliteal artery for both de novo atherosclerotic disease and restenosis.[43] With a mean lesion length of 58.4 mm they found impressive primary and secondary patencies of 94.6%/97.9% at 6 months and 87.7%/96.5% at 12 months, respectively.

Whilst much research has been conducted with a focus on PAD of the SFA, the popliteal artery is often ignored or included in smaller numbers within those SFA trials. PTA remains the cornerstone for endovascular treatment; however, there are a host of new devices broadly suited to the popliteal territory. Whilst results from registry data evaluating new stent technology in the popliteal artery are encouraging, further randomised trials are necessary to confirm their safety and long-term durability.

Infrapopliteal artery disease

Intervention for occlusive disease of the infrapopliteal (IP) arteries is performed almost exclusively for critical limb ischaemia. Therefore, there is no evidence by which to recommend infrapopliteal intervention for patients with claudication. The practice of treating IP arteries to improve patency after a more proximal intervention (surgical or endovascular), whilst intuitive, also lacks supportive evidence.

There are several revascularisation options to achieve in-line blood flow to the periphery to facilitate wound healing or pain relief in the patient with CLI. These include a variety of different percutaneous interventions, including balloon angioplasty with uncoated or drug-coated balloons, cutting balloons, cryoplasty, atherectomy, laser atherectomy, stenting with bare-metal, bioresorbable or drug-eluting stents, as well as surgical bypass. Many of these endovascular technologies suffer from poor-quality, retrospective datasets to support their use. Relatively few have sufficient supporting evidence to withstand evidence-led, scientific interrogation.

Surgical bypass for infrapopliteal disease

✅ There is an extensive body of literature to attest to the efficacy of lower extremity bypass to treat occlusive IP disease.[44] In these smaller distal vessels, venous conduit is preferred. This is normally great saphenous vein in an in situ or reversed configuration; however, spliced small saphenous and arm vein may be used. Synthetic grafts with a vein cuff have also been used in the past, with inferior results. As with bypass for femoropopliteal lesions the proximal anastomosis site may vary depending on the extent of disease. Whilst bypass from the CFA may be performed, the proximal anastomosis can also be taken from a more distal location, such as the SFA or popliteal artery, which may reduce the length of conduit required. The distal anastomosis can be to any of the crural arteries, or indeed to the proximal pedal arteries themselves. If the surgery is distal to the proximal thigh the use of a pneumatic tourniquet may avoid clamping of the tibial arteries, which are often small and calcified.

There are no large RCTs that have evaluated surgical bypass in isolated IP disease; however, both the BASIL and PREVENT III trials included a significant proportion of subjects with disease in that location, with the tibial or pedal arteries the site of distal anastomosis in 31% and 65% of participants in those two trials, respectively.[9,28] In PREVENT III, 12-month primary patency, limb salvage and patient survival were 61%, 88% and 84%, respectively, with no observed difference for bypass above or below the knee. In BASIL, 12-month amputation-free survival was 68%, and overall survival 71%; patency was not evaluated. Major morbidity in those two trials is particularly relevant, with 30-day mortality 5.5% and 2.7%, myocardial infarction 7% and 4.7%, stroke 1.5% and 1.4% and wound complications seen in 22% and 4.8% of subjects in

BASIL and PREVENT II, respectively. These results clearly demonstrate that bypass surgery in patients with CLI carries a significant risk.

In a meta-analysis of autologous, popliteal-to-distal bypass grafts from 31 published series between 1981 and 2004 the authors found 1-, 3- and 5-year primary patency of 81.5%/72.3%/63.1%, secondary patency 85.9%/76.7%/70.7% and limb salvage rates of 88.5%/82.3%/77.7%, respectively.[44] This demonstrates the durability and limb preservation efficacy of a good-quality, infrapopliteal bypass graft.

Percutaneous treatment for infrapopliteal disease

The use of endovascular techniques for the treatment of occlusive IP disease has gained widespread acceptance and is now undertaken by many as the first-line treatment for patients with critical limb ischaemia. In the past, tibial artery intervention was plagued by low rates of immediate technical success. This was due to a paucity of dedicated endovascular devices and purpose-built guidewires, as well as rudimentary technique. There has been a rapid increase in the availability of dedicated guidewires designed to cross chronic total occlusions, support catheters, angioplasty balloons and re-entry devices, which have steadily increased those rates of success. Moreover, advanced refinements of technique to perfect the bidirectional approach with retrograde (pedal/tibial) access, introduce coronary techniques such as CART (controlled antegrade–retrograde subintimal tracking) and reverse CART (where an inflated balloon creates a target space for the opposite wire), and the double balloon technique (where overlapping balloons are positioned from antegrade and retrograde before simultaneous inflation to connect bidirectional subintimal guidewires) have concurrently laid the foundation for success. As a result, most contemporary series now have technical success rates in the high 90% range.[45]

Percutaneous Transluminal Angioplasty

✅ There are many case series reporting outcomes of PTA performed to the crural arteries. Romiti et al. performed a meta-analysis comparing 30 published articles reporting outcomes of 2693 crural artery PTAs from 1990–2006.[46] They found an immediate technical success rate of 89%, 1- and 3-year primary patency of 58.1% and 48.6% and secondary patency rates of 68.2% and 62.9%, respectively. Despite those rates of success and patency, which are poor by today's standards, limb salvage rates remained acceptable at 86% and 82.4% after 1 and 3 years. Furthermore, those limb salvage rates were comparable with another meta-analysis conducted to evaluate results of distal bypass surgery over that same period.[44]

Drug-coated balloon angioplasty

A large number of retrospective studies and small, single-centre, randomised trials emerged between 2010 and 2013, with results that suggested DCB may have the potential to limit restenosis and improve patency for angioplasty to the arteries below the knee.[47–49] However, following that period the In.Pact Deep trial published results from 358 patients with infrapopliteal lesions who were randomised 2:1 to DCB or PTA.[50] This large, multicentre study was well adjudicated, using independent, blinded core labs and a clinical events committee. At 12 months they found no difference in late lumen loss (0.61 mm vs 0.62 mm; $P=0.95$), or clinically driven TLR rates (17.7% vs 15.8%; $P=0.66$). There was also a trend toward higher amputation rates in the DCB arm compared to PTA (8.8% vs 3.6%; $P=0.08$), which did not reach statistical significance. This led to a complete withdrawal of the device and a root cause analysis, performed to determine the reasons for its failure. This result leaves us uncertain as to whether drug-coated balloon technology has any benefit over PTA and some have questioned its safety in patients with CLI.

There is one randomised study currently evaluating drug-coated balloons in the infrapopliteal arterial circulation. It is designed to assess an alternative paclitaxel-coated balloon with different active drug dose and excipient. The Lutonix BTK trial (NCT01870401) aims to recruit 480 patients through 59 global sites and is well on the way to achieving that goal. No results have yet been released.

Bare-metal stents

Even though simple angioplasty has become technically achievable in the majority of patients it remains relatively common to achieve a suboptimal outcome with PTA alone. The goal of stenting has been to treat an unsatisfactory result due to elastic recoil, residual stenosis, flow-limiting dissection or perforation.

A single RCT has compared a variety of BMS (balloon- and self-expanding) to PTA in 38 limbs. In this small and underpowered study, there was no statistical advantage to BMS over PTA in survival (74.7 vs 69.3%), limb salvage (91.7 vs 90%), primary (56 vs 66%) or secondary (64 vs 79.5%) patency rates after 12 months.[51] In a 2009 systematic review, 18 non-randomised studies comprising 640 patients who had infragenicular stent implantation at experienced centres had data pooled.[52] Of those, 232 had balloon-expandable BMS, 116 self-expanding BMS, 272 balloon expandable DES and 20 bioresorbable stents. They found that bailout stenting after unsatisfactory PTA in this region derived satisfactory angiographic results but no patency advantage. Balloon- and

self-expanding stent types were unable to be separated in terms of primary patency (73 vs 79%; $P=0.18$) and clinical outcomes (TLR 18 vs 6%, $P=1.0$; limb salvage 98 vs 96%, $P=1.0$) after a median follow-up of 12 months.

It is apparent that BMS are effective at treating residual stenosis, elastic recoil and dissection after PTA, thus improving the immediate technical result, but they are not able to achieve improved long-term patency as they also suffer from significant restenosis.

Drug-eluting stents

✅✅ Drug-eluting stents (DES) are known to reduce the neointimal proliferation response to vascular wall injury which in turn leads to reduction in the luminal area (negative remodelling), recurrent stenosis and loss of patency. In contrast to the low-level evidence which exists for the use of other endovascular technologies below the knee, the use of coronary drug-eluting stents is supported by results from four RCTs[53–56] (Table 4.2) and four meta-analyses.[57–60]

The YUKON-BTK trial was the first to publish, after randomising 161 patients with CLI (47%) and intermittent claudication (53%) to treatment with a polymer-free, 2% sirolimus-coated stent or the same stent uncoated.[54] The drug-eluting stent achieved a superior primary patency at the 12-month follow-up of 80.6% versus 55.6% for the BMS ($P=0.004$). Target lesion revascularisation was also improved upon with the use of the DES (9.7% vs 17.5%; $P=0.29$) but not significantly so. At a longer follow-up of mean 2.8 years, limb salvage was higher in the CLI patients; however, this was not statistically significant (97.4% vs 87.1%; $P=0.10$); the primary endpoint of freedom from amputation, TVR, AMI and death found in favour of the DES (65.8% vs 44.6%; $P=0.02$).

Following that study, the DESTINY trial randomised 140 CLI patients to primary treatment with an everolimus eluting stent or BMS comparator.[53] At the 12-month follow-up primary patency was higher in the DES group (85.2% vs 54.4%; $P=0.0001$), and late lumen loss was significantly lower (0.78 mm vs 1.41 mm; $P=0.001$), as was TLR (8% vs 35%; $P=0.005$). Once again, these results found in favour of the DES.

The ACHILLES (Angioplasty and DES in the Treatment of Subjects with Ischemic Infrapopliteal Arterial Disease) trial randomised 200 patients with CLI and occlusive tibial disease (<120 mm; mean length 27 mm) to treatment with a sirolimus-eluting stent or standard PTA.[55] The primary endpoint was 12-month, in-segment, binary restenosis determined by quantitative angiography, which once again found in favour of the DES (22.4% vs 41.9%;

Table 4.2 • Randomised controlled trials that have evaluated drug-eluting stents in the infrapopliteal circulation

Trial	Year	Study design		Patients (n)	Mean lesion length (mm)	Endpoints
YUKON-BTK (Rastan et al.[54])	2011 and 2012	RCT	Sirolimus-eluting stent (polymer free) vs Bare-metal stent	161 (75 CLI; 86 IC)	31	Primary patency(12 mth); 81% vs 56% (P=0.004) Secondary patency (12 mth); 92% vs 71% (P=0.005) TLR (12 mth); 9.7% vs 17.5% (P=0.29) Limb salvage in CLI (2.8 yr); 97.4% vs 87.1% (P=0.10) Freedom from amputation, TVR, AMI and death (2.8 yr) 65.8 vs 44.6% (P=0.02)
DESTINY (Bosiers et al.[53])	2012	RCT	Everolimus-eluting stent vs Bare-metal stent	140 (all CLI)	17	Primary patency (12 mth); 85% vs 54% (P=0.0001) LLL (12 mth); 0.78 mm vs 1.41 mm (P=0.001) TLR (12 mth); 8% vs 35% (P=0.005) Limb salvage (12 mth); 99% vs 97% (NS) Death (12 mth); 18% vs 16% (P=0.06)
ACHILLES (Scheinert et al.[55])	2012	RCT	Sirolimus-eluting stent vs Angioplasty	200 (CLI and IC)	27	Primary patency (12 mth); 78 vs 58% (P=0.019) TLR (12 mth); 10% vs 17% (P=0.257) Limb salvage (12 mth); 86% vs 80% (P=0.3) Death; 10% vs 12% (P=0.82)
IDEAS (Siablis et al.[56])	2014	RCT	Zotarolimus-, sirolimus- or everolimus-eluting stents vs Paclitaxel-coated balloon	50 (CLI and IC)	148/127	Binary restenosis (6 mth); 28% vs 57.9% (P=0.0457) TLR (6 mth); 7.7% vs 13.6% (P=0.65)

$P=0.019$). This result was even more pronounced when diabetic patients were analysed separately (17.6% vs 53.2%; $P<0.001$), however, there was no significant difference seen in; clinically driven TLR (10% vs 16.5%; $P=0.257$) or limb salvage (86.2% vs 80%; $P=0.3$), reflecting the multiple factors that impact those endpoints.

Finally, the IDEAS trial compared paclitaxel DCB with DES (zotarolimus-, sirolimus- or everolimus-eluting stents) for longer lesions (>70 mm), in patients of Rutherford category 3 to 6.[56] Randomisation took place over 52 limbs in 50 patients and found that the 6-month angiographic restenosis rate was lower in the DES group (28% vs 57.9%; $P=0.046$). There were no differences observed in clinically driven TLR, major amputation or survival rates.

✔✔ Together these studies demonstrate a consistent 12-month primary patency result with DES for short lesions below the knee, clearly superior to standard therapy of PTA or BMS. Furthermore, the IDEAS trial result suggests that DES may have advantages over DCB, both in terms of immediate angiographic results and mid-term patency.

Choice of revascularisation method for the infrapopliteal arteries

There is currently no published RCT dedicated to determining the superiority of open surgery or endovascular treatment for infrapopliteal disease. However, BASIL 2 is a multicentre RCT designed to find out if a 'vein bypass-first' or a 'best endovascular-first' revascularisation strategy derives superior clinical outcomes and cost-effectiveness for the treatment of patients with severe limb ischaemia. It is currently enrolling and plans to recruit 600 patients from England, Scotland and Northern Ireland, over a 3-year period. Patients will be randomised 1:1, to have either vein bypass or endovascular intervention as their first treatment. They will be followed up for an average of just over 3 years following intervention. This trial should provide valuable insights into the differing treatment options for this challenging region.

The angiosome concept

✅ The angiosome concept is that each foot is divided into distinct blocks of tissue fed by source arteries that interconnect through functional arterio-arterial communications (**Fig. 4.4**). When tissue loss occurs due to critical limb ischaemia, proponents of the concept suggest that performing a direct revascularisation procedure to the source artery may lead to superior rates of tissue healing and limb salvage compared with indirect revascularisation.

There are no randomised studies which have compared direct to indirect revascularisation. However, a 2015 meta-analysis identified nine non-randomised studies, three of which used comparative analysis techniques to compare the two strategies.[61] The authors evaluated 779 lower limbs and found that direct revascularisation significantly improved the overall survival of limbs (HR 0.61; 95%CI 0.46–0.80; P <0.001) and time to wound healing (HR 1.38; 95%CI 1.13–1.69; P =0.002). Insufficient data were available to compare mortality rates. The authors concluded that based on these data direct revascularisation was preferred and that a randomised controlled study was necessary to confirm the results and eliminate bias.

Whilst the angiosome concept is a useful method of considering the vascular supply of the foot the reality is that anomalous variation in the infrapopliteal vascular circulation is common and occlusive disease within the pedal arch may make the revascularisation of a non-angiosomal artery more effective at optimising perfusion to the region of tissue loss. We advocate a dedicated foot angiogram in orthogonal planes to determine the preferred target vessel for revascularisation as a practical approach before tibial interventions, both surgical and endovascular.

Primary amputation

Despite a movement towards aggressive revascularisation and limb-salvage 'centres of excellence', major amputations are still performed for a variety of indications. These include extensive

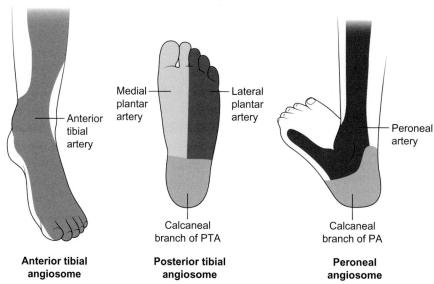

Figure 4.4 • The six angiosomes of the foot and calf, arising from the three crural arteries. The anterior tibial artery supplies the anterior calf and then crosses the ankle as the dorsalis pedis artery which supplies the dorsum of the foot. The posterior tibial artery (PTA) supplies the posterior calf then goes on to supply the plantar surface of the foot, toes and web spaces after splitting into medial and lateral plantar arteries. It also gives off a calcaneal branch which supplies the medial aspect of the heel. The peroneal artery (PA) supplies the lateral aspect of the calf and ankle. It also has a calcaneal branch that supplies the lateral aspect of the heel. It is noteworthy that the heel has dual supply with crossover between the calcaneal branches of the posterior tibial artery and peroneal artery.

pedal gangrene, overwhelming sepsis arising from the foot, exhausted treatment options for critical limb ischaemia, late presentation of acute limb ischaemia and non-ambulatory status. The most common cause is chronic critical limb ischaemia with no option left for revascularisation. This is often exacerbated by late referral to a specialist centre.

Major amputation incurs a considerable survival penalty, with mortality rates of approximately one-third at 12 months, 50% at 24 months and almost 75% at 5 years.[62] It also carries a significant financial burden, of more than $US 500 000 per amputation[63] – a

lifetime healthcare cost which is borne by the community. It therefore remains preferable to salvage a limb wherever feasible and reserve major amputation for when extensive gangrene has devitalised the weight-bearing surface of the foot beyond salvage.

Disclosure

No financial support from grants or industry was provided for this manuscript. The author has no relevant conflicts of interest to declare.

Key points

- Best medical therapy is mandatory, and supervised exercise programmes should be considered for initial treatment in patients with claudication. Exercise programmes are underutilised, as they take time, persistence and are often under-resourced by healthcare providers.
- There is a global trend towards an endovascular-first approach to revascularisation, but few robust data support this approach, other than demonstrating its safety compared with open surgery.
- Extensive aorto-iliac occlusive disease can now be safely treated with endovascular techniques, which have acceptable mid- to long-term patency.
- Iliac occlusions should be treated with primary stenting, with the use of covered stents determined by the extent of disease and other individual factors.
- Suprainguinal surgery remains a useful treatment option with durable patency; however, the high risk of major complications makes it most suitable for patients with few comorbidities.
- Autologous vein remains the conduit of choice particularly for a distal anastomosis at the infrapopliteal level.
- There are a multitude of technologies available for the percutaneous treatment of disease within the femoropopliteal segment; however, most comparative trials have used the historical treatment of PTA as a control rather than comparing with an endovascular gold standard.
- Stents and angioplasty balloons coated with the antiproliferative drug paclitaxel show promise in the femoropopliteal region. Trial data are emerging.
- Advancements have been made in the endovascular treatment of infrapopliteal disease, both with regards to increased technical success rates and durable patency in short- to moderate-length lesions; however, long lesions continue to demonstrate poor patency.
- Drug-eluting stents have been proven to be the most durable therapy for short- to moderate-length lesions below the knee.
- The angiosome concept of direct revascularisation for tissue loss in CLI has promise; however, further evidence is required.
- Primary amputation has a diminishing role in the treatment of CLI with expansion of endovascular techniques now available to revascularise even the most challenging of patients and disease processes.

🌐 Full references available at **http://expertconsult. inkling.com**

Key references

2. Tendera M, Aboyans V, Bartelink M-L, et al. ESC Guidelines on the diagnosis and treatment of peripheral

artery diseases. Eur Heart J 2011;32(22):2851–906. PMID: 21873417.

3. Anderson JL, Halperin JL, Albert NM, et al. Management of patients with peripheral artery disease (compilation of 2005 and 2011 ACCF/AHA guideline recommendations). Circulation 2013; 127(13):1425–43. PMID: 23457117.

4. Norgren L, Hiatt WR, Dormandy JA, et al. Inter-Society Consensus for the Management of

Peripheral Arterial Disease (TASC II). J VascSurg 2007;45(Suppl S):S5–67. PMID: 17223489.

Comprehensive guidelines for the treatment of peripheral arterial disease.

5. Murphy TP, Cutlip DE, Regensteiner JG, et al. Supervised exercise, stent revascularization, or medical therapy for claudication due to aortoiliac peripheral artery disease: the CLEVER study. J Am Coll Cardiol 2015;65(10):999–1009. PMID: 25766947.

A RCT of patients with aorto-iliac occlusive disease comparing a structured exercise programme with endovascular revascularisation. Functional walking improvement and QoL were improved in both and the two groups could not be separated in their effectiveness.

6. Fakhry F, Rouwet E, Den Hoed P, et al. Long-term clinical effectiveness of supervised exercise therapy versus endovascular revascularization for intermittent claudication from a randomized clinical trial. Br J Surg 2013;100(9):1164–71. PMID: 23842830.

A RCT comparing structured exercise with endovascular therapy for aorto-iliac or femoropopliteal disease.

9. Bradbury A, Ruckley C, Fowkes F, et al. Bypass versus angioplasty in severe ischaemia of the leg (BASIL): multicentre, randomised controlled trial. Lancet 2005;366(9501):1925–34. PMID: 16325694.

Whilst now representing a historical period, the BASIL trial remains the only RCT to have made a direct comparison between open and endovascular revascularisation for the treatment of patients with severe limb ischaemia. They found equivalence in amputation-free and overall surivival between the two techniques over the first two years; however, a late overall survival advantage was seen in the open surgery arm for those who survived beyond that time.

15. Klein WM, Graaf Y, Seegers J, et al. Dutch iliac stent trial: long-term results in patients randomized for primary or selective stent placement 1. Radiology 2006;238(2):734–44. PMID: 16371580.

This randomised trial compared primary stent placement or PTA for aorto-iliac occlusive disease (1993-1997). There was no difference between the group who ultimately received stents versus those who underwent uncomplicated PTA.

16. Goode S, Cleveland T, Gaines P. Randomized clinical trial of stents versus angioplasty for the treatment of iliac artery occlusions (STAG trial). Br J Surg 2013;100(9):1148–53. PMID: 23842828.

A multicentre randomised controlled trial where 118 patients with iliac artery occlusions underwent either PTA or primary iliac stenting. They found that primary stent placement resulted in increased technical success rates and reduced major complication rates compared with simple PTA, with no difference in primary patency at mid-term follow-up.

18. Mwipatayi BP, Thomas S, Wong J, et al. A comparison of covered vs bare expandable stents for the treatment of aortoiliac occlusive disease. J Vasc Surg 2011;54(6):1561–70 e1. PMID: 21906903.

A multicentre, randomised trial comparing PTFE-covered- or bare-metal stents for the treatment of aorto-iliac occlusive disease. They found a patency advantage to the TASC C and D lesions treated with covered stents, with no such difference observed in the TASC B subgroup.

28. Conte MS, Bandyk DF, Clowes AW, et al. Results of PREVENT III: a multicenter, randomized trial of edifoligide for the prevention of vein graft failure in lower extremity bypass surgery. J Vasc Surg 2006;43(4):742–51 e1. PMID: 16616230.

The largest prospective, randomised, double-blind, multicentre trial to have performed a rigorous, objective evaluation of patency rates for venous bypass surgery in patients with critical limb ischaemia. They found a 12-month graft primary patency rate of 61%, with no difference when the bypass was performed at a distal anastomotic site above or below the knee.

32. Anderson JL, Halperin JL, Albert N, et al. Management of patients with peripheral artery disease (Compilation of 2005 and 2011 ACCF/AHA Guideline Recommendations) a report of the American College of Cardiology Foundation/American Heart Association Task Force on Practice Guidelines. J Am Coll Cardiol 2013;61(14):1555–70. PMID: 23473760.

Comprehensive guidelines for the treatment of peripheral arterial disease.

33. Acin F, De Haro J, Bleda S, et al. Primary nitinol stenting in femoropopliteal occlusive disease: a meta-analysis of randomized controlled trials. J Endovasc Ther 2012;19(5):585–95. PMID: 23046322.

A meta-analysis with results from 17 randomised clinical trials which used either primary nitinol stenting or PTA for symptomatic femoropopliteal occlusive disease. They found that the nitinol stent group had higher rates of technical success, and at 12-month follow-up lower rates of both target lesion revascularisation and binary restenosis, with similar safety outcomes.

36. Giacoppo D, Cassese S, Harada Y, et al. Drug-coated balloon versus plain balloon angioplasty for the treatment of femoropopliteal artery disease: an updated systematic review and meta-analysis of randomized clinical trials. JACC: Cardiovasc Intervent 2016;9(16):1731–42. PMID: 27539695.

A meta-analysis of data from eight multicentre, randomised controlled trials which compared DCB to PTA for femoropopliteal lesions. They found that paclitaxel-coated balloons were superior to PTA in reducing TLR over mid- to long-term follow-up.

37. Dake MD, Ansel GM, Jaff MR, et al. Durable clinical effectiveness with paclitaxel-eluting stents

in the femoropopliteal artery 5-year results of the Zilver PTX randomized trial. Circulation 2016;133(15):1472–83. PMID: 26969758.

This RCT randomised patients with symptomatic femoropopliteal disease to DES or PTA, and then performed a secondary randomisation between DES and BMS for those that failed PTA. After 5 years, DES was superior to PTA in freedom from persistent or worsening symptoms of ischaemia, primary patency, and freedom from TLR. Provisional DES also had superior clinical and patency outcomes over provisional BMS.

41. Rastan A, Krankenberg H, Baumgartner I, et al. Stent placement versus balloon angioplasty for the treatment of obstructive lesions of the popliteal artery: a prospective, multicenter, randomized trial. Circulation 2013;127(25):2535–41. PMID: 23694965.

A prospective, multicentre trial conducted on isolated popliteal artery lesions. They randomised subjects to either nitinol stent placement or PTA. Twelve-month primary patency was significantly higher in the nitinol stent group compared to PTA and clinically driven TLR was significantly lower; however, this difference was solely accounted for by a 25.2% acute failure rate in the PTA group. The authors concluded that primary PTA with provisional bailout stenting for short lesions of the popliteal artery is a reasonable strategy.

44. Albers M, Romiti M, Pereira C, et al. Meta-analysis of allograft bypass grafting to infrapopliteal arteries. Eur J Vasc Endovasc Surg 2004;28(5):462–72. PMID: 15465366.

A meta-analysis of autologous, popliteal-to-distal bypass grafts from 31 published series between 1981 and 2004 found excellent 5-year patency and limb salvage rates. Demonstrating the durability and limb preservation efficacy of autogenous, infrapopliteal bypass graft.

50. Zeller T, Baumgartner I, Scheinert D, et al. Drug-eluting balloon versus standard balloon angioplasty for infrapopliteal arterial revascularization in critical limb ischemia: 12-month results from the IN.PACT DEEP randomized trial. J Am Coll Cardiol 2014;64(15):1568–76. PMID: 25301459.

This large, well-adjudicated RCT evaluated patients with infrapopliteal lesions randomising 2:1 to DCB or PTA. At 12 months they found no difference in late lumen loss or clinically driven TLR rates, with a trend toward higher amputation rates in the DCB arm compared to PTA.

52. Biondi-Zoccai GG, Sangiorgi G, Lotrionte M, et al. Infragenicular stent implantation for below-the-knee atherosclerotic disease: clinical evidence from an international collaborative meta-analysis on 640 patients. J Endovasc Ther 2009;16(3):251–60. PMID: 19642789.

A systematic review, combining 18 non-randomised studies which evaluated patients who had infragenicular

stent implantation. They found that bailout stenting after unsatisfactory PTA in this region derived satisfactory angiographic results but no patency advantage over simple angioplasty.

53. Bosiers M, Scheinert D, Peeters P, et al. Randomized comparison of everolimus-eluting versus bare-metal stents in patients with critical limb ischemia and infrapopliteal arterial occlusive disease. J Vasc Surg 2012;55(2):390–8. PMID: 22169682.

The DESTINY RCT randomised patients with infrapopliteal disease to primary treatment with an everolimus-eluting stent or BMS comparator. At the 12-month follow-up primary patency was higher in the DES group, and late lumen loss and TLR significantly lower.

54. Rastan A, Brechtel K, Krankenberg H, et al. Sirolimus-eluting stents for treatment of infrapopliteal arteries reduce clinical event rate compared to bare-metal stents: long-term results from a randomized trial. J Am Coll Cardiol 2012;60(7):587–91. PMID: 22878166.

The YUKON-BTK trial was the first RCT to publish a comparison between DES and BMS in the infrapopliteal circulation. The DES achieved a superior primary patency at 12 months. Target lesion revascularisation was also improved with the use of the DES but not significantly so. At a longer follow-up of 2.8 years the primary endpoint of freedom from amputation, TVR, AMI and death also found in favour of the DES.

55. Scheinert D, Katsanos K, Zeller T, et al. A prospective randomized multicenter comparison of balloon angioplasty and infrapopliteal stenting with the sirolimus-eluting stent in patients with ischemic peripheral arterial disease: 1-year results from the ACHILLES trial. J Am Coll Cardiol 2012;60(22):2290–5. PMID: 23194941.

This RCT randomised patients with CLI and occlusive tibial disease to treatment with a DES or standard PTA. The primary endpoint was 12-month, in-segment, binary restenosis determined by quantitative angiography, which once again found in favour of the DES. However, there was no significant difference seen in clinically driven TLR or limb salvage, reflecting the multiple factors which impact those endpoints.

61. Huang T-Y, Huang T-S, Wang Y-C, et al. Direct revascularization with the angiosome concept for lower limb ischemia: a systematic review and meta-analysis. Medicine 2015;94(34). PMID: 26313800.

A meta-analysis of nine non-randomised studies, three of which used comparative analysis techniques to compare direct (angiosomal) and indirect revascularisation strategies for patients with CLI. The authors found that direct revascularisation significantly improved the overall survival of limbs and time to wound healing, concluding that it was preferred and that a randomised controlled study was necessary to confirm the results.

5

The diabetic foot

Fran Game

Introduction

Foot problems are one of the most common complications of diabetes, with 15% of patients developing a foot ulcer in their lifetime.[1] Foot complications account for more hospital admissions than other complications of diabetes[2] and are associated with high mortality, worse than many common forms of cancer.[3]

The term diabetic foot disease actually encompasses a number of different conditions, including peripheral sensory neuropathy and/or neuropathic pain, peripheral artery disease, ulceration, infection including osteomyelitis, Charcot neuroarthropathy and possibly even lower limb amputation. Unfortunately, people with diabetes are still eight to 24 times more likely than those without diabetes to have a lower limb amputation,[4] and it is suggested that about 85% of those amputations could be avoided by early detection and involvement of a specialist foot team, as the majority of lower limb amputations are preceded by ulceration.[5]

Epidemiology

The estimated global prevalence of diabetes in 2010 was 285 million, expected to rise to 438 million by 2030,[6] and, in the UK alone in 2014–15, there were 3.5 million people diagnosed with diabetes, an increase of 65% over the last decade[6] and, as such, the burden of foot ulceration is also highly likely to increase in parallel. In 2002 in a study from the north-west of England, the annual incidence of foot ulceration was reported to be 2.2% among 10 000 community-based patients with type 2 diabetes,[7] a similar incidence to an earlier US study.[8]

The main risk factors for the development of foot ulcers in diabetes are peripheral neuropathy and peripheral artery disease, either alone or in combination with deformity.[5] In the UK, new Public Health England data show that the annual number of diabetes-related amputations in England is now over 7000 a year[9] and it is now estimated that every 27 seconds, a leg is lost to diabetes somewhere in the world.[10]

Development of foot ulceration

Diabetic peripheral neuropathies

The prevalence of diabetic peripheral sensory neuropathy (DPSN) is approximately 30% in hospitalised diabetes patients and 20–30% in community-based patients.[11] It is now increasingly accepted that it is one of the earliest complications to develop, being seen in patients even with prediabetes.[12] The main clinical features of DPSN include symmetrical, predominantly sensory deficits in the distal lower extremities, and neuropathic pain.[13] The development of neuropathy is linked to the duration of diabetes and poor glycaemic control over many years[13] as well as height, hypertension, dyslipidaemia, obesity and possibly smoking.[14] Annual foot examination is recommended to identify this as it is a risk factor for ulceration in all patients with diabetes, and appropriate regular foot review should be instituted depending on the result.[5]

Not every patient with sensory diabetic neuropathy will describe symptoms of painful peripheral neuropathy (PPN). Although the two conditions may coexist this is not inevitable, with one study showing painful symptoms occurring in 26% of patients without neuropathy (Neuropathy Disability Score (NDS) ≤2) and 60% of patients with severe neuropathy (NDS >8).[15] The symptoms of PPN can be extremely disturbing, and include symptoms such as burning, altered temperature perception, paraesthesia or allodynia (touch perceived as a painful stimulus), or numbness or deadness in the limb. Symptoms of neuropathy can be differentiated from intermittent claudication by the nocturnal exacerbations, lack of relationship to exercise and location of symptoms, although this is not always straightforward.

Coexistent autonomic neuropathy causes a reduction in sweating in the skin and open arteriovenous shunts.[16] Although this appears to increase blood flow to the limb, with easily bounding pulses, the consequence of the shunting of blood away from skin capillaries results in functional local skin ischaemia. The neuropathic foot therefore appears warm with bounding pulses but has dry, often cracked, skin.

Motor neuropathy mainly affects the intrinsic muscles of the foot, causing wasting (guttering between the metatarsals) and altered foot shape, with clawed toes and prominent metatarsal heads (**Fig. 5.1**). The subsequent deformity, particularly in conjunction with DPSN, may lead to unnoticed trauma from ill-fitting footwear. Neuropathy is responsible for a high proportion of foot ulcers. In the Eurodiale study, which looked at 1232 patients across 14 European centres, peripheral neuropathy was present in 86% of patients undergoing treatment for foot ulcers.[17]

Diagnosis of neuropathy

The diagnosis of DPSN, particularly for the assessment of foot ulceration risk, is usually done by clinical examination, which reveals a 'stocking' distribution of sensory loss to one or more of pain,

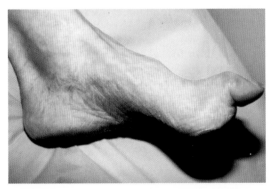

Figure 5.1 • Typical appearance of a neuropathic foot, with clawed toes, dry skin, callouses and prominent metatarsal heads.

pressure, temperature and vibration modalities. Quantitative sensory testing can be performed for perception of vibration, pressure and temperature thresholds, but the perception of pressure threshold is the simplest and most commonly used in clinical practice. A nylon monofilament is used; by pressing against the skin until it buckles by about 1 cm, a load of 10 g of pressure can be accurately applied. Patients unable to feel this at a number of pre-specified sites of the foot are at approximately fourfold increased risk of ulceration.[7] This test can be simplified further by using the Ipswich Touch test,[18] a test with a good sensitivity and specificity compared with the monofilament and dispensing with the requirement for specific equipment.

Peripheral artery disease (PAD)

Atherosclerotic vascular disease is probably present (at least in a subclinical form) in all patients with a long-standing history of diabetes.[19]

The distribution of vascular disease in the lower limb is thought to be different in patients with diabetes from those without the disease, with more frequent involvement of vessels below the knee. One study of patients referred for angiography showed no difference in proximal disease (iliac, femoropopliteal vessels) but distal disease (calf vessels) was twice as high in patients with diabetes as those without.[19] In clinical practice it is not uncommon to see patients with extensive PAD of the posterior and anterior tibial arteries. Long calcified occlusions of these vessels are typical. There is frequently relative sparing of the peroneal artery and digital vessels. The distribution of disease has important consequences for revascularisation strategies. Bypasses are often required into the foot and angioplasty may be difficult due to the long length of occlusion and calcified nature of the atherosclerotic plaques.

Patients with diabetes and PAD may present with intermittent claudication; however, due to coexistent sensory peripheral neuropathy, the symptoms of vascular disease are frequently absent. The first clinical presentation may unfortunately therefore be foot ulceration.

Peripheral neuropathy, and other comorbidities, also have an influence on the results of investigations recommended to investigate PAD. The ankle–brachial pressure index is recommended by both NICE[5] and the International Working Group of the diabetic foot.[20] Care needs to be taken, however, with the interpretation of the results as arterial calcification secondary to peripheral neuropathy and/or chronic kidney disease will falsely elevate the measurement even within the normal range[21] (**Fig. 5.2**). Toe pressures may also prove useful to

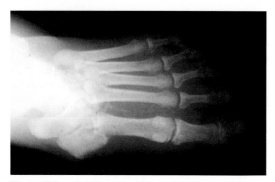

Figure 5.2 • Calcification of the foot arteries in a patient with diabetes and neuropathy. This may falsely elevate Doppler pressures even within the normal range.

reliably exclude PAD but can also be affected by digital calcification. In this situation, the Doppler waveform seems useful, as loss of the normal triphasic waveform suggests vascular disease. Transcutaneous oxygen tension (measured by an electrode placed on the foot) accurately reflects skin oxygenation and can be used to determine the severity of ischaemia and the likelihood that an ischaemic ulcer will heal; however, as the result depends on the assumption of capillary dilatation when the sensor is heated to a pre-specified temperature, then once again the presence of neuropathy may affect the result as capillary dilatation may be affected in the presence of autonomic neuropathy.[21]

Biomechanical aspects

The most important cause of foot ulceration is loss of protective pain sensation, permitting 'painless' repetitive trauma and tissue injury particularly in those with deformity, as above. Plantar pressures can be measured by a number of methods, both dynamic and static. Patients with peripheral neuropathy and particularly patients with foot ulcers have high plantar pressures, although high pressures alone in the absence of insensitivity do not lead to ulceration. Frykberg et al.[22] used an F-scan pressure mat system, and identified patients at risk of ulceration with foot pressures >6 kg/cm^2. Stacpoole-Shea et al.[23] studied an in-shoe pressure analysis system, and demonstrated its ability to predict potential sites for foot ulceration with a sensitivity of 83% and a specificity of 69%.

Neuropathy and altered proprioception, and small-muscle wasting, can, in themselves, lead to alteration of the foot architecture and shape, resulting in clawing of the toes, prominent metatarsal heads and a high arch, all of which result in changes in foot pressures.[24] To some extent, this can be reviewed clinically and raises suggestions as to where ulcers are likely to occur on the foot. The more severe deformities associated with Charcot neuroarthropathy, with joint dislocation and bony deformities, can also result in increased foot pressures and subsequent ulceration.

Limited joint mobility is a further contributing factor to elevated plantar pressures. Chronic hyperglycaemia results in glycosylation of proteins and, when collagen is involved, the collagen bundles become thickened and cross-linked. This alters the mechanics of walking and is strongly associated with high plantar pressures.[25]

Neuropathy alone does not usually lead to spontaneous ulceration, the precipitating factor commonly being from some traumatic event, including rubbing from inappropriate or ill-fitting footwear. In the North West diabetes study[7] approximately half the ulcers were precipitated by problems with footwear. The presence of callus (produced in response to pressure) may exacerbate the problem by increasing pressure further.[26] Removal of callus significantly reduces foot pressures,[27] and should be done regularly by an experienced podiatrist.

Although measurement of foot pressures can predict risk of ulceration with a degree of accuracy it requires equipment that may not be available in all centres. Good clinical examination that inspects foot shape and identifies the presence of callus can provide very valuable information, however. In particular, the presence of haemorrhage into callus is a pre-ulcerative phenomenon and requires urgent attention. Footwear, and the wear pattern of the footwear, should also be inspected as part of this assessment.[5]

Other risk factors

Impaired vision and immobility make it difficult for patients to inspect and care for their feet on a daily basis as recommended in most guidelines, and are therefore additional risk factors. By far and away the most important additional risk factor, however, is end-stage renal disease, particularly if the patient is receiving renal replacement therapy (RRT). The development of foot ulcers increases exponentially in the first year after the onset of RRT.[28,29] It is not clear exactly why this is, although a small study has noted a marked drop in the transcutaneous pressure of oxygen (TcPO$_2$) throughout and for at least 4 hours after a standard haemodialysis session.[30] Additionally, there may be a risk to patients' heels from being stationary for prolonged periods of time during RRT and greater risks from shoe rubbing given the variation in peripheral oedema which may occur between dialysis sessions. Recent guidance has emphasised the need for extra podiatric input to this extremely high-risk group.[31]

Management

The management of diabetic foot problems requires input from a number of different healthcare professionals, and evidence strongly suggests that specialist diabetic foot clinics can significantly reduce ulceration and amputation rates. One retrospective study showed an approximate 75% reduction in major amputation after introduction of a multidisciplinary foot team (MDFT).[32]

National Institute for Health and Care Excellence (NICE) Guidelines 2015 have suggested that the MDFT should consist of specialists with skills in the following areas for optimal patient care:[5]

- Diabetology
- Podiatry
- Diabetes specialist nursing
- Vascular surgery
- Microbiology
- Orthopaedic surgery
- Biomechanics and orthoses
- Interventional radiology
- Casting
- Wound care.

The 'at-risk' foot

NICE recommends[5] that the identification of patients at risk of foot ulceration should be done on an annual basis for all patients with diabetes. Screening does not require expensive equipment and testing can be done in an ordinary clinic setting. In addition to 10 g monofilament testing and palpation of pulses, as described above, skin should be checked for the dryness and cracking associated with autonomic neuropathy, any signs of tinea pedis, which may cause fissuring between the toes, and shoes should be examined. Symptoms of neuropathic pain (burning, paraesthesiae, etc.) should be actively sought.

Risk status – low, moderate or high (**Fig. 5.3**) – should be ascertained,[5] the patient advised of this and any necessary care of their feet explained along with the requirement for follow-up in a foot protection service.

Patients also need to know how to gain rapid access to advice and treatment from the footcare team, and in the event of a new foot ulcer, urgent assessment by a multidisciplinary team should be made within 24 hours.[5]

Regular podiatry is needed for most at-risk patients. Callus needs to be debrided regularly; although it develops in response to pressure and friction, its removal can reduce pressure, as stated previously. Callus can sometimes hide ulceration, which will

Low risk: no risk factors present except callus alone
Moderate risk: deformity **or** neuropathy **or** non-critical limb ischaemia
High risk: previous ulceration **or** previous amputation **or** on renal replacement therapy **or** neuropathy and non-critical limb ischaemia together **or** neuropathy in combination with callus and/or deformity

Figure 5.3 • Risk classification for the development of diabetic foot ulceration.

only be revealed when the callus is removed. Without removal, infection and abscess formation are more likely, but it is important to explain to the patient that the podiatrist has not caused the underlying ulcer revealed when the callus is removed. The presence of callus should always prompt a search for its cause, and shoe modification may be necessary.

The surgical correction of specific foot deformities is sometimes necessary to prevent ulceration. This should be done only after confirming that there is good peripheral circulation and it is important to remember that correction deformities may create pressure problems elsewhere; for example, correction of a hallux valgus may leave a rigid hallux with resultant high plantar pressures on the plantar hallux. Correction of deformity is usually only performed in patients with a history of ulceration, rather than for primary prevention.

Ulcer management

All patients with diabetes presenting with foot ulcers need a full examination of the foot, including peripheral sensation and circulation in order to classify and understand the main aetiology of the ulcer. They also need assessment of footwear and deformities.

A number of classification systems have been published but none has been universally accepted[33] and few have been fully validated outside the population from which they were drawn. Classifications have been designed for the purposes of research, e.g. PEDIS,[34] audit, e.g. SINBAD[35] (Table 5.1) as used in the National Diabetes Foot Audit of the UK,[36] or description in clinical practice, e.g. University of Texas (Table 5.2).[37] A classification designed for research purposes need not be able to classify every ulcer in a community, only those to be included in a particular research protocol, and may be much more detailed than one used in clinical practice. A classification used

Table 5.1 • The SINBAD classification

	Score = 0	Score = 1
Site	Forefoot	Midfoot, hindfoot
Ischaemia	At least one pulse palpable	Clinical evidence of reduced pedal blood flow
Neuropathy	Protective sensation intact	Protective sensation lost
Bacterial infection	None	Present
Area	<1 cm^2	≥1 cm^2
Depth	Ulcer confined to skin and subcutaneous tissue	Ulcer reaching muscle, tendon or deeper

Table 5.2 • The University of Texas score

	0	1	2	3
A	Skin intact	Superficial not involving tendon, capsule or bone	Penetrates to tendon or capsule	Penetrates to bone
B	Infection	Infection	Infection	Infection
C	Ischaemia	Ischaemia	Ischaemia	Ischaemia
D	Infection and ischaemia	Infection and ischaemia	Infection and ischaemia	Infection and ischaemia

for audit, or comparison of outcome between centres, needs to be able to classify all ulcers, but needs to be simple in order to be performed in everyday practice. A classification that generates prognostic information for clinical practice, on the other hand, needs to be able to classify all ulcers, but also be sufficiently detailed to distinguish ulcers that heal from those that don't.

Being very simplistic, ulcers can also be classified by their dominant aetiology into neuropathic or ischaemic.

Neuropathic ulcers

Typically, the foot is warm and well perfused, with bounding pulses and distended veins. The ulcer is usually at the site of repetitive trauma and, as ulcers are most commonly due to a shoe rub, on the dorsum of the toes or a high-pressure area under the metatarsal heads. Due to dense sensory neuropathy, a patient may walk on a foreign body for hours or even days without realising it, for example a nail through the sole of a shoe, or an old dressing or sock stuffed in the end of a shoe, and these may easily cause quite significant ulcers before the patient is aware.

The key to management of neuropathic ulcers is pressure relief or offloading.[38] With shoe-induced ulcers, new footwear must be provided to prevent future ulcers in the longer term. Merely providing the shoes may not be enough; patients often fail to wear the shoes due to appearance, or a belief that they are only to be used outside the home, and so continued support must be provided to encourage the patient to carry on with this form of therapy.

To relieve sufficient pressure from a plantar ulcer to allow it to heal, however, shoes are insufficient and a more aggressive approach is required. Bed rest is simple, but expensive in hospital and difficult to enforce in a patient who feels well and is pain free, so ambulatory methods have been designed. The total contact cast was originally used for patients with neuropathic ulcers due to leprosy, and modified for use in patients with diabetic neuropathic ulcers. The cast extends from below the knee and encases the whole foot and works by transferring load from the forefoot to the heel, and directly to the leg via the cast wall, as well as reducing oedema and shear forces. Excellent healing rates have been described in randomised controlled trials[39] compared with other forms of offloading if the ulcers are on the plantar forefoot; the results for heel ulcers have been less impressive.[40] The main disadvantage is that it is labour-intensive and requires a high level of skill. It may need frequent changes, and signs of wound infection or new ulceration secondary to the cast may not be seen. A number of commercially produced pressure-relieving boots are now available, with proven capacity to reduce pressure. However, since these alternative devices are removable, patients may take them off whilst at home, and therefore impede further healing. These can be made non-removable by wrapping the removable cast with fibreglass casing material, or using plastic tags. Evidence suggests that healing with this form of offloading is almost on a par with total contact casting.[41]

The second important element of management of neuropathic ulcers is debridement of callus. Wounds heal from the margins and callus prevents the migration of epidermal cells from the wound margin, and encourages and masks wound infection.

Debridement of callus and necrotic tissue may be required as often as weekly, and continued presence or rapid re-accumulation of callus should prompt a review of the pressure relief used.

Ischaemic and neuroischaemic ulcers

Purely ischaemic ulcers are relatively rare and most are, in fact, neuroischaemic as the majority of patients have neuropathy.[36] Typical sites include the toes, heel and medial aspect of the first metatarsal head. Callus is usually absent and the ulcer is often surrounded by a rim of ischaemia and may have a necrotic centre. The presence of pain depends on the degree of neuropathy. Ulceration is often precipitated by minor trauma; again, the most common culprit is ill-fitting shoes. Prompt vascular assessment is crucial. Revascularisation should be performed whenever possible, both for ulcer healing (ischaemic and neuroischaemic ulcers only rarely heal without improvements in blood flow) and to prevent future ulceration.

Gangrene and amputation are among the most feared complications of diabetes. Although gangrene may complicate neuropathic ulceration (micro-organisms in infected digital ulcers may produce necrotising toxins, which lead to thrombotic occlusion of digital arteries and subsequent gangrene), it usually only occurs when significant vascular disease is present.

Infection

Infection in diabetic foot ulcers can vary from superficial cellulitis to deeper infection of the soft tissues and bones. All ulcers are colonised with bacteria but when a species invades and there is a local response to this then it is said that the ulcer is infected. The distinction between colonisation and infection cannot be made with microbiological investigations,[42] and must be made by assessment of the clinical signs. Infection can be classified as mild, moderate or severe[42] dependent on the degree of erythema or the development of systemic symptoms (severe) (Table 5.3). Treatment decisions,

particularly the choice of antibiotics, will vary depending on the severity of the infection and particularly whether bone infection is suspected.[42] Mild infection in superficial ulcers is usually caused by Gram-positive organisms such as *Staphylococcus aureus* or streptococcal species. Deeper ulcers or ischaemic ulcers, or an ulcer that has been present for a longer period of time, may be colonised with more Gram-negatives and/or anaerobic organisms and antibiotic protocols should reflect this.[42] Microbiogical sampling should be done before antibiotic therapy is instituted and ideally should consist of tissue rather than surface swabs which may just grow colonisers rather than invading pathogens.[43] Newer molecular biological techniques may in future overcome the problem of fastidious organisms failing to grow in standard culture, but the role of these techniques in routine practice has not yet been fully evaluated.[44]

Osteomyelitis is an important predisposing factor for amputation, and occurs in about 20% of patients with diabetes and a foot ulcer[45] and should be suspected in any deep infected ulcer, particularly if bone is palpable.[42] Plain radiography is often used as the first-line test, but the characteristic changes of bone destruction (**Fig. 5.4**) can take 2 weeks or longer to develop and do not occur until 30–50% of the bone has been destroyed.[46]

Other imaging modalities include three-phase bone scans, and indium-labelled white cell scans or Leucoscan, along with magnetic resonance imaging. Guidelines from the Infectious Diseases Society of America recommend magnetic resonance imaging and bone sampling.[42] Magnetic resonance imaging can also prove useful by showing marrow oedema before cortical bone loss occurs, although there may be difficulty differentiating osteomyelitis from Charcot neuroarthropathy, particularly where the two coexist. The use of the simple clinical test 'the probe to bone test' (the ability to probe to bone with a blunt instrument at the base of the ulcer) in diagnosing osteomyelitis

Table 5.3 • The IDSA classification of diabetic foot infection

Clinical manifestations of infection	Infection severity
Wound lacking purulence or any manifestation of inflammation	Uninfected
Presence of ≥2 manifestations of inflammation (purulence, or erythema, pain, tenderness, warmth, or induration), but any cellulitis/erythema extends ≤2 cm around the ulcer, and infection is limited to the skin or superficial subcutaneous tissues; no other local complications of systemic illness	Mild
Infection (as above) in a patient who is systemically well and metabolically stable but which has ≥1 of the following characteristics: cellulitis extending >2 cm, lymphangitic streaking, spread beneath the superficial fascia, deep tissue abscess, gangrene and involvement of muscle, tendon, joint or bone	Moderate
Infection in a patient with systemic toxicity or metabolic instability (e.g. fever, chills, tachycardia, hypotension, confusion, vomiting, leukocytosis, acidosis, sever hyperglycaemia or azotaemia)	Severe

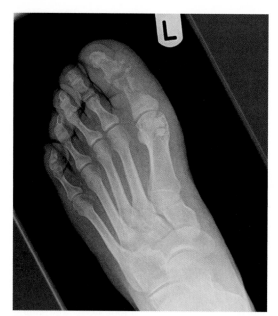

Figure 5.4 • Osteomyelitis of the hallux in a patient with diabetes.

infections require urgent hospitalisation, bed rest, relevant surgical debridement and broad-spectrum antibiotics.

Topical wound healing agents

There are now innumerable topical agents, applications and dressings that are marketed to accelerate wound healing in the diabetic foot. Few of these have been subject to rigorous controlled trials which prove their efficacy and/or cost-effectiveness, and of those that have, the evidence to suggest benefit is poor.[48] Their availability should not obscure the fact that most ulcers respond to simple care, comprising pressure relief, debridement and control of infection, and must not be seen as a replacement, but as an addition to good wound care

Medical problems on the surgical ward

Patients with diabetes on the vascular surgical ward will often have multiple comorbidities and other complications related to their diabetes. Apart from peripheral neuropathy and peripheral artery disease, they may have evidence of ischaemic heart disease, diabetic nephropathy and autonomic neuropathy, all of which can affect their eventual outcomes. These comorbid conditions need to be considered and addressed – for example, patients with significant renal impairment may need a renal review prior to any procedures, particularly angiography with contrast media, as this carries a risk of worsening renal function. Metformin must be stopped for 48 hours prior to elective angiography due to a risk of worsening renal failure and consequent lactic acidosis. Coronary artery disease and cardiac autonomic neuropathy increase the risk of intraoperative cardiac events, and should be addressed prior to surgery. The hormonal and metabolic changes associated with surgery create a particular problem in diabetes, and intravenous insulin infusions (with dextrose and potassium) are usually needed for the perioperative period, unless the duration of anaesthesia is short (<45 minutes) and the patient is not usually on insulin.

Patients with neuropathy are at great risk of developing heel ulcers whilst lying immobile in bed for several days.[49] These can be difficult to heal, are entirely preventable and medicolegally indefensible. The simple provision of foam or padded heel protectors is often all that is needed to relieve pressure on the heels whilst the patient is in bed, and should be routine in patients at risk.

has been controversial. Latest guidance suggests that in the presence of an infected ulcer the ability to probe to bone can support the diagnosis of osteomyelitis, whilst the inability to probe to bone in a clinically uninfected ulcer can virtually rule out the diagnosis.[47]

Antibiotics are only required for clinically infected wounds or osteomyelitis. They do not aid wound healing *per se*. When choosing an antibiotic regimen, the severity of infection and whether osteomyelitis is suspected are important, as well as the spectrum of antibiotic activity, the intended duration of treatment, local policy and patients' other comorbidities, particularly renal disease. Mild infections can often be treated with relatively narrow-spectrum antibiotics with coverage against Gram-positive cocci, for example oral flucloxacillin or a tetracycline. Ciprofloxacin or co-amoxiclav can be used if Gram-negative infection is suspected, although the potential for these particular antibiotics to be implicated in *Clostridium difficile* diarrhoea should be considered.

There are a number of other factors that must be addressed to ensure healing of an infected foot wound. Attention must be paid to the patient's general medical condition, and it is important to correct any accompanying hyperglycaemia, renal failure or electrolyte disturbance. Regular debridement is important to remove necrotic and devitalised tissue, pus should be drained and the foot offloaded. The principles of dressing a healing wound include keeping it moist, managing exudates and protecting the surrounding intact skin.[27] Limb-threatening

Charcot neuro-osteoarthropathy

Charcot neuro-osteoarthropathy (the Charcot foot) is a complication of neuropathy characterised by inflammation, bone and joint destruction, fragmentation and remodelling.[50] It can be one of the most devastating foot complications of diabetes, and was first described as a complication of tabes dorsalis. It can develop in any joint, and has been reported in most sensory neuropathies, but diabetes is now the commonest cause. The exact prevalence is unknown and estimates vary from 0.04/1000 patients with diabetes[51] to about 3/1000 patients[52] and was present in 1% of those patients registered with ulcers in the UK national diabetes footcare audit.[36] Charcot foot can be triggered by trauma to the foot (of which the patient may be unaware as they have sensory neuropathy), including surgical interventions or preceding ulceration and/or infection trauma of the foot.[53] In the early stages, the foot becomes swollen, warm and erythematous, and may be incorrectly diagnosed as being due to a sprain, gout, cellulitis or deep vein thrombosis. If not treated promptly, osteolysis and osteopenia can occur; ligaments can become lax and gradual remodelling of the foot occurs, with chronic deformity and fusion of the bones in abnormal positions.

Most textbooks describe this as a painless condition, but there is frequently some discomfort, although usually not enough to prevent walking. The presentation may be several weeks after the onset of symptoms and, because of the lack of significant pain, plain radiographs are not always performed. Plain radiography may be sufficient to make the diagnosis once fracturing/dislocations have occurred but in the early stages when the architecture of the foot is still preserved (and it is preferable to make the diagnosis at this stage) then magnetic resonance imaging can be used to demonstrate marrow oedema.[50] Treatment is aimed at minimising weight-bearing to reduce potential bone and joint destruction and reduce the inflammatory phase. The midfoot is the commonest site of Charcot neuroarthropathy[53] and, when affected, can result in midfoot collapse, with a plantar bony prominence and 'rocker-bottom deformity', which has a very high risk of ulceration (**Fig. 5.5**). The mainstay of treatment is rest and immobilisation, usually in a total contact cast, which may need to be continued for many months until disease activity has subsided. In one UK study the median time in offloading before the

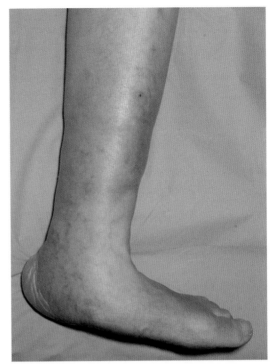

Figure 5.5 • 'Rocker bottom foot' associated with Charcot foot.

patient was fully able to mobilise in orthotic or other footwear was 10 months.[53] Disease activity is usually judged by measuring the temperature of the skin with an infrared thermometer and comparison with the contralateral (non-affected foot). A 2° difference is often quoted as being significant although the evidence behind this is weak.[50] Once the temperature difference is <2° then the patient can be weaned out of offloading devices/casts into orthotic footwear manufactured to fit any deformity.

Trials of bisphosphonates have been undertaken in the past in an attempt to improve the outcome of the disease. A recent systematic review concluded, however, that there is no current evidence to support their use in this disease process.[54]

If the Charcot is in the fore- or mid-foot then surgery is usually avoided in the active stage, due to the gross oedema of the involved bone, and the risk that it (like trauma) will trigger further bone resorption. In the hindfoot/ankle immediate surgery may be necessary, however, to stabilise the joint.[51] However, corrective surgery may also be useful at a later stage in order to remove bony prominences, which may increase risk of ulceration.

Key points

- The management of the diabetic foot is challenging and requires a multidisciplinary approach, ideally coordinated by a specialised clinic.
- Identification of at-risk patients requires screening that must be both comprehensive and regular, supported by appropriately trained staff.
- If ulcers develop, early aggressive management can achieve good results with a significant reduction of both amputation and re-ulceration rates.
- Future research may ultimately enable the prevention of foot ulcers and predisposing factors that lead to ulceration and may demonstrate superior ways of healing ulcers. However, the dissemination of current 'best practice' should have the greatest impact on the outlook for this condition.

🌐 Full references available at **http://expertconsult. inkling.com**

Key references

17. Prompers L, Huijberts M, Apelqvist J, et al. High prevalence of ischaemia, infection and serious comorbidity in patients with diabetic foot disease in Europe. Baseline results from the Eurodiale study. Diabetologia 2007;50:18–25. PMID: 17093942.
   A large multicentre study looking at the outcomes of 1232 patients from 14 large European centres.

27. Schaper NC, Van Netten JJ, Apelqvist J, et al. International Working Group on the Diabetic Foot (IWGDF). Prevention and management of foot problems in diabetes: A summary guidance for daily practice 2015, based on the IWGDF guidance documents. Diabetes Res Clin Pract 2017;124:84–92. PMID: 28119194.
   First of a series of guideline papers from the International Working Group of the Diabetic Foot, based on systematic reviews.

42. Lipsky BL, Berendt AR, Cornia PB, et al. Infectious Diseases Society of America clinical practice guideline for the diagnosis and treatment of diabetic foot infections. Clin Infect Dis 2012;54(12):132–73. PMID: 22619242.
   Guidelines on the management of infection in the diabetic foot based on a systematic review.

50. Rogers LC, Frykberg RG, Armstrong DG, et al. The Charcot foot in diabetes. Diabetes Care 2011;34(9):2123–9. PMID: 21868781.
   Review of diagnosis and management of the Charcot foot in diabetes.

6

Amputation, rehabilitation and prosthetic developments

Ramesh Munjal
Gillian Atkinson

Introduction

For some patients with lower limb ischaemia, amputation may be the only interventional option because revascularisation is not possible, has failed or the leg is unsalvageable. Amputation may also be a better option than complex revascularisation when patients are bed-bound and/or have severe cognitive impairment. Amputation should not be regarded as 'failure' of treatment but should be seen by patients as well as clinicians as a positive procedure. Amputation should aim to relieve pain, remove dead, severely ischaemic or infected tissue, and improve quality of life. This is true even for those who may not be able to walk with a prosthesis.

The planning and process of rehabilitation for amputees should start prior to amputation and continue into the community. Expert and holistic assessment of the patient leading to careful selection of the level of amputation, good surgical technique and optimal postoperative management are all vital in the initial stage of amputee rehabilitation. The process then dovetails into postamputation early rehabilitation, e.g. use of early walking aids, wheelchair and home assessments, prosthetic rehabilitation where appropriate, and continuing follow-up and support to patients and their families in the community.

This chapter concentrates on the rehabilitation of patients undergoing amputation due to peripheral artery disease, although the principles involved are similar for amputations due to other causes, such as trauma.

Epidemiology

Peripheral artery disease (PAD) and diabetes account for the vast majority of lower limb amputations in high-income countries. More than 80% of all amputations carried out in the UK are due to vascular disease, with an increasing proportion having diabetes mellitus (with or without PAD).[1] The overall risk of amputation is six times higher in insulin-dependent people with diabetes compared with non-insulin-dependent people with diabetes. A global study group also reported a marked difference in the incidence of amputation between 10 centres in six different countries. Rates were highest in the North American and Northern European centres and lowest in Spain, Taiwan and Japan. In the Navajo population, a very high prevalence of diabetes was thought to be the explanation for their high amputation rates.[2]

The National Amputee Statistical Database for the UK reported that 'dysvascularity' is the most common reason for referral to prosthetic services centres following a lower limb amputation, accounting for 70% of all lower limb referrals in 2006–7.[3] In this group referred to the prosthetic centres in the UK, 53% were transtibial and 39% were trans-femoral amputees. In this 1-year period there were a total of 4957 referrals to prosthetic services in the UK, of which 4574 were following lower limb amputation (92% of the total).[3]

There is some evidence that the impact of modern vascular surgery may reduce the incidence of amputation.[4] The Danish National Amputation Register has demonstrated a 27% fall in the number of major amputations due to peripheral artery disease in the decade 1980–90. This decline was attributed to the increased use of infrainguinal bypass operations.[5] A paper from Finland also reported that it was possible to reduce amputation rates with an aggressive reconstruction policy in critical limb ischaemia.[6] However, the West Coast Vascular Surgeons Study Group in Sweden failed to demonstrate a negative correlation between amputation and revascularisation rates.[7]

Survival rates after an amputation depend upon the cause of the amputation rather than the amputation itself. Those who have amputations following trauma tend to have good long-term survival, but those from vascular disease (including diabetes) face a 30-day mortality rate reported to be between 9% and 15% and a long-term survival rate of 60% at 1 year, 42% at 3 years and 35–45% at 5 years.[8] Of people with diabetes who have lower limb amputation, up to 55% will require amputation of the second leg within 2–3 years.[9]

Indications for amputation

The decision to perform amputation seems straightforward where there is extensive tissue loss or no reasonable prospect of revascularisation. However, the precise role of amputation in the management of critical limb ischaemia (CLI) remains controversial. If it is predicted that vascular reconstruction is likely to be unsuccessful, then primary amputation perhaps offers the best outcome in terms of quality of life and cost benefit.[10] Chapter 3 discusses the treatment of chronic lower limb ischaemia and covers the issues of economics and quality of life in more detail. Where patients with CLI also have coexisting disabilities or other medical conditions that would render them unable to make use of a salvageable limb, then primary amputation with appropriate rehabilitation offers the best option. Examples of such patients include those with severe dementia, dense hemiplegia or spinal paralysis, severe arthritis and severe cardiorespiratory disease.

Level selection

Selection of the ideal level of amputation depends on the healing potential, rehabilitation potential and prosthetic considerations. The potential for rehabilitation and likely goals can only be set by a holistic assessment of the patient by the specialist amputee rehabilitation team. This assessment should include other illnesses and disabilities, cognitive state and motivation, likely discharge destination, lifestyle, as well as the patient's own aspirations and wishes.

In general terms, the more proximal the level of amputation, the more difficult it will be for the patient to achieve independent walking. Therefore, the more distal the amputation site, the better the rehabilitation potential for walking, as this preserves more joints and hence more control of the prosthesis. **Figure 6.1** is an algorithm dealing with amputation level selection.

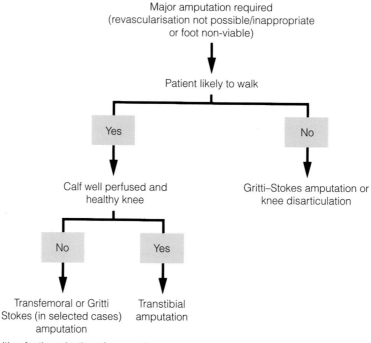

Figure 6.1 • Algorithm for the selection of amputation level.

Minor amputations (below the level of the ankle joint) require a good blood supply. Local amputation of single or multiple toes generally does not heal unless the foot can be revascularised. Transmetatarsal or ray amputations, if technically feasible, produce excellent functional results. Chopart's mid-tarsal amputation and Symes' through-ankle amputation are rare in CLI and are not recommended because of the risks of developing an equinus deformity (in Chopart's), movement of the distal flap (in Symes'), poor long-term flap viability and considerable technical difficulties in prosthetic fitting. Thus, the commonest major levels of amputation in limb ischaemia are transtibial, knee disarticulation, Gritti–Stokes and transfemoral. Hip disarticulation and hindquarter amputation are rare and in 2006–7 accounted for just over 1% of all cases of lower limb amputations referred to the prosthetic centres in the UK. Dysvascularity was given as the cause for this level of amputation in only 19% of cases.[3] In our experience this level of amputation is mainly considered for people with neoplasia (usually sarcoma) or intravenous drug users (IVDUs). Preservation of the knee joint has enormous advantages in terms of mobility. In one study, 80% of transtibial amputees achieved unlimited household mobility or better, compared with 40% of above-knee amputees.[11] In a Sheffield study of amputees who underwent prosthetic rehabilitation, only 26% of transfemoral vascular amputees achieved community ambulation at 1 year follow-up, compared with 50% of transtibial amputees. Household mobility was achieved in 48% and 63%, respectively.[12]

Transcutaneous oximetry (tcP_{O2}),[13] photoplethysmography,[14] laser Doppler velocimetry,[15] thermography[16] and isotope clearance rates[17] have all been shown to correlate with subsequent stump healing. However, while all these methods seem superior to Doppler ankle pressures,[18] a review concluded that sensitivities and specificities were inadequate to recommend their use in routine clinical practice.[19]

The energy cost of walking with prostheses for vascular amputees is increased by 63% for transtibial and 117% for transfemoral amputees compared with non-amputees. In patients who have undergone bilateral transfemoral amputation the energy cost is 280% higher.[20] Therefore, it should not seem surprising that even in a selected group of bilateral transfemoral amputees who were successfully trained to walk with prostheses in an inpatient rehabilitation facility, the majority of them abandoned walking when they returned home and preferred to be wheelchair-dependent.[21]

Thus, for patients in whom major lower limb amputations are necessary, the following points should be remembered:

- Preserve the knee joint whenever possible if it is anticipated that the patient has the potential to achieve prosthetic walking or has the potential to use a prosthetic limb for assisting transfers (from chair, bed, etc).
- In patients likely to remain chair- or bed-bound following amputation, a transtibial amputation risks non-healing and may become a hindrance to transfers if flexion contractures of the knee and hip joints develop. In such patients, knee disarticulation or Gritti–Stokes amputation seems a better option.
- Where there is a fixed knee flexion deformity of 25% or more and/or severe arthropathy, satisfactory fitting of a transtibial prosthesis for walking may not be possible. In such cases, a more proximal amputation should be undertaken.
- For patients likely to remain wheelchair- or bed-bound, including bilateral amputees, knee disarticulation or Gritti–Stokes amputation is preferable to transfemoral or transtibial as the longer lever lengths and larger surface areas are more conducive to transferring and provide a much better seating balance.
- In patients where a transtibial amputation is not possible but the patient has the potential to walk, most amputee rehabilitation units prefer a transfemoral rather than knee disarticulation or Gritti–Stokes amputation. This is because of problems of prosthetic fitting, which may compromise cosmetic appearance and function. Cosmesis is affected because the prosthetic knee joint extends beyond the length of the femur. Therefore for those with a through-knee amputation, the femoral component is longer. Functionally, this may mean that sitting in small spaces is restricted due to this increased length of the femoral component. Conversely some studies have demonstrated better functional outcomes in patients with a through-knee amputation. This is attributed to a longer, stronger stump as more muscle length and distal proprioception is maintained.

Surgical considerations

All amputations should be carried out by surgeons experienced in the procedure and should not be delegated to unsupervised and inexperienced junior staff.

NCEPOD (National Confidential Enquiry into Patient Outcome and Deaths) have published a document on major lower limb amputations and the standards for quality improvements for major amputation surgery. The details are available from www.ncepod.org.uk. In the light of this, a dedicated multidisciplinary team for care planning of amputees and access to other medical specialities and health professionals, both pre- and postoperatively, are recommended for best outcomes. It also recommends that a consultant vascular surgeon should be present in the operating theatre for all major amputations performed by a trainee. The following important general principles should be followed:

- tissues must be handled with care and meticulous haemostasis;
- flaps should be oversized initially and then shaped and trimmed as required;
- there should be good-quality sensate skin coverage of stump without any tension;
- bone edges should be smoothed off and bevelled;
- skin and muscle flaps should be trimmed and shaped to prevent dog-ears, redundant tissue or a bulbous stump;
- creating the correct shape of the stump is the responsibility of the surgeon at the time of surgery;
- the use of a thigh tourniquet can reduce blood loss significantly during fashioning of muscle flaps.

Transfemoral amputation

Ensure adequate muscle (myoplastic) cover over the cut end of the femur to prevent pain and discomfort and allow balanced action of flexors and extensors.[22] The technique of myodesis, where drill holes are made in the bone to fix muscles, may not be applicable in ischaemic limbs due to poor tissue quality. However, this minimises the risk of the muscles slipping off the end of the femur. The myoplasty and myodesis need to be performed with the hip joint in the neutral and naturally adducted position.

Allow at least 12 cm of clearance from the distal end of the stump to knee-joint level in order to allow space for incorporating a prosthetic knee joint. This will prevent an unacceptable cosmetic and functional disability of a lowered knee centre in the prosthetic limb. The exact level of bone section will depend on the thickness of the thigh muscles and subcutaneous tissue. With this in mind, a through-knee level should be considered in morbidly obese patients.

Through-knee amputation

Historically, this level of amputation was considered in those patients who were deemed incapable of walking. The longer stump assists transfers, sitting balance and maintains muscle attachment and proprioception. However, recent research articles including a systematic review and meta-analysis suggest that the primary outcome measure of Physical Component Score (PCS) of the short-form-36 measure of quality of life (SF-36) are much higher for through-knee amputation than transfemoral amputation. A significantly greater proportion of patients with through-knee amputation were able to walk 500 metres than those with transfemoral amputation. However, patients with a through-knee amputation wore their prosthesis significantly less and had significantly more pain than those with a transfemoral amputation.[23] Another study[24] has concluded that the through-knee amputation is associated with an acceptable primary healing rate and satisfactory functional outcome in patients with peripheral artery disease. This study concluded that the advantages of through-knee amputation over transfemoral amputation make it the preferred alternative for patients with vascular disease who are candidates for prosthetic rehabilitation.

The conventional through-knee amputation is associated with problems caused by the bulbous femoral condyles and leakage of synovial fluid. The modified Gritti–Stokes amputation avoids these problems and has fewer problems with wound healing than the alternative Mazet technique (**Fig. 6.2**). Limitations in prosthetic fitting due to a lowered knee centre, and limited availability of stance and swing phase control mechanisms in the prosthetic knee joint at this level, make the through-knee level unpopular with prosthetists, and further research is needed to develop suitable prosthetic devices. This may be prompted by the increasing use of the through-knee level for soldiers and

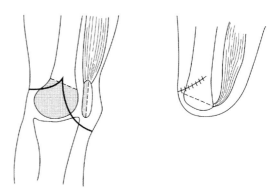

Figure 6.2 • Transection of the femur with a backward angle results in a more stable attachment of the patella in the modified Gritti–Stokes amputation.

civilians with extensive lower leg injuries caused by antipersonnel mines or improvised explosive devices (IEDs).

Transtibial amputation

Many surgeons now favour the skew flap technique[25] rather than the traditional Burgess long posterior flap.[26] The skewed skin flaps are based on the arteries that run with the great and small saphenous veins, which provide the main blood supply to the skin. In a small study of posterior flap and skew flap techniques, evaluation of flap hypoxia demonstrated that the posterior flap was associated with greater and more persistent reduction in $tcPo_2$.[27]

> ✔✔ Randomised trials have shown little difference in healing between the skew flap and traditional Burgess long posterior flap, although exposure of the tibia occurs less often with skew flaps.[28] The time to limb-fitting and early mobility was shorter in the skew flap group due to a less bulbous stump (**Fig. 6.3**).

The Burgess amputation still seems useful when skew flaps might be compromised by the medial skin incision of a failed femorodistal bypass graft or following fasciotomies (**Fig. 6.4**).

A tibial section at about 15 cm is considered ideal. The fibula should be divided around 1.5 cm proximal to the level of the tibial section. A short bevel and rounding off the sharp corners of the tibia must be undertaken. Much shorter transtibial stumps (up to 8 cm), though not ideal, can be fitted with additional suspension systems, e.g. pin and liner.

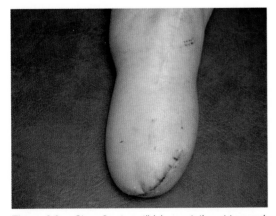

Figure 6.3 • Skew flap transtibial amputation at two and a half weeks showing a nicely shaped stump suitable for early limb fitting.

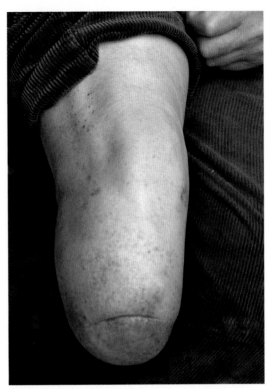

Figure 6.4 • An excellent transtibial amputation stump with a long posterior flap myoplasty.

Foot amputation

Digital amputation is most commonly performed in people with diabetes because of their susceptibility to infection. As a useful rule of thumb a digital amputation will only heal if foot pulses are present or can be restored. Therefore it is better to leave toes with partial dry gangrene alone. Amputation is best performed through the base of the proximal phalanx, leaving the wound open to heal by secondary intention. When infection extends beyond the proximal phalanx, a 'ray amputation' is indicated, especially in people with diabetes. After excision of the relevant toes, the line of excision is carried back through the infected tissue until healthy tissue is reached. The underlying metatarsal head is excised and the wound left open like a 'fish mouth'. Infection of the first or fifth metatarsophalangeal joint requires a 'tennis-racquet' incision; the handle of the racquet can usually be closed after excision of the metatarsal head. If osteomyelitis is present, a sample of the excised and retained bone should be sent for microbiological culture as the organisms causing the osteomyelitis are often different from those in the ulcer.

A transmetatarsal amputation can be useful when all the toes are gangrenous but when the plantar skin is still viable. A dorsal skin incision is made at mid-metatarsal level with a long plantar flap and bone transection through the metatarsal bases. As much soft tissue as possible should be preserved and consideration given to leaving the flaps open with delayed closure, as infection and gangrene of the flaps may occur if primary closure is attempted. Negative pressure wound therapy may facilitate the healing of such open-foot amputations.

Rehabilitation

The process of rehabilitation for vascular amputees, who are usually elderly and often have a number of other concurrent disabilities and illnesses, can pose a considerable challenge. A 'team approach' to amputee rehabilitation throughout the inpatient and prosthetic care pathway has now become the standard within the UK. The core members of the team should include a vascular surgeon, a specialist in rehabilitation medicine, a specialist physiotherapist, an occupational therapist and a prosthetist. Ready availability of a social worker, community nurses and a clinical psychologist is invaluable. Other services include wheelchair personnel, housing and adaptation officers, social services and orthotists. Close liaison and cooperation between all members of the team are vital. Counsellors and amputee volunteers, if available, can be very valuable.

> ✅ The British Society of Rehabilitation Medicine has recently updated and published standards and guidelines in amputee and prosthetic rehabilitation based on national consensus.[29]

Planning

A pre-amputation consultation by specialists in rehabilitation medicine and their team is ideal but impractical for every patient for whom an amputation is planned. However, a member of the amputee rehabilitation team (usually a therapist) should see all patients prior to amputation in order to make an initial assessment and prepare the patient for the likely programme to be implemented, instil realistic expectations and resolve any specific questions or anxieties. Other members of the multidisciplinary team may be involved at this stage if specially required. In our unit, specialist physiotherapists cover the boundary between the vascular and rehabilitation units and we find that this works extremely effectively. In the case of elective amputation, once the decision to amputate has been made, a referral is made to the therapists so the rehabilitation process can commence prior to admission. The therapists would contact the patient and either speak to them on the phone, or arrange

to see the patient and carers either in the hospital clinic or in the home environment. Their needs can be identified and information given along with realistic expectations. Their discharge from hospital can be planned, and any equipment they may need for a successful discharge, including provision of a wheelchair, can be put in place to prevent delays in discharge. In cases where amputation is a treatment option rather than a necessity, and in situations where there is some uncertainty regarding level selection, we recommend that the surgical team obtain advice from an appropriate consultant in rehabilitation medicine. In the Sheffield Limb Service Catchment area, of the 208 patients triaged following major amputation in 2015, 33% were suitable for prosthetic rehabilitation.

Stump management

Tight or elasticated stump bandaging should not be used in vascular amputees as it can generate unacceptable pressures causing tissue breakdown.[30] Rigid dressings of plaster of Paris are not generally used for vascular amputees in the UK, although some studies have suggested that they reduce the knee contracture rate following transtibial amputation. Adhesive clear-plastic film dressing applied postoperatively can be very useful as this allows easier and regular wound inspection. This type of dressing makes life easier for the physiotherapist when inspecting wounds before and after application of early walking aids. Where a more conventional dressing for the wound is required, an elasticated tubular bandage (e.g. Tubifast) is usually placed on the stump to hold these dressings in place. If the wound is healed or healing satisfactorily, then elasticated and graduated pressure stump shrinker socks (e.g. Juzo) are applied to the stump (**Fig. 6.5**). A survey of amputee physiotherapists in the UK (unpublished) revealed that the current practice is moving forward using the stump shrinker socks earlier than previously. In Sheffield, if the vascular surgeons are satisfied with the below-knee stump wound and the patient is able to tolerate it, the Juzo sock is applied on the fourth postoperative day. On the first day it is applied for 1 hour and then the wearing time is gradually increased over the next few days until the patient is wearing it all day and night. This process is carefully monitored by experienced staff. Stump supports are fitted to the wheelchair so that the patients can keep their below-knee stump elevated to prevent oedema and knee flexion. Sometimes stump supports may also be necessary for long transfemoral or through-knee stumps. Specialist footwear may be required to protect the other foot from damage if it is vulnerable. In our centre we

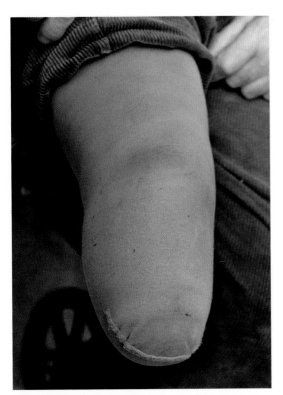

Figure 6.5 • A stump shrinker sock applied over a transtibial amputation stump.

find pressure-relieving ankle–foot orthoses are effective for this purpose and also relieve pressure on the heel whilst lying down.

Pain management

The use of a continuous local anaesthetic infusion to the sciatic nerve via a catheter placed intraoperatively may be beneficial in reducing postoperative pain. The catheter remains in place for a minimum of 3 days. Controlling stump and phantom pain is vital for the patient to participate successfully in a rehabilitation programme. Houghton et al.[31] found a significant relationship between pre-amputation pain and phantom pain in the first 2 years after amputation in vascular amputees. Nikolajsen et al.,[32] in a study of mostly vascular amputees, found a relationship between preoperative pain and incidents of phantom pain at 1 week and 3 months after amputation, but not after 6 months. Early involvement of the 'pain team' in such cases is most beneficial. Numerous medical interventions have been proposed over the years but tricyclic antidepressants and sodium channel blockers are currently considered to be the drugs of choice for neuropathic pain.[33] The anticonvulsant carbamazepine, a non-specific sodium channel blocker, has been reported to be effective in phantom pain.[34,35] The newer drug, pregabalin, has been found to be clinically effective in severe phantom pain.

In addition to the medical treatment of stump and phantom pains, various non-invasive treatments such as transcutaneous electrical nerve stimulation, vibration therapy, acupuncture, hypnosis and biofeedback can prove useful, although evidence of efficacy is limited.

Early postoperative rehabilitation

The occupational therapist and physiotherapist should work closely together to ensure an effective and timely rehabilitation programme. Following amputation, the physiotherapist usually sees the amputee on the first postoperative day and will begin a programme of bed mobility, joint movements, transferring and wheelchair mobility, depending on the patient's general condition and pain control. Stump exercises, exercises for the remaining limb and upper limbs, muscle strengthening, maintaining range of movements of the proximal joints, sitting balance and improvement of general cardiovascular fitness will all be incorporated into the programme. Each amputee will be assessed for an appropriate wheelchair and cushion as early as possible to facilitate discharge. The amputee will be taught the skills necessary for independent use of the wheelchair. By around the 1-week assessment, the therapist is usually reasonably sure of a patient's potential ability to use a prosthesis or not. However, some amputees are too unwell at the early postoperative stage but later may recover sufficiently to benefit from prosthetic rehabilitation. Therefore appropriate follow-up assessment may need to be arranged for this group of amputees.

Extreme frailty, severe dementia, severe cardiorespiratory disease, gross fixed flexion contractures and severe arthritis are contraindications to prosthetic rehabilitation. In our experience, elderly, vascular, bilateral transfemoral amputees do not achieve the ability to walk with a prosthesis. Assessing the home environment and adaptations, advice regarding driving, hobbies and employment also need addressing as an integral part of the rehabilitation.

✔ Evidence-based guidelines on the early rehabilitation phase have been published by the British Association of Chartered Physiotherapists in Amputee Rehabilitation.[36]

Primary prosthetic rehabilitation

All amputees who receive a prosthesis should undergo prosthetic rehabilitation to achieve the best prosthetic outcome. The role of the prosthetist in the fitting of a comfortable and functional prosthesis cannot be overemphasised. Prosthetic rehabilitation should aim to establish an energy-efficient gait based on normal physiological walking patterns. The physiotherapist should teach efficient control of the prosthesis through postural control, weight transfer, use of proprioception, and specific muscle strengthening and stretching exercises to prevent and correct gait deviations. Prosthetic rehabilitation will work towards the individual's own realistic goals, and should include functional activities relevant to that person and his or her lifestyle. All encouragement should be given to enable the individual to resume hobbies, sports, social activities, driving and return to work.

> ✔ The British Association of Chartered Physiotherapists in Amputee Rehabilitation have published useful evidence-based clinical guidelines for the physiotherapy of adults with lower limb prostheses.[37]

Sport activities for amputees

Amputation should not prevent an individual actively participating in sport. We often think of running, cycling, swimming and football, but there are others that may be more appropriate for the older, vascular amputee, including darts, snooker, bowls, fishing and golf.

Most sports will not require special prostheses and can be played alongside the able-bodied. Specialised componentry/prostheses are available for amputees who may want to run or swim. They may enable amputees to participate in more comfort and at a higher level than previously. Beach/water activity limbs do not assist the user to swim but allow an amputee to access in and around the water for activities such as windsurfing, sailing and canoeing, where not having the limb may prevent the activity. Previous and current fitness, concurrent disabilities/comorbidity and determination will all be important factors in the individual returning to or engaging in a new sport. Amputees may seek advice from professionals at their amputee rehabilitation centre, from peers, from groups such as British Amputee Les Autres Sports Association (BALASA) and, ever increasingly, the internet. Many local areas have groups who specialise in disabled sport and leisure that the amputee could access. The English Federation of Disability Sports (EFDS) keeps a list of all the disabled clubs nationally who deal with sports and leisure.

Prostheses

There are two main types of early walking aids used in the UK (**Figs 6.6** and **6.7**). The best known is the pneumatic post-amputation mobility aid

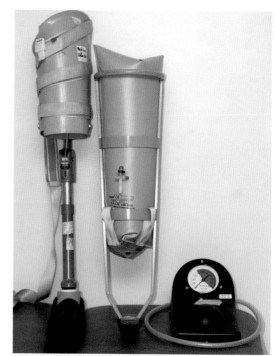

Figure 6.6 • A selection of early walking aids: Femurette (*left*) and pneumatic postamputation mobility aid (PPAM Aid; *centre*). A foot pump to inflate the PPAM Aid is shown on the right.

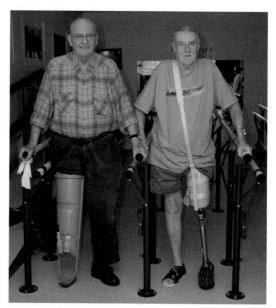

Figure 6.7 • A patient wearing Femurette (*right*) and a patient wearing PPAM Aid (*left*).

(PPAM Aid). The PPAM Aid is widely used and can be used for transtibial, through-knee and transfemoral levels of amputation. The Femurette is an excellent early walking aid for transfemoral amputees as it mimics a definitive transfemoral prosthesis in terms of an ischial tuberosity-bearing socket configuration and knee joint and it also has a foot.[38] The early walking aids are excellent morale boosters and are also used as assessment tools to estimate an amputee's potential for walking. They allow stump desensitisation, assist in reduction of stump oedema and may promote wound healing, and allow re-education of postural reflexes, balance and gait. The early walking aids should be considered around 1 week after amputation, under the judicious supervision of experienced therapists. However, in some cases where wound healing is poor, introduction of early walking aids needs to be delayed.

Prosthetic developments

The lower limb prostheses used in the UK are mainly of endoskeletal modular construction (**Fig. 6.8**). This system allows much speedier manufacture, socket change, adjustments and repairs compared with old conventional exoskeletal prostheses. A new limb, from measurement to delivery, is usually available within 5 working days for new patients. The standard prostheses usually incorporate thermoplastic materials like polypropylene or laminated plastics as socket materials and carbon fibre or lightweight alloy for fabrication of the weight-bearing components. Usually, vascular amputees are measured for their first prosthesis at about 6–8 weeks from amputation, although earlier fitting can take place subject to wound-healing status and the general condition of the stump. It is not imperative that the stump be completely healed before a prosthesis can be provided.

The traditional methods of casting have been superseded by scanning technology.

Younger dysvascular transfemoral amputees may have good musculature of the stump and adequate hand function and agility to benefit from prostheses with suction socket fitting and sophisticated 'free knee' mechanisms like pneumatic or hydraulic swing phase controls. Microprocessor knee joints providing swing and stance phase control are also available for transfemoral amputees, although often the price is prohibitive in many NHS centres.[39] In the UK, most elderly and dysvascular transfemoral amputees, if they are accepted for a prosthetic rehabilitation programme, are provided with non-suction prostheses with some form of waist-belt suspension and a 'locked' knee (bends only to sit down). More active dysvascular transfemoral amputees may benefit from free knee designs, including four-bar hydraulic, pneumatic or microprocessor knee units with suspending sockets.

For knee disarticulation, Gritti–Stokes or long transfemoral amputees, prosthetic options are limited. Use of polycentric knee joints like four-bar linkage knee mechanisms has eased some of the difficulties, though prostheses at these levels still create cosmetic as well as functional difficulties (**Fig. 6.9**). A polycentric knee, often a 4-bar linkage knee, has inherent stability due to the centre of rotation of the knee being behind the ground reaction force. It gives an improved cosmetic effect because the joint folds back on itself at 90 degrees flexion, e.g. when sitting.

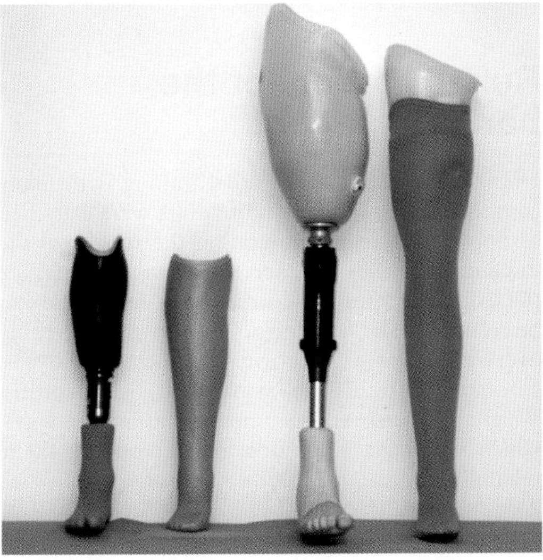

Figure 6.8 • Modular endoskeletal prostheses for transfemoral and transtibial amputation, with and without cosmetic covers.

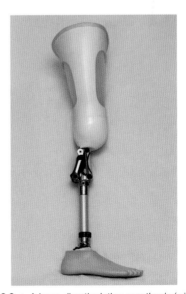

Figure 6.9 • A knee disarticulation prosthesis (without cosmetic cover) incorporating a four-bar linkage polycentric knee joint.

Osseointegration is a newer way of attaching the prosthesis to the stump. A metal rod is inserted into the distal bone, i.e. femur, and the prosthesis is fixed to the metal end. However this has not been trialled on vascular amputees and has only been trialled on young healthy, traumatic amputees with some success. The major risk has been the risk of infection in the bone, and loosening of the insert.

For transtibial amputees there are various socket systems available to the prosthetist to achieve optimum fit and suspension. In addition to the anatomical system utilising a pelite liner (a soft foam that is heat- and pressure-resistant) and supracondylar suspension, the introduction of silicone or gel suspension systems using pin or valve locking mechanisms has improved suspension as well as reducing friction and shear forces at the stump–socket interface[40] (**Fig. 6.10**). This type of prosthesis uses a silicone or gel sleeve directly on the stump, which is then locked into the prosthetic socket or uses a suction valve for suspension. There are many commercially available liners for use with pin suspension systems. Much shorter transtibial amputation stumps can now be fitted successfully, which was not possible previously with the traditional patellar tendon-bearing prosthesis.

Rehabilitation of those with very-high-level amputations (e.g. hip disarticulation and hemipelvectomy) due to cancer surgery, intravenous drug use causing major arterial thrombosis and major trauma, has improved with new socket designs (bikini socket), new prosthetic hip joint components and intensive multidisciplinary team input.

Similar to prosthetic knee joints, there is a wide variety of commercially available prosthetic feet. They are categorised by their function. The most commonly prescribed foot in the UK is the multi-axis multiflex foot (www.blatchford.co.uk), which provides movement through weight-bearing in the anteroposterior and mediolateral directions. Energy-return feet can be considered for patients with higher activity levels and include Flexfoot, Elite, Epirius, Blade and Seattle. Energy-storing feet are known to be less energy-consuming for ambulant amputees.

☑☑ More recently, energy-return feet have also been found to offer significant help to transfemoral amputees.[41,42]

One of the problems with wearing a prosthesis is excessive sweating, particularly with the silicone type liners. To combat that, prosthetic manufacturing companies have developed sweat management liners which allow the sweat to evaporate, thus providing the skin with a safer environment inside the socket. These enable the patient to keep their skin more healthy and improve the comfort and suspension of the prosthesis.

Other useful components include a patient-adjustable heel height device when shoes with different heel height are to be worn, torsion devices and vertical shock absorber in the shin of a prosthesis that absorb vertical forces and rotational torque, turntables that allow sitting cross-legged on the floor, or individually created, highly life-like silicone cosmetic cover, swimming or shower legs. Selection of the prostheses and components will be determined by clinical assessment and with consideration of the amputee's wishes, realistic goals, progress in rehabilitation and ability to benefit from a prescribed device.

Rehabilitation for the bariatric patient

Obesity is increasing in the UK, along with many countries. In 2014, 25.6% of adults were classified as obese. Following amputation the weight of the missing limb needs to be accounted for when making the calculation for the correct body mass index to be recorded. The health risks associated with being overweight are well known and include diabetes, coronary heart disease, stroke and osteoarthritis. Weight gain also affects amputees in unique ways, which will have a negative impact on prosthetic rehabilitation.

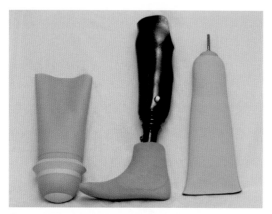

Figure 6.10 • (*Left to right*) An ICEROSS liner with a distal locking pin which is applied by rolling onto the stump; a transtibial prosthesis on which the stump with the liner is inserted and locked in; and a Seal-in silicone liner that provides excellent suspension by suction without the necessity of a locking pin.

- **Osteoarthritis.** Wearing a prosthesis puts an excessive strain on the joints of the residual limb and contralateral limb, causing pain and increased likelihood of osteoarthritis.

- **Cardiovascular effects.** As already discussed, there is a greater energy expenditure when walking following amputation and any additional body weight would further compromise cardiac and pulmonary function.
- **Component selection.** There are currently many dozens of prosthetic components on the market, each having its own upper weight limit. As a person's weight increases, the choice of components will become limited. The heavy-duty components tend to be heavier, costlier and more difficult to obtain, and will increase the overall weight of the prosthesis.
- **Socket fit.** The comfort of the socket is vital; however, where there is an excess of soft tissue and the bony prominences are less well defined, it is difficult to obtain a firm stable fit with good suspension. Consequently the soft tissues are more prone to inflammation and ulceration.

Key points

- In the UK, 80% of all amputations carried out are due to peripheral artery disease, and an increasing proportion have diabetes.
- Revascularisation may reduce the incidence of amputation.
- Selection of the ideal level of amputation depends on healing potential, rehabilitation potential and prosthetic considerations.
- Transtibial amputees have a much higher potential to achieve prosthetic mobilisation compared with those undergoing transfemoral amputation.
- For patients who are not likely to achieve prosthetic walking, a Gritti–Stokes amputation is preferable to amputation at the transfemoral level.
- A comprehensive and holistic assessment of amputees or prospective amputees, followed by multidisciplinary rehabilitation, is likely to provide the optimal outcome.
- Amputation surgery should be considered as a constructive procedure to create the best possible amputation stump and should therefore be carried out by surgeons who have had proper training in these procedures.
- Stump bandaging with elasticated bandages is not recommended.
- Appropriate use of early walking aids during the early postamputation period is an essential part of rehabilitation.
- Modern prostheses are modular and can be made quickly using modern materials technology.
- Increasingly, more sophisticated components are becoming available, although they tend to be applicable only for the more active amputee.
- The types of prostheses and their components will be determined by the amputee's realistic goals, progress in rehabilitation and ability to benefit.

🌐 Full references available at **http://expertconsult. inkling.com**

Key references

19. Savin S, Sharni S, Shields DA, et al. Selection of amputation level: a review. Eur J Vasc Surg 1991;5:611–20. PMID: 1756874.

   The authors reviewed the evidence for many tests (Doppler indices, segmental pressures, skin blood flow, skin perfusion pressure, tcP_{O_2}, thermography) to predict the likelihood of successful healing of an amputation stump. They concluded that the foremost requirement to raise the below-knee/above-knee ratio is to promote awareness among surgeons of the value of medical management and encourage the use of routinely available tests such as ankle–brachial pressure index and Doppler segmental pressures. The value of more specialised tests remains to be established.

28. Ruckley CV, Stonebridge PA, Prescott RJ. Skewflap versus long posterior flap in below-knee amputations: multicenter trial. J Vasc Surg 1991;13:423–7. PMID: 1999863.

   A multicentre trial – 191 patients with end-stage occlusive vascular disease needing transtibial amputation were randomised to skew flap technique in 98 and long posterior flap technique in 93 patients.

The two groups were well matched: 30-day mortality rate, state of wound at 1 week and need for surgical revision at the same or higher level were not statistically significant between the groups. Follow-up information at 6 months showed 64 (84%) of the skew flaps and 50 (77%) of the long posterior flaps were fitted with prostheses. Walking, alone or with support, was achieved in 59 (78%) and 46 (71%), respectively. None of these differences reached statistical significance.

41. Graham LE, Datta D, Heller B, et al. A comparative study – oxygen consumption and energy storing prosthesis in transfemoral amputees. Clin Rehabil 2008;22(10,11):896–901. PMID: 18955421.

This experimental crossover trial established transfemoral amputees wearing Multiflex foot initially and then Variflex foot and concluded that a high functioning transfemoral amputee who wears an energy-storing prosthetic foot may have significantly reduced oxygen consumption at normal walking speed.

42. Graham LE, Datta D, Heller B, et al. A comparative study of conventional and energy storing prosthetic feet in high functioning transfemoral amputees. Arch Phys Med Rehab 2007;88(6):801–6. PMID: 17532907.

In this study of the same subjects as in reference 41 it was shown that a transfemoral amputee who wears an energy-storing foot can have a more symmetrical gait in regard to some measures of spatial symmetry, kinetics and kinematics than one who wears a conventional prosthetic foot.

7

Revision vascular surgery

Jan Brunkwall
Michael Gawenda

Introduction

Revision of vascular reconstructions and interventions is frequently required beyond the first 6 weeks because of progressive atherosclerosis, graft occlusion, aneurysm formation or infection. Up to 40% of femorodistal bypass surgery grafts require reintervention within 5 years.[1] The same is true for endovascular intervention where it has been shown that up to 30% of patients need a reintervention within 5 years after endovascular aortic aneurysm reconstruction (EVAR).[2–7] Revision surgery requires experience and judgement; it is technically more difficult because of fibrosis and the loss of easily definable tissue planes, which necessitate careful sharp dissection to gain arterial control. The anatomy might be altered by previous operations or interventions and operating times, blood loss, infection rates and operative risk are therefore increased.

Graft occlusion

Graft thrombosis usually presents with acute limb ischaemia but is occasionally foreshown by increasing ischaemic symptoms, ranging from mild claudication to critical ischaemia. Nevertheless, asymptomatic graft occlusion can also occur. Occasionally, simultaneous distal embolisation causes digital ischaemia (blue toe syndrome or gangrene). Graft thrombosis with loss of run-off due to distal embolisation is associated with a high risk of limb loss. Whereas graft thrombosis in the first 6 weeks is generally due to technical error or poor run-off, most late occlusions result from intimal hyperplasia within the bypass or progressive inflow or run-off disease (see Chapter 4). Graft stenoses are usually asymptomatic and occur in 20–30% of infrainguinal vein grafts, mostly in the first year.[8,9] Stenoses of greater than 70% (velocity >3 m/s or velocity ratio >3.0) compromise flow and often occlude if left untreated.[10]

Factors influencing graft occlusion

Local factors

These are essentially for the quality of the inflow, the run-off and the conduit itself (see Chapter 4).

Patency is better for suprainguinal than infrainguinal grafts and graft occlusion is more frequent in femorotibial than in femoropopliteal bypasses.[11]

Infrainguinal bypass patency of autologous vein is better than Dacron, polytetrafluoroethylene (PTFE) or human umbilical vein.[12] For Dacron and PTFE used in femoropopliteal bypass graft patency at 5 years is similar.[13] The 1-year-results of a Scandinavian multicentre randomised trial revealed that a heparin-bonded PTFE graft significantly reduced the overall risk of primary graft failure by 37%. Risk reduction was 50% in femoropopliteal bypass cases and in cases with critical ischaemia.[14] However, follow-up to 5 years demonstrated that there was no difference in primary graft patency between Hb-PTFE and standard PTFE grafts. Patients receiving heparin bonded-PTFE grafts for critical limb ischaemia were more likely to have a patent graft at 5 years than those with standard PTFE grafts.[15]

✔✔ The results of reversed and in situ vein grafts are equivalent.[16,17] In a meta-analysis on the long-term primary and secondary patency and foot preservation following popliteal-to-distal bypass grafts there was a superiority trend favouring reversed vein grafts.[18]

The outcomes from well selected arm vein conduits are similar to great saphenous vein provided that angioscopically detected defects are corrected.[19] Preoperative ultrasound mapping seems to be crucial to use the best autogenous conduit available.[20] A recent published retrospective study of infrainguinal bypasses for critical leg ischaemia (CLI) using arm vein conduit or prosthetic grafts revealed that arm vein conduits, even when spliced, are superior to prosthetic grafts in terms of midterm assisted primary patency, secondary patency and leg salvage in infrapopliteal bypasses for CLI.[21]

✔✔ A Cochrane Review published in 2010 demonstrated a clear primary patency benefit for autologous vein when compared to synthetic materials for above-knee bypasses. In the long term (5 years) Dacron confers a small primary patency benefit over PTFE for above-knee bypass. PTFE with a vein cuff improved primary patency when compared to PTFE alone for below-knee bypasses.[22]

The risk for ischaemic complications and the need for emergency limb revascularisation are greater with occlusion of prosthetic grafts compared to venous grafts. This is because the thrombus in the prosthetic graft extends into the outflow artery. Vein cuffs at the distal anastomosis reduce the risk of outflow impairment after thrombosis of PTFE grafts (**Fig. 7.1**).[23]

✔✔ The Dutch BOA Study found no difference between venous and prosthetic graft material in the risk of amputation after infrainguinal bypass occlusion.[24]

The quality and number of run-off vessels appear to potentially identify patients at high risk for a poor initial outcome by predicting patency in infrainguinal bypass reconstructions.[25,26] Bypasses for gangrene occlude more frequently than for ulceration, rest pain or claudication.[27] This is probably related to the inferior run-off associated with worsening ischaemia.

General factors

✔ Continued smoking after lower limb bypass surgery results in an at least threefold increased risk of graft failure.[2] Diabetes and renal failure compromise patient survival but not graft patency.[28–30]

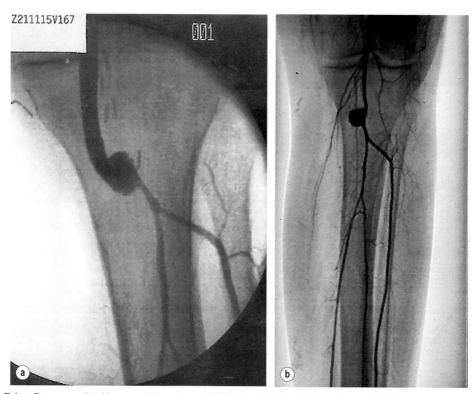

Figure 7.1 • Femoropopliteal bypass with venous cuff (Miller cuff) at the distal anastomosis. Perioperative angiography **(a)**. Preservation of outflow vessels after thrombosis at 3 years **(b)**.

Raised fibrinogen, hyperlipidaemia, thrombophilias (e.g. protein C, protein S or antithrombin III deficiency, antiphospholipid antibodies), and increased platelet aggregation favour graft thrombosis,[31] whereas factor V Leiden mutation is debatable.[32,33]

> ✅ Black race and female gender are risk factors for adverse outcomes after vein bypass surgery for limb salvage, with graft failure and limb loss being more common events in black patients, and black women being a particularly high-risk group.[34]

Even white women have more graft occlusions and recurrent stenosis, and hormone replacement therapy potentiates this.[35,36]

Prevention of graft thrombosis

> ✅✅ Antiplatelet therapy with aspirin had a slight beneficial effect on the patency of peripheral bypass grafts but seemed to have an inferior effect on venous graft patency compared with artificial grafts.[37] The Dutch BOA trial revealed that aspirin is more effective for infrainguinal prosthetic grafts, whereas warfarin is better for vein grafts.[38]
>
> In the CASPAR trial the combination of clopidogrel plus aspirin did not improve limb or systemic outcomes in the overall population of peripheral artery disease patients requiring below-knee bypass grafting. A subgroup analysis suggested that clopidogrel plus aspirin may benefit patients receiving prosthetic grafts without significantly increasing major bleeding risk.[39]

Surveillance for suprainguinal bypass grafts does not seem to be cost-effective. Occlusion is far more frequent after infrainguinal bypass grafting and since most of the occlusions occur within 2 years after the implantation, patients should be carefully followed during this time period. This includes medical history, clinical examination and Doppler pressure measurements. Duplex scanning after prosthetic bypass appears ineffective.

> ✅✅ Some published reports tend to argue in favour of Duplex surveillance on the basis of patency alone.[40] In a randomised trial with 596 patients, intensive surveillance with Duplex scanning did not show any additional benefit in terms of limb salvage rates for patients undergoing femoropopliteal or femorocrural vein bypass graft operations.[41]

Management of graft stenosis (the failing graft)

Although there is some discussion about asymptomatic stenosis, symptomatic graft stenosis should be treated by either angioplasty or surgical revision. Open surgical revision of infrainguinal vein grafts provides an increased freedom from further reinterventions or major amputation; however, early success rates for endovascular procedures were similar, particularly for non-occluded grafts. And percutaneous transluminal angioplasty of infrainguinal vein grafts is safe and effective in the treatment of failing grafts. Graft angioplasties do not appear to lose effectiveness when repeated and have shown cumulative benefit in prolonging graft survival.[42] With time, endovascular revisions require an increasing number of reinterventions and manifested higher rates of failure.[43] Surgical revision is probably more durable in the long term, but an endovascular approach is actually preferred because of the acceptable short-term patency and a low rate of complications, particularly for late graft stenosis (>3 months), short (<2 cm) and single stenosis.[43–45]

Short graft stenosis, whether midgraft or anastomotic, commonly responds well to angioplasty with high inflation pressures (**Fig. 7.2**). Cutting angioplasty balloons have been advocated, but seem to offer only a small benefit at the expense of an elevated complication rate.[46–48] Stents are an option but should be used only selectively given their poor long-term durability.[49]

> ✅✅ A recently published randomised clinical study demonstrated that implantation of a polymer-free, paclitaxel-coated nitinol drug-eluting stent (DES) in patients with moderate-length lesions of the superior femoral artery and proximal popliteal artery was safe and associated with a superior 12-month patency compared with both percutaneous transluminal angioplasty (PTA) and provisional bare-metal stent (BMS) placement. The proportion of treated re-stenoses in both cohorts was only 5.5% and 5.9%, respectively.[50] Two-year and 5-year outcomes with the paclitaxel-eluting stent support its sustained safety and effectiveness in patients with femoropopliteal artery disease, including the long-term superiority of the DES to PTA and to provisional BMS placement.[51,52] Unfortunately, there is a paucity of data on limb salvage and amputation-free survival rates with these new technologies.

Longer graft stenoses are best treated by open surgery and may be bypassed using the contralateral long saphenous or superficial femoral vein.[19] Tibial or distal popliteal anastomotic stenoses resistant to angioplasty are best treated by a jump graft to a fresh run-off vessel to avoid the scar tissue or adherent tibial veins (**Fig. 7.3**). If autogenous venous conduit has been exhausted radial artery is a useful alternative, especially where a short jump graft may be required.

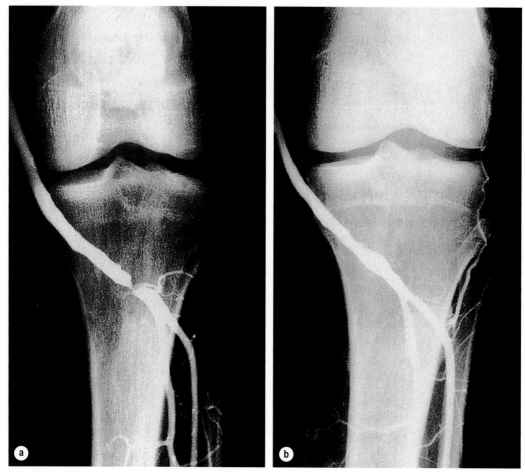

Figure 7.2 • Vein graft stenosis near the below-knee popliteal anastomosis **(a)** successfully treated by balloon angioplasty **(b)**.

Management of the occluded (failed) graft

If graft occlusion causes non-disabling claudication, a conservative approach might be preferred. Acute subcritical ischaemia allows time for thrombolysis or elective surgery but an insensate paralysed limb demands emergency revascularisation within a few hours (see Chapter 8).

Role of thrombolysis

> ✅ Local catheter-directed thrombolysis might be a valuable tool for a viable limb within 14 days of prosthetic graft occlusion provided that the patient has undergone surgery within 3 months.[53]

Thrombolysis is suitable for prosthetic and suprainguinal grafts. It is less frequently used for femorodistal graft occlusion. Vein graft occlusion often presents late when the limb may not be salvageable.. The exact mechanism why vein grafts appear to respond poorly to thrombolyisis has been speculated to be due to ischaemia of the endothelium.

The advantages of thrombolysis are that redo surgery may be avoided and the graft will be cleared of thrombus, unmasking the underlying cause of thrombosis, which can often be treated endovascularly during the same session. The outflow vessels might also be cleared more effectively than with open surgery. Percutaneous mechanical thrombectomy or the use of high bolus therapy can reduce the duration of the procedure.[54-56] If thrombolysis is unsuccessful or reveals a problem that is not amenable to endovascular treatment, then open surgery can be performed with a clear knowledge of the cause of the problem and the state of the runoff. Although thrombolysis has a high initial success rate, it is also characterised by a number of contraindications, resource use (multiple trips to the interventional suite), haemorrhagic complications (especially in

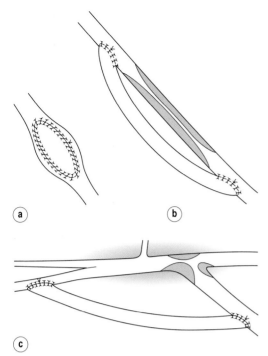

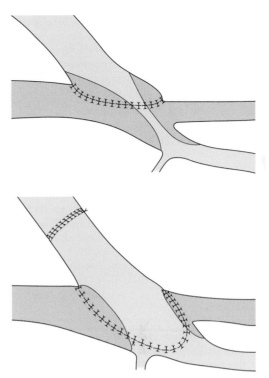

Figure 7.3 • **(a)** Vein patch angioplasty, **(b)** bypass of long vein graft stenosis and **(c)** jump graft around stenosed distal anastomosis of a femoropopliteal bypass graft to the popliteal artery.

Figure 7.4 • Extension graft to one limb of an aorto-bifemoral graft to treat a stenosis at the profunda femoris origin. In this case the superficial femoral artery is occluded.

those over 80 years), poor long-term patency and persistent ischaemia.[57,58] This explains the reduced popularity of thrombolysis, and why the pragmatic solution to reserve thrombolysis for patients with associated extensive thrombosis of the outflow vessels is often applied.[59]

Suprainguinal graft thrombosis

A unilateral limb thrombosis of an aorto-bifemoral graft can be thrombectomised through the groin even months after the occlusion. Thrombectomy is performed with Fogarty embolectomy catheters, an adherent clot catheter or a ring stripper. During these manoeuvres, the contralateral groin is compressed to avoid contralateral embolisation. The underlying cause is most frequently a stenosis at the distal anastomosis, which should be repaired by extension of the graft, mostly into the profunda femoris artery (**Fig. 7.4**). Graft thrombectomy by a femoral approach is usually not possible in cases of bilateral graft occlusion, as the problem is more likely to be in the proximal region (inflow problem). Here the graft should be replaced in situ instead or by an extra-anatomical bypass (axillo-bifemoral bypass).

The underlying cause of the occlusion in cases of axillofemoral grafting is most frequently an anastomotic stenosis or stenosis of the inflow vessel.[60] Thrombectomy can then be performed from the groin,

but frequently an additional incision along the graft is needed. The underlying cause needs to be managed. The inflow vessels (subclavian artery for axillofemoral graft) are checked pre- or perioperatively and inflow stenosis is treated if necessary. A new graft in clean tissues offers the best solution in cases of long-standing thrombosis or when thrombectomy is insufficient. For an occluded femorofemoral graft the same principles apply. In this situation it is not uncommon to encounter bilateral stenoses so that both groins need repair.

Infrainguinal graft thrombosis

In cases of chronic occlusion, the decision regarding revascularisation should be taken in light of the clinical examination and results of investigations.

In patients with acute ischaemia, an immediate decision should be taken regarding thrombolysis or open surgery. Prosthetic grafts can usually be thrombectomised by a groin approach if the occlusion is less than 1 week old. Anastomotic stenosis must be corrected, and inflow and outflow vessels need to be checked by perioperative angiography. If necessary, outflow vessels can be selectively approached by an infragenicular approach, and intraoperative thrombolysis might be an adjunct in selected cases (see Chapter 8).[61] Venous grafts are usually more difficult to thrombectomise. Here it is usually more appropriate to place a new graft. If at all possible, a venous graft should be used. Following thrombectomy for acute ischaemia, four-compartment fasciotomy should be considered to relieve pressure and improve distal perfusion, especially if there is any calf swelling or tenderness preoperatively.[62,63]

Graft infection

Graft infection is relatively uncommon (1–5%) but has a high amputation and mortality risk.[64] In a recent multicentre audit of 55 graft infections, 32% died, 33% underwent amputation and only 45% left the hospital alive without amputation.[65] Treatment has therefore to focus on patient survival, eradication of infection and revascularisation by a method that is durable and does not become infected itself.

Causes

Graft infection is thought to occur most commonly by inoculation of bacteria from the patient's skin at the time of surgery (e.g. skin commensals) or by direct spread in the perioperative period, often secondary to wound breakdown.[66] Surgical site infection (SSI) after open surgery for lower extremity revascularisation is a serious complication that is associated with a more than twofold-increased risk of early graft loss and re-operation.[67]

Patients with gangrene, the elderly, obese and those undergoing re-operation during the same hospital admission have a higher risk. Preoperative shaving, open surgical drainage for more than 3 days, operations lasting over 4 hours, emergency surgery, redo-surgery, female gender, diabetes, steroids, renal failure, recent angiography and wound haematoma are all risk factors.[67,68] Blood-borne bacteria from intravenous lines or systemic infections may also cause graft inoculation and sepsis.

Venous grafts are more resistant to infection than prosthetic, but direct bacterial erosion can occur, especially when exposed in an open wound.

Prevention

Patients should be admitted as near to surgery as possible and isolated from patients with known infections, especially methicillin-resistant *Staphylococcus aureus* (MRSA). Many hospitals have a policy of screening elective surgical patients for MRSA colonisation before admission and eradicating any infection before proceeding with surgery.

Strict aseptic technique and laminar air-flow theatres minimise infection rates. Iodine-impregnated adhesive drapes help isolate the operative field. Prophylactic antibiotics (cephalosporin or co-amoxiclav) reduce wound and graft infection. There is no evidence for using more than a single preoperative dose of prophylactic antibiotics. Some surgeons add a further two postoperative doses of antibiotics. A single dose of gentamicin is active against many strains of MRSA. Vancomycin should be used if the patient is MRSA-positive. Evidence for new generation antibiotics is still lacking.

A recently published RCT of a silver-eluting alginate dressing placed over incisions after leg arterial surgery showed no effect on the incidence of wound complications.[69]

✅✅ Prophylactic systemic antibiotics reduced the risk of wound infection and early graft infection. Antibiotic prophylaxis for more than 24 hours appears to be of no added benefit. Rifampicin bonding of Dacron grafts does not appear to reduce graft infection.[70] The same is true for the more recent silver-coated grafts.[71,72] There was no evidence of a beneficial or detrimental effect on rates of wound infection with suction groin-wound drainage[70] or of any benefit from a preoperative bathing or shower regimen with antiseptic agents over unmedicated bathing.[73]

There is also little evidence regarding the need for prophylactic antibiotics before other surgical or dental procedures in the presence of prosthetic grafts.

Presentation

Wound infections after vascular surgery are classified according to the Szilagyi system of depth of tissue involvement: type 1 involves the skin only, type 2 the subcutaneous tissue and type 3 the graft itself.[74] Prosthetic graft infection can present at any time from days to years after surgery with pyrexia, systemic sepsis, local abscesses and sinuses, graft exposure, thrombosis or anastomotic haemorrhage. On rare occasions septic emboli can be the first sign (**Fig. 7.5**). Septic erosion of exposed vein grafts can occur at any point.

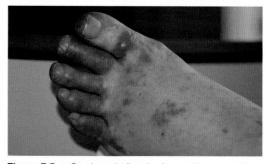

Figure 7.5 • Septic emboli at the foot as the presenting sign of aortofemoral graft infection.

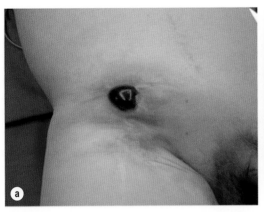 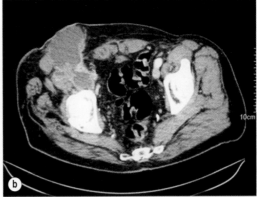

Figure 7.6 • Aortoenteric fistula leading to retroperitoneal and groin abscesses: **(a)** aspect of the groin; **(b)** CT scan.

Infrarenal aortic grafts can erode the third or fourth part of the duodenum causing an aortoduodenal fistula, which may present with one or two sentinel gastrointestinal bleeds before the inevitable catastrophic haemorrhage. Occasionally, an aortic graft can also erode any other part of the bowel, including the appendix, and also the ureter. Such aortoenteric erosion will lead to localised peritonitis with retroperitoneal or groin abscesses (**Fig. 7.6a,b**) and ultimately catastrophic bleeding. The mortality rate of aortoenteric complications is high (>50%), with recurrent infection or aortic stump blowout in over 25%.[75]

Bacteriology

Most graft infections are due to skin commensals.[76] *Staphylococcus epidermidis* is the least virulent, producing a biofilm or an infected seroma months or years after the procedure. It is difficult to culture, requiring homogenisation of explanted graft material to dislodge adherent bacteria. *Staphylococcus aureus* is more virulent and usually presents earlier. MRSA infections have a particularly high morbidity and mortality and the incidence is unfortunately increasing. Apart from staphylococci, there is a wide variety of organisms that can cause graft infection. Gram-negative species include *Escherichia coli* and *Pseudomonas aeruginosa*, the latter being recognised by a high tendency of anastomotic disruption and bleeding. It may be difficult or even impossible to culture the causative organism, particularly after prolonged periods of antibiotic therapy.

Diagnosis

In most cases there is a perigraft collection or sinus. Aspiration of frank pus or turbid fluid from around the graft and the subsequent culture of a causative organism are diagnostic. Computed tomography (CT), magnetic resonance imaging (MRI) or ultrasound usually demonstrate perigraft fluid and inflammation but can underestimate the extent of infection, especially if a sinus is present, and in this regard sinography may be useful. For wholly intra-abdominal prostheses there may be few signs of infection, therefore diagnosis of aortic graft infection is often difficult, requiring a high index of suspicion and comprehensive investigation. Leucocyte count, erythrocyte sedimentation rate and C-reactive protein are often raised. Persistence of perigraft fluid or perigraft soft-tissue attenuation beyond 3 months or perigraft gas (**Fig. 7.7**) beyond 4–7 weeks should be presumed to be infection and perigraft fluid should be aspirated using an image-guided technique and characterised for pathogens.[77] One in four anastomotic aneurysms results from graft infection, but this is not always evident from CT. Where doubt exists, indium-labelled leucocyte or positron-emission tomography (PET) scanning is occasionally helpful. In aortoenteric fistula, the graft may be seen eroding the duodenum

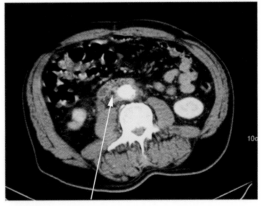

Figure 7.7 • Perigraft gas bubbles in between duodenum and aortic graft.

at endoscopy (**Fig. 7.8**). Definitive confirmation of an infection is sometimes made only at the operation by the presence of pus around the graft and the absence of tissue incorporation (**Fig. 7.9**).

Management

General principles

Once infection is confirmed, semi-urgent treatment is required to pre-empt catastrophic haemorrhage, graft thrombosis or systemic sepsis. An infected prosthesis acts as a foreign body, rendering bacteria inaccessible to antibiotics. Conservative measures (including prolonged antibiotic therapy, drainage and irrigation of abscesses, muscle flaps) may be helpful and can buy time, but they are rarely curative.

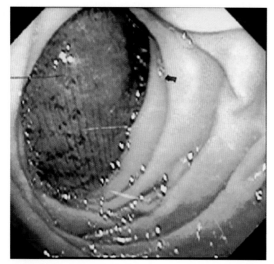

Figure 7.8 • Aortic graft, eroding the duodenum as seen during endoscopy.

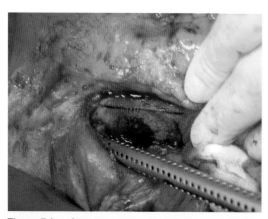

Figure 7.9 • Situs intraoperatively with absence of tissue incorporation of the graft and discolouration by duodenal secretion.

The mainstay of vascular graft infection management is as follows: First, excision of the graft, as this as a foreign body may potentiate the infection. Second, wide and complete debridement of devitalised and infected tissue to provide a clean wound in which healing can occur. Third, establishment of vascular flow to the distal bed. Fourth, the intensive and prolonged treatment with antibiotics, in order to reduce the risk for sepsis and secondary graft infection.[78]

Complete graft excision might be mandatory. Partial graft resection commonly requires later replacement.[79] Although contrary to conventional concepts, partial or complete graft preservation combined with aggressive drainage and groin wound debridement is an acceptable option for treatment of infection involving an entire aortic graft in selected patients with prohibitive risks for total graft excision.[80,81]

Simple graft excision without revascularisation can eradicate infection but usually results in major amputation, even in patients operated on initially for claudication.

Revascularisation is traditionally performed by extra-anatomic bypass (axillofemoral graft for infrarenal aortic graft infection, obturator bypass for infection at the groin, lateral bypass for infection of a femoropopliteal graft).[64]

✔ There is growing evidence that in situ reconstruction produces equal or better results than graft excision and extra-anatomical bypass, with regard to reinfection rate and particularly late patency and amputation rates.[82,83]

✔ An autologous conduit is preferable for in situ reconstruction.[84]

Arterial allografts are an alternative but they might dispose to late complications such as stenosis, occlusion or aneurysmal degeneration.[82,85] There are a few encouraging reports on the use of rifampicin-bonded grafts or silver-impregnated grafts, but they should be reserved for patients with low-grade infections (e.g. *Staphylococcus epidermidis*).[86,87]

The duration of postoperative antibiotic therapy is a matter for debate. Most authors will accept a period of 2–6 weeks depending on the causative organism.[88]

Infrarenal aortic graft infection

Extra-anatomic bypass, specifically axillo-bifemoral bypass, with complete removal of the infected aortic graft, has constituted traditional management of aortic graft infection. During the last two decades, methods have included debridement of infected tissue, with in situ replacement using cryopreserved allograft, autogenous vein, or rifampicin-bonded prostheses (**Fig. 7.10**).

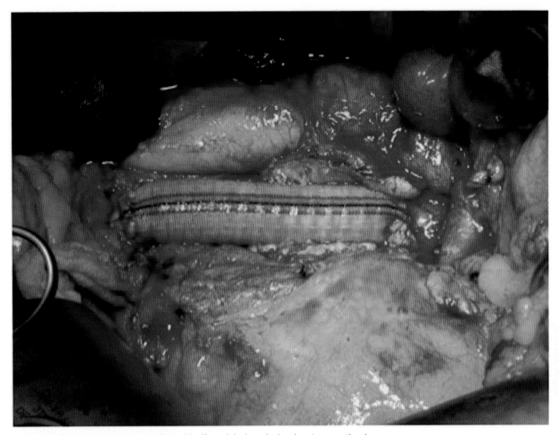

Figure 7.10 • In situ reconstruction with rifampicin-bonded polyester prosthesis.

✅✅ A recent meta-analysis of in situ replacement methods found these alternative techniques overall to be superior to the traditional method in terms of rates of reinfection, conduit failure, and early and late mortality and amputation rates.[83] Rifampicin-bonded prosthetics were found to have the lowest rates of amputation, conduit failure and early mortality. The reinfection rate with rifampicin-impregnated grafts was higher than that of other methods. Autogenous vein had the lowest rate of reinfection, followed by cryopreserved allograft. Later mortality was lowest for autogenous vein and cryopreserved allograft reconstruction. When all outcomes were considered, in situ options for aortic graft infection have shown considerable promise.

An early study of silver-coated prosthetic grafts had encouraging results for in situ management of aortic graft infection. That study showed the method to be safe and effective, with a 3.7% reinfection rate at 16 months. A later study showed results similar to other in situ methods. The use of silver to prevent infection is commonplace; however, in treatment of aortic graft infection, this modality requires further study.[86,89]

As an alternative, in aortic in situ reconstruction restoration with the superficial femoral veins following total graft excision is commonly used.[90,91] The basic steps in this operation are as follows.

1. Harvesting of the superficial femoral vein. The patency of the femoral veins is checked preoperatively by duplex scanning. The superficial femoral vein itself is approached by an incision anteromedially on the thigh, commonly used for harvesting of the greater saphenous vein. After incision of the fascia the vein is identified just next to the superficial femoral artery. The bifurcation with the profunda femoris vein is situated in the groin a couple of centimetres below the arterial bifurcation. When working from medially, this means that the venous bifurcation can be approached without entering the original and mostly infected groin incision. Distally the adductor canal is opened and the dissection is continued to the level of the mid-popliteal artery. The vein is transected at the level of the knee joint and then freed upwards with ligation of the different side branches (**Fig. 7.11**).

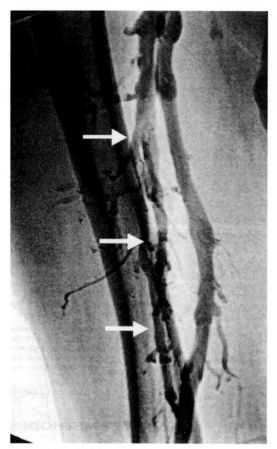

Figure 7.11 • Phlebography showing the femoral vein. Important collaterals by the profunda femoris vein (*white arrows*) protect from venous hypertension after harvest.

At the level of the adductor canal there are usually dense adhesions with the artery and multiple fragile side branches. Proximally the excision should be extended to the level of the venous confluence and the profunda femoris vein is carefully preserved since it receives important collateral circulation from the popliteal vein.

Excision of one superficial femoral vein will usually be sufficient for aorto-(bi)-iliac reconstruction. In the event of an aorto-(bi)-femoral reconstruction the veins need to be harvested from both lower limbs. After excision, the veins are preserved in cold (4°C) solution and the wounds are closed.

2. Excision of the infected graft.

   The preferred approach is median xyphopubic laparotomy. The retroperitoneal approach might be an alternative in selected cases but the disadvantage is that it hampers a complete debridement and coverage of the new reconstruction with healthy tissue (omentoplasty). In addition, it renders the approach to the femoral vessels and reconstruction in this area more difficult. The infrarenal aorta is approached in the traditional way, but in case of dense adhesions, the right retrocolic approach can be a good option. It is frequently necessary to obtain aortic control at the suprarenal or supracoeliac level. Once the aorta has been freed, the distal anastomoses at the iliac or femoral level are exposed. The aorta is clamped after systemic heparinisation and the infected graft is excised completely. The periaortic tissues and any other sites of infection are generously debrided in order to achieve a healthy bed for the new graft. Existing retroperitoneal tunnels are irrigated and mechanically debrided by pulling open gauze sponges through them. Finally the aorta itself and the femoral vessels are debrided to achieve a clean anastomotic site.

3. In situ reconstruction with the deep vein (**Fig. 7.12**).

   The veins can be used in reversed or non-reversed position, this after fracture of the valves with a valvulotome. The proximal aortic anastomosis is simply sutured with one vein end-to-end to the aorta. Taking into account the diameter discrepancy between the aorta and the veins, it is frequently necessary to downsize the aortic cuff somehow with two or three separate through-and-through stitches. The second vein graft is anastomosed afterwards to the first one some 5 cm below this proximal anastomosis. When replacing an infected aorto-bifemoral bypass, the vein grafts are brought to the groin through the old tunnels and anastomosed to the femoral vessels in the usual way. Afterwards, the vein grafts are covered both in the abdomen and at the femoral level with viable tissues, leaving no residual cavities. Omentoplasty is generally used at the proximal anastomosis and muscle flaps are provided in the groin in case of extensive infection.

It is agreed that in situ reconstruction with the superficial femoral veins represents a technically demanding and time-consuming operation. The operation has also been criticised because of the risk of venous hypertension in the lower limbs and an increased need for fasciotomy.[92] In one study 4.5% of the patients required a fasciotomy within 30 days of the operation.[93]

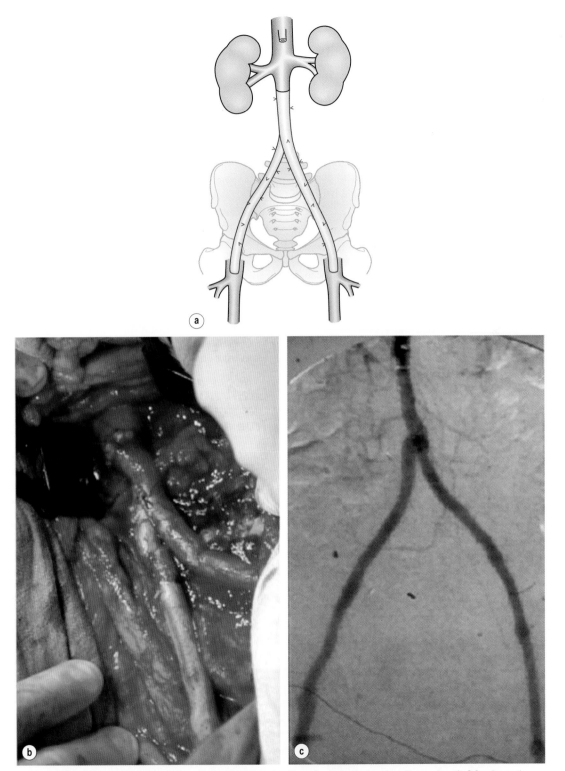

Figure 7.12 • The reversed Y technique for in situ reconstruction of an infected aorto-bifemoral graft: **(a)** schematic drawing; **(b)** perioperative view; **(c)** postoperative angiography.

As an alternative to the aortic in situ reconstruction with the superficial femoral veins, allogeneic vessel transplants might be used (**Fig. 7.13**). Depending upon availability, one might use a fresh homograft or a cryopreserved one. We have almost exclusively used cryopreserved ones from the German Transplant Donor Organisation (DSO).

As we rarely get any homografts as aortic bifurcations, the thoracic aorta is more often provided. In such a case, we conduct a new bifurcation (**Fig. 7.13**a), as when the first polyester grafts were produced. The homograft is often larger in diameter than the aorta, but by using a purse-string technique an appropriate anastomosis can be fashioned. It is wise to check for bleeding along the suture line before the graft is being tunnelled. Furthermore, the length is more appropriate when the allograft is stressed with arterial pressure. If the section from the renal arteries to the femoral junction is to be replaced, it might not always suffice lengthwise with an allograft and then it is possible to extend with saphenous vein segments or a part of an artery that has been thromboendarterectomised (**Fig. 7.13**b).

The role of endovascular reconstruction in graft infection, and particularly infrarenal aortic graft infection, seems limited.

Endovascular repair is often successful in the short term, achieving favourable immediate outcome. In the presence of systemic infection, however, EVAR alone as an ultimate solution is often followed by repeat infection and bleeding.[94] A staged combination of EVAR treatment for acute bleeding and aggressive infection treatment with systemic and local antibiotics, surgical abscess revision and fistula tract closure might be an option in fragile patients. For patients fit for open repair, EVAR can be used as a bridging procedure to definitive repair, particularly in the setting of systemic infection.[95]

Endograft infection occurs in less than 1% of endovascular grafts implanted[96–100] (**Fig. 7.14**). Approximately one-third of patients present with evidence of an aortoenteric fistula (although less than half of these present with gastrointestinal haemorrhage), one-third present with non-specific signs of low-grade sepsis (malaise, weight loss) and the remainder with

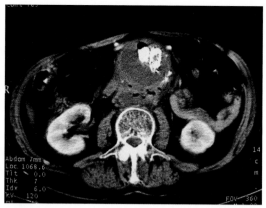

Figure 7.14 • CT scan demonstrating gas bubbles inside the aneurysm sac following EVAR with concomitant retroaortic abscess formation.

evidence of severe systemic sepsis.[99] Mortality was 18% overall, 36.4% after conservative treatment and 14% after surgical treatment. Mortality was 16% after surgical treatment with extra-anatomical bypass versus 5.8% for surgical treatment with in situ reconstruction.[98,100,101]

Graft aneurysms

True aneurysms

Following repair of a true aneurysm, the adjacent artery may also become aneurysmal. Aneurysms were frequent within some early PTFE grafts but manufacturing improvements have almost eliminated this. Biological grafts such as the human umbilical vein graft frequently became aneurysmal before the addition of a Dacron wrap.[102] Xenografts such as bovine mesenteric vein and cryopreserved venous or arterial allografts are particularly subject to aneurysmal degeneration.[82,85] Dacron undergoes late degradation and dilatation, which becomes clinically significant in 2–3% of the cases. After 5–10 years, disruption can occur at points of stress (e.g. under the inguinal ligament)

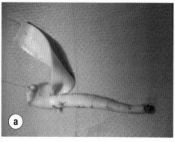
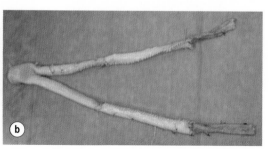

Figure 7.13 • Cryopreserved allograft from thoracic aorta: (**a**) suturing a new bifurcation; (**b**) peripheral extension with thrombendarterectomised superficial femoral arteries.

causing false aneurysms,[103] which may present with haemorrhage or thrombosis. Distraction during shoulder abduction may cause spontaneous rupture or axillary anastomotic disruption of PTFE axillofemoral grafts.[104] Vein graft aneurysms are rare but are more frequent in bypasses for popliteal aneurysms than for occlusive disease (perhaps as part of a systemic disease process).[105] Information on the natural history of untreated graft aneurysms is lacking but repair is generally recommended and is essential to prevent rupture, thrombosis, or embolism. Treatment is either with a covered endovascular stent or by graft replacement.

False aneurysms

False aneurysms are essentially pulsating haematomas, which may occur at the arterial puncture site after angiography (or intervention), following intra-arterial injection by intravenous drug users (IVDU), after trauma (usually penetrating), due to primary arterial infection (e.g. salmonella and HIV) and at disrupted arterial anastomoses. Puncture-site aneurysms often thrombose spontaneously.

✓✓ Although limited, the present evidence appears to support the use of thrombin injection as an effective treatment for femoral pseudoaneurysm. This has been done when the aneurysms are 2 cm or larger. The prerequisite though is that there is a compressible neck and that the thrombin is not spilled over into the distal arterial circulation. A pragmatic approach may be to use compression (blind or ultrasound-guided) as first-line treatment, reserving thrombin injection for those in whom the compression procedure fails.[106]

Some pseudoaneurysms that are small may thrombose on their own but at the moment there are few data to inform what size of pseudoaneurysm will spontaneously thrombose.

Ultrasound-guided compression occludes over 80% and most others will thrombose following thrombin injection.[107] Direct surgical repair or a covered stent are rarely necessary. The management of infected (mycotic) aneurysms is dealt with in Chapter 13.

The incidence of anastomotic aneurysms is increasing, due primarily to the increased frequency of prosthetic vascular reconstructions involving groin anastomosis. The overall incidence following vascular anastomoses is about 2%, but this increases to 3–8% when the anastomosis involves the femoral artery. Although they are most common after prosthetic bypass, anastomotic aneurysms occasionally occur after vein bypass, semi-closed endarterectomy, and open endarterectomy with a vein patch. Anastomotic aneurysms can occur anywhere, but they frequently develop near to a joint. About 80% occur at the groin, presumably due to movement-related strains.[108]

Aortic anastomotic aneurysms are not easily discovered by clinical examination, but when followed by CT, the incidence may be as high as 4%.[109] Some feel this justifies the need for life-long follow-up after aortic reconstruction,[110] but many patients who develop an aneurysm above a previous aortic graft never come to revision because they are too old or the repair is too complex (involving the renal/visceral arteries).

Anastomotic aneurysms at the femoral level are best handled by open surgery and graft interposition,[110] although there are anecdotal reports of endovascular reconstruction.[111] The treatment of choice for iliac anastomotic aneurysms is now stent graft placement by the groin (**Fig. 7.15**). The procedure can be done under local anaesthesia and mortality and morbidity is minimal. Late complications include endoleak and occlusion in a minority of the cases.[112,113] Preoperative embolisation of the internal iliac artery is frequently required, which may lead to gluteal claudication[114] and other pelvic complications (see Chapter 13).

Graft interposition for aortic anastomotic aneurysms is done by laparotomy or, preferentially, retroperitoneal approach. It is, however, associated with a higher surgical risk than a primary vascular operation: perioperative mortality in the elective setting ranges from 0% to 17% and is definitely higher than 50% in the case of rupture.[115,116]

✓ Endovascular reconstruction is actually preferred if the patient has a suitable morphology (Fig. 7.16).[117–122] A comparative study confirmed reduced blood loss, procedural time and a shorter hospital stay in the endovascular group. The operative mortality was 19% in the surgical group versus 10% in the endovascular series.[123]
A recently published study demonstrated that endovascular repair of para-anastomotic aortic and iliac aneurysms after initial prosthetic aortic surgery is safe and durable in patients with an appropriate anatomy. The long-term follow-up demonstrated that fewer complications occurred after procedures with bifurcated stent grafts compared with procedures with tube grafts, aorto-uni-iliac, or iliac extension stent grafts.[124] Although a tubular stent graft from a technical point of view can exclude most of these aneurysms from the circulation, there are indications that a bifurcated stent graft might be more effective at mid-term follow-up.[125]

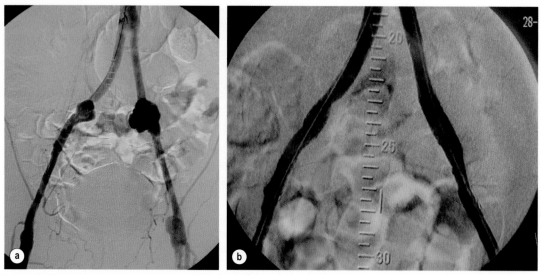

Figure 7.15 • Preoperative angiography with bilateral para-anastomotic iliac artery false aneurysm: **(a)** preoperative angiography; **(b)** angiography after placement of tubular endoprostheses.

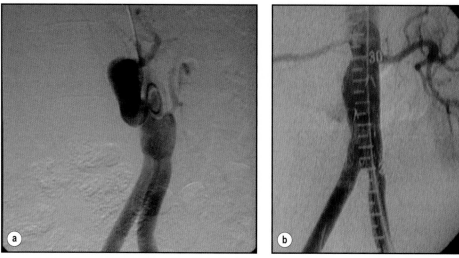

Figure 7.16 • Preoperative angiography with para-anastomotic false aneurysm in aortal localisation after interval of 4 years: **(a)** preoperative angiography; **(b)** angiography after placement of tubular endoprosthesis.

Carotid artery

Infection

Revision of the carotid artery surgery is either required postoperatively during the first 48–72 hours due to acute bleeding, emboli or thrombosis leading to hemispheric symptoms. These complications are extensively dealt with in Chapter 10 and will not be focused on here. During follow-up, the risk for patch infection is generally <1%[126,127] and is highest when foreign material has been used (**Fig. 7.17**). The patient normally presents with neck swelling

or a sinus with a positive bacterial isolate. In cases of infection carotid surgery should be performed under general anaesthesia because surgery is more extensive. Frequently the scar tissue is so dense that one may not be able to have the external carotid artery dissected free but a balloon is necessary to occlude it. In order to gain full access to the healthy part of the internal carotid artery it might be wise to use the Pruitt–Inahara shunt to prevent back bleeding from the internal carotid artery and thus secure the perfusion of the brain early in the operation. A further advantage of the shunt is that it permits access to an extra 1 cm of the carotid to use

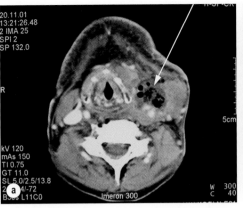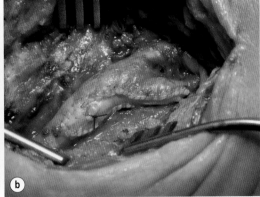

Figure 7.17 • Infection following CEA with patch: **(a)** CT scan; **(b)** situs intraoperatively with vein patch.

for the patch because a carotid clamp is not needed. We normally shift from polyester to a saphenous vein patch from the groin rather than the ankle.[128]

Stents or stent grafts do not seem to play any definite role in the treatment of carotid artery infection, but may play a bridging role to temporarily stop bleeding.

Aneurysm formation

The carotid artery aneurysm after carotid endarterectomy (CEA) that is most frequently encountered is usually due to a 'low-grade' infection or pseudoaneurysm (**Fig. 7.18**). Owing to the turbulent flow, it is recommended that these aneurysms are operated upon when they have reached a 2 cm diameter or if they have been producing symptoms. The surgical exposure technique does not differ from the one using standard CEA but it might be necessary to resect the artery and use a venous interposition graft instead. There are few data on the use of carotid artery stenting (CAS) to treat aneurysm formation after CEA but it may be possible with covered stents if surgery for some reason should not be possible.

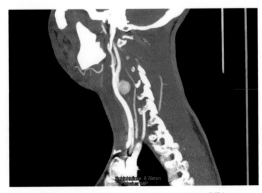

Figure 7.18 • Carotid artery aneurysm after CEA.

Revision after CAS

The risk for complications might be higher when doing CEA after CAS for occlusive disease and especially if longer segments have been stented. The operative treatment should therefore generally be reserved for patients that are neurologically symptomatic. The surgical exposure is as per the standard one as described in detail in Chapter 10. The dissection of the common and carotid artery, though, is often more difficult as there is often considerable inflammation around the stented artery. Should the stent penetrate the arterial wall, it is often necessary to insert an interposition graft instead of doing a thrombendarterectomy (**Fig. 7.19**).

Revision surgery after EVAR

EVAR is associated with a significant risk of late complications, which may occur at a rate of 5–10% per annum. Endoleaks are the most frequent complication and are described in more detail in Chapter 13. Most complications can be treated by endovascular re-intervention, if necessary.[129] Surgical techniques such as laparoscopic clipping of the side branches and remodelling of the aneurysm have not attracted much enthusiasm (see Fig. 7.12).[130,131] Open surgery, on the other hand, is a good alternative to endovascular interventions for iliac limb thrombosis with graft thrombectomy or femorofemoral crossover grafting.[129]

✔ A recently published review revealed that the rate of early conversion (from EVAR to open surgery) ranged from 0.8% to 5.9%; the latest studies carried lower rates of early conversion. Mortality rates of early conversion varied between 0% and 28.5%, with an average mortality of 12.4%. The rates of late conversion ranged from 0.4% to 22% with a total average of 1.9%; the mortality rate was 10%.[132]

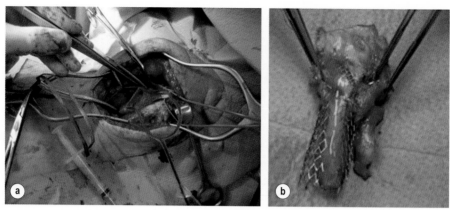

Figure 7.19 • CEA after CAS: **(a)** situs intraoperatively; **(b)** specimen following thrombendarterectomy.

Although the operation is more challenging, open conversion is essentially performed according to the principles used in primary aneurysm surgery. Dissection of the proximal infrarenal aortic neck might be more difficult because of periaortic inflammation caused by the stent graft. Suprarenal and preferably supracoeliac clamping is frequently required, particularly in stent grafts with suprarenal fixation. Endografts with infrarenal fixation are easily removed once the aneurysm sac has been opened and the aorta is clamped below the renal arteries. In grafts with suprarenal fixation, particularly in those with hooks and barbs, it might be wise to leave the suprarenal portion in place and to amputate the infrarenal portion of the endoprosthesis by cutting the metal frame of the suprarenal attachment system.[133] The suprarenal fixation system is then incorporated into the proximal anastomosis, which is performed under supracoeliac aortic clamping. By preference, the graft should be removed completely. In the usual case of a bifurcation graft this means that the iliac arteries have to be dissected and that the external and internal iliac arteries have to be clamped selectively in order to perform a reconstruction to the iliac bifurcation.

Although it is understood that conversion is associated with increased risk of mortality and morbidity, different teams have reported a 0% mortality rate for elective late conversion. Mortality rates for early conversion range from 7% to 25%, rising to 40% in patients with a ruptured abdominal aortic aneurysm (AAA) post EVAR.[134–136]

Revision surgery after infected EVAR

EVAR as a primary treatment modality for AAA is associated with a low risk of endograft infection, of between 0.4% and 3%.[97,98,101,137,138] However, this does confer a very significant postoperative mortality, as high as 40%, comparable to infection of open aortic grafts.[139–141] Explantation is the only technique that can potentially result in cure of an aortic stent graft infection.[139] Preservation of the stent graft followed by appropriate antibiotic therapy and percutaneous drainage or surgical debridement has been described as an alternative treatment in selected high-risk patients who are unfit for extensive open repair.[96,141] A recently published extensive electronic health database search documented an overall mortality of 45% at 11.4 months. Patients with aortoenteric fistula have the worst outcome and there was evidence for lower mortality in patients who undergo an additional procedure, such as drainage, surgical debridement, sac irrigation and/or omentoplasty. The authors concluded that surgical debridement or CT-guided percutaneous drainage followed by appropriate antibiotic therapy should be reserved for physically capable patients who are, however, poor candidates for major aortic reconstructive surgery.[142]

Revision after TEVAR

Although most of the complications after thoracic endovascular aortic repair (TEVAR) are confined to endoleaks or migration of the stent graft, which may be dealt with endovascularly (see Chapter 14), there are some situations that are more complicated and these are aortobronchial fistula, aorto-oesophageal fistula and stent graft infection.

Aortobronchial fistula

Aortobronchial fistula after TEVAR is rare. Statistically robust data are not available, but according to a national survey of 1113 TEVARs, there appears to be a less than 2% rate when combined with aorto-oesophageal fistula.[143] Analysis of an international multicentre registry (European Registry of Endovascular Aortic Repair Complications) between 2001 and 2012 with a total caseload of 4680 TEVAR procedures (14 centres) revealed a prevalence of either central airway (aortobronchial) or pulmonary parenchymal (aortopulmonary) fistulation (ABPF) in the entire cohort after TEVAR in the study period was 0.56% (central airway 58%, peripheral parenchymal 42%) The incidence was 0.40/1000 interventions/year (range: 0.08–2.36).[144]

The symptoms prior to presentation with haemoptysis and a frank fistula are usually vague. The typical patient will have some episodes of minor bleeding before the major one and the diagnosis is therefore often delayed.

Although a bronchoscopy might theoretically show the graft, sometimes the fistula is more peripheral in the lung tissue.

A new stent graft might serve as a bridge solution to get the patient into a stable position, but the more radical solution with open surgery and replacement by a standard graft or an allograft is most likely a more long-lasting solution. In case of a new prosthetic graft, long-term therapy with antibiotics is needed. We prefer to use an allograft instead, if time allows (Fig 7.20).

Aorto-oesophageal fistula

The stent graft and its hooks or bare stent may penetrate the oesophagus due to mechanical reasons, but an aorto-oesophageal fistula (AEF) might also appear even in patients where the stent graft is not in contact with the oesophagus. Aorto-oesophageal arterial branches might be occluded by the stent graft, thereby leading to an ischaemic necrosis. TEVAR could serve as a bridge to surgery for emergency cases of AEF only, with definitive open surgical correction of the fistula undertaken as soon as possible.[145] In addition to the aforementioned principles for the aorta, it is needed to resect the oesophagus and later perform a new gastro-oesophageal anastomosis for restoring the normal tract.

Infection

Stent graft infection occurs in 0.2–3% of endovascular grafts implanted.[80,99] The infected stent graft is a challenge where the definite treatment is normally

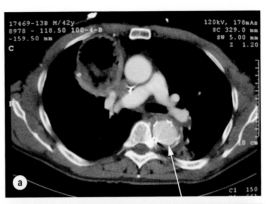
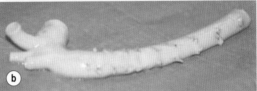
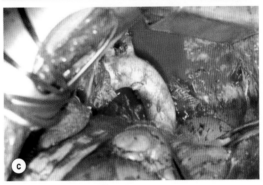

Figure 7.20 • Infection following TEVAR in case of traumatic transection 4 years before: **(a)** CT scan; **(b)** cryopreserved thoracic allograft; **(c)** thoracic aortic reconstruction with allograft.

containing explantation of the stent graft. Although the antibiotic therapy over a long time might be an alternative for 'no surgery candidates', it might withhold the infection but rarely eradicates it. As for several of the thoracic entities, there are no robust data but more case reports on one or some cases.[100]

Allografts do seem to be a good choice if available, otherwise a polyester graft soaked in rifampicin is used.

Key points

- Late graft occlusion is caused by intimal hyperplasia or progression of atherosclerosis of the inflow or outflow.
- Graft stenoses occur in 20–30% of infrainguinal vein grafts. Symptomatic stenoses require treatment. Angioplasty offers excellent early results. In the long term, open surgery is probably better.

- Thrombolysis of occluded infrainguinal grafts may be attempted in patients aged under 80 years with critical ischaemia provided that limb viability is not severely threatened, that the patient has not undergone surgery within 3 months and that the occlusion is less than 14 days old. For vein grafts this time period is shortened to 24-48 hours as the endothelium gets destroyed after a longer period of time.
- Graft infection results from a breakdown of sterility at surgery, by extension from a superficial wound infection or from blood-borne bacteria.
- Prosthetic graft infections cause perigraft abscesses, sinuses and anastomotic haemorrhage, including aortoenteric fistula and erosion. Vein grafts may be eroded by infection, particularly in open wounds.
- *Staphylococcus epidermidis* is the most frequent cause of low-grade infection. *Staphylococcus aureus* and Gram-negative infections tend to present early and are more virulent. The incidence of MRSA infection is increasing.
- Any fluid around a graft after 3 months or gas beyond 4–7 weeks on CT or ultrasound suggests infection. Aspiration or perigraft fluid pus can usually secure the diagnosis.
- Conservative measures, such as prolonged antibiotic therapy, drainage and irrigation, or covering exposed grafts with muscle or omental flaps, are rarely curative. The same goes for partial graft excision.
- Simple graft excision without revascularisation usually causes severe ischaemia leading to amputation or death.
- Extra-anatomical revascularisation has been the gold standard in the past. In situ revascularisation with autologous vein (e.g. femoral vein) has better patency and recurrent infection is rare. Arterial allografts are an alternative. In situ reconstruction with silver-bonded or rifampicin-bonded Dacron grafts is still semi-experimental.
- Endoprostheses can buy time in case of bleeding aortoduodenal fistula but recurrence of infection is high.
- True aneurysms can occur within prosthetic or vein grafts or adjacent to previous aneurysms.
- False aneurysms may result from anastomotic distraction or infection. Treatment of femoral false aneurysms is surgical. Endovascular treatment offers an excellent alternative in case of non-infected iliac or aortic false aneurysms.
- Surgical conversion is rarely needed after endovascular treatment of abdominal aortic aneurysms. If necessary, surgery can be performed with excellent results.

▶ Recommended video

- Carotid endarterectomy – https://vimeo.com/14521575

🌐 Full references available at **http://expertconsult.inkling.com**

Key references

16. Moody AP, Edwards PR, Harris PL. In situ versus reversed femoropopliteal vein grafts: long-term follow-up of a prospective, randomized trial. Br J Surg 1992;79:750–2. PMID: 1393459.

17. Wengerter KR, Veith FJ, Gupta SK, et al. Prospective randomized multicenter comparison of in situ and reversed vein infrapopliteal bypasses. J Vasc Surg 1991;13:189–97; discussion 97–9. PMID: 1990160.

18. Albers M, Romiti M, Brochado-Neto FC, et al. Meta-analysis of popliteal-to-distal vein bypass grafts for critical ischemia. J Vasc Surg 2006;43:498–503. PMID: 16520163.

22. Twine CP, McLain AD. Graft type for femoro-popliteal bypass surgery. Cochrane Database Syst Rev 2010; CD001487. PMID: 20464717.

37. Brown J, Lethaby A, Maxwell H, et al. Antiplatelet agents for preventing thrombosis after peripheral arterial bypass surgery. Cochrane Database Syst Rev 2008; CD000535. PMID: 18843671.

38. Dutch BOA trial. Efficacy of oral anticoagulants compared with aspirin after infrainguinal bypass surgery (The Dutch Bypass Oral Anticoagulants or

Aspirin Study): a randomised trial. Lancet 2000; 355:346–51. PMID: 10665553.

39. Belch JJ, Dormandy J, Biasi GM, et al. Results of the randomized, placebo-controlled clopidogrel and acetylsalicylic acid in bypass surgery for peripheral arterial disease (CASPAR) trial. J Vasc Surg 2010;52:825–33 33 e1-2. PMID: 20678878.

40. Golledge J, Beattie DK, Greenhalgh RM, et al. Have the results of infrainguinal bypass improved with the widespread utilisation of postoperative surveillance? Eur J Vasc Endovasc Surg 1996;11:388–92. PMID: 8846169.

41. Davies AH, Hawdon AJ, Sydes MR, et al. Is duplex surveillance of value after leg vein bypass grafting? Principal results of the Vein Graft Surveillance Randomised Trial (VGST). Circulation 2005;112:1985–91. PMID: 16186435.

50. Dake MD, Ansel GM, Jaff MR, et al. Paclitaxel-eluting stents show superiority to balloon angioplasty and bare metal stents in femoropopliteal disease: twelve-month Zilver PTX randomized study results. Circ Cardiovasc Interv 2011;4:495–504. PMID: 21953370.

51. Dake MD, Ansel GM, Jaff MR, et al. Durable clinical effectiveness with paclitaxel-eluting stents in the femoropopliteal artery: 5-year results of the Zilver PTX randomized trial. Circulation 2016;133:1472–83; discussion 83. PMID: 26969758.

52. Dake MD, Ansel GM, Jaff MR, et al. Sustained safety and effectiveness of paclitaxel-eluting stents for femoropopliteal lesions: 2-year follow-up from the Zilver PTX randomized and single-arm clinical studies. J Am Coll Cardiol 2013;61:2417–27. PMID: 23583245.

70. Stewart A, Eyers PS, Earnshaw JJ. Prevention of infection in arterial reconstruction. Cochrane Database Syst Rev 2006;3:CD003073. PMID: 16855996.

71. Gao H, Sandermann J, Prag J, et al. Prevention of primary vascular graft infection with silver-coated polyester graft in a porcine model. Eur J Vasc Endovasc Surg 2010;39:472–7. PMID: 20060756.

72. Larena-Avellaneda A, Russmann S, Fein M, et al. Prophylactic use of the silver-acetate-coated graft in arterial occlusive disease: a retrospective, comparative study. J Vasc Surg 2009;50:790–8. PMID: 19660894.

73. Webster J, Osborne S. Preoperative bathing or showering with skin antiseptics to prevent surgical site infection. Cochrane Database Syst Rev 2007; CD004985. PMID: 17943905.

83. O'Connor S, Andrew P, Batt M, et al. A systematic review and meta-analysis of treatments for aortic graft infection. J Vasc Surg 2006;44:38–45. PMID: 16828424.

8

Management of acute lower limb ischaemia

Lucinda Frank

Robert J. Hinchliffe

Introduction

✓✓ The revised (2007) TASC Inter-Society Consensus defines acute leg ischaemia (ALI) as any sudden decrease in limb perfusion causing a potential threat to limb viability.[1]

Presentation is usually less than 2 weeks' duration. However, some overlap with chronic critical leg ischaemia is inevitable. The severity of ischaemia is best defined according to the SVS/ISCVS guidelines (Table 8.1),[2] which group patients into the following categories:

- I Viable
- IIa Threatened (salvageable if promptly treated)
- IIb Threatened (salvageable if immediately treated)
- III Irreversible

Data on the incidence of acute limb ischaemia are sparse. Epidemiological surveys would suggest that the incidence is in the region of 140 per million of the general population.[1] A study investigating the incidence of hospitalisation for acute limb ischaemia among the US Medicare population has demonstrated that the incidence is decreasing from 45.7 per 100 000 in 1998 to 26.0 per 100 000 in 2009.[3] However, the US Medicare population is not necessarily comparable to the UK population. The Oxford Vascular Study found that the incidence of acute limb ischaemia was 10 per 100 000 per year between 2002 and 2012.[4]

The COhorte des Patients ARTeriopathes (COPART) is a prospective multicentre registry of patients from three academic hospitals in Southwest France. They recorded the reason for referral among patients hospitalised for lower limb peripheral artery disease (PAD) and found that acute limb ischaemia was responsible for 9.3% of hospitalisations compared to chronic limb ischaemia (90.8%).[5]

There is evidence that the outcome is improved when patients are managed by a vascular service providing 24-hour cover.[6] ALI is associated with a high cost to the community because of the risk of amputation (10–30% at 30 days) and prolonged hospitalisation. Costs are minimised and outcome optimised by accurate clinical assessment and an understanding of the available therapeutic options.

Aetiology

ALI is the result of occlusion of a native artery or vascular/endovascular prosthesis. In situ thrombosis or embolism can cause native arterial occlusion (Box 8.1).

Embolism

Until about 30 years ago, embolism was the underlying cause of most cases of ALI. Emboli large enough to occlude major vessels usually arise in the heart. Rheumatic mitral valve disease was the most common cause, with large emboli forming in a dilated left atrium. Atrial fibrillation due to ischaemic heart disease is now the cardiac origin in

Table 8.1 • Suggested classification of acute limb ischaemia

Category	Description	Capillary return	Muscle paralysis	Sensory loss	Doppler signals Arterial	Venous
I Viable	Not immediately threatened	Intact	None	None	Audible	Audible
IIa Threatened	Salvageable if promptly treated	Intact/slow	None	Partial	Inaudible	Audible
IIb Threatened	Salvageable if immediately treated	Slow/absent	Partial	Partial/complete	Inaudible	Audible
III Irreversible	Primary amputation	Absent staining	Complete tense compartment	Complete	Inaudible	Inaudible

Reproduced from Rutherford RB, Flanigan DP, Gupta SK, et al. Suggested standards for reports dealing with lower extremity ischemia. J Vasc Surg 1986;4:80–94, with permission from Society for Vascular Surgery.

Box 8.1 • Aetiology of acute lower limb ischaemia

Thrombosis
* Atherosclerosis
* Popliteal aneurysm
* Bypass graft occlusion
* Endovascular stent or stent graft occlusion
* Iatrogenic (localised arterial dissection post endovascular intervention, e.g. arterial closure device failure)
* Thrombotic conditions

Embolism
* Atrial fibrillation
* Mural thrombosis
* Vegetations
* Proximal aneurysms
* Atherosclerotic plaque

Rare causes
* Dissection
* Trauma (including iatrogenic)
* Illicit drug use
* External compression
* Popliteal entrapment
* Cystic adventitial disease
* Iliac endofibrosis

80% of embolic cases; mural thrombus following acute myocardial infarction causes most of the remainder.[7] Less commonly, embolisation from mural thrombi of the aorta, aortic aneurysms and iliac arteries is observed. Large emboli typically lodge at an arterial bifurcation, particularly in the common femoral or popliteal arteries (**Fig. 8.1**). Patients with cardiac embolism may also suffer from peripheral vascular disease as a result of the underlying process of atherosclerosis. This increases the difficulty in establishing the cause of the ischaemia and in planning revascularisation.

In 20% of patients with ALI, a source for the embolus cannot be found.

Atheroembolism

Less common sources of emboli include proximal aneurysms or atherosclerotic plaques, usually located in the thoracic or abdominal aorta. Whereas cardiac embolism usually consists entirely of platelet thrombus, embolism from proximal arteries can include atherosclerotic plaques or cholesterol-rich emboli. This has a much worse prognosis than cardiac embolism because embolectomy is less effective. Small particles of atheroembolism can pass to very distal vessels in the foot. This digital embolism can result in the 'acute blue toe syndrome'. In this condition, the embolic source should be identified and treated if possible. Often this is a proximal arterial plaque that has ruptured and the emboli are a mixture of platelet thrombus and cholesterol (**Fig. 8.2**). Embolisation of cholesterol-rich atheroma can occur spontaneously, but also follows intravascular manipulation by endovascular intervention, or occasionally surgery (trash foot). This can be disastrous, since both large and small arteries are occluded and cannot be reopened with either surgery or thrombolysis. This often results in limb or end-organ damage, and is sometimes fatal (**Fig. 8.3**).

Thrombosis

In situ thrombosis in a native artery is now the commonest cause of ALI. It may be the result of rupture of an atherosclerotic plaque or critical flow arrest at the site of an atherosclerotic stenosis. The advancing age of the population and the commensurate increase in atherosclerosis have increased the proportion of

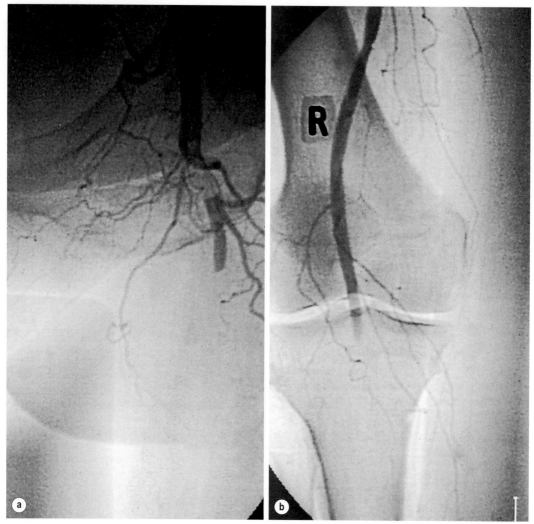

Figure 8.1 • Arteriogram demonstrating an embolus lodged in the bifurcation of the common femoral artery **(a)** with further emboli occluding the distal profunda and popliteal artery **(b)**.

ALI caused by thrombosis. Acute native vessel arterial occlusion may be compounded by surgery (e.g. knee replacement destroying geniculate collateral vessels formed around a popliteal occlusion), heart failure or a thrombotic tendency (polycythaemia, dehydration, malignancy, etc.). Acute thrombosis of a popliteal aneurysm poses the highest risk to the leg. Typically, this occurs in elderly men in association with aneurysms elsewhere (50% have an aortic aneurysm) or generalised arterial ectasia. Popliteal aneurysms usually commence in the above-knee popliteal artery and extend distally to the tibial trifurcation. As they enlarge they can fill with lamellar thrombus, which may cause either acute thrombosis or distal embolisation that occludes the tibial vessels. The latter will place the leg in extreme jeopardy (50% limb loss).

Other causes

The increasing use of both open and endovascular techniques to revascularise ischaemic limbs means that surgeons often have to deal with acute thrombosis of bypass grafts and arteries that have previously undergone endovascular treatment. Grafts occlude for a variety of reasons. Graft occlusion within 1 month of insertion is usually the result of technical problems at the time of surgery or poor distal run-off. Graft occlusion within 1 year of placement is often caused by myointimal hyperplasia at an anastomosis or the development of stenoses within a vein graft. Occlusion after 1 year is usually due to progression of distal atherosclerosis. Prosthetic grafts have a higher occlusion rate than autogenous vein grafts (see Chapters 3 and 7).

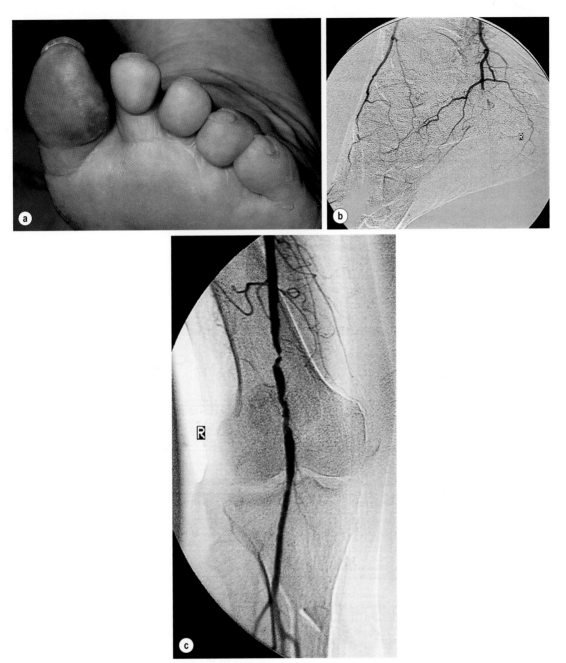

Figure 8.2 • **(a)** 'Blue toe syndrome' due to digital and pedal arterial atheroembolism **(b)** from a proximal atherosclerotic stenosis **(c)**. Note the acute cut-off of the posterior tibial artery. Ultrasonography excluded a popliteal aneurysm and the lesion was treated by balloon angioplasty.

Iliac limb occlusions are observed after aorto-bifemoral bypass surgery if limbs become kinked or have poor outflow. Endovascular stent grafts used to repair abdominal aortic aneurysms (EVAR) have similar modes of failure. Occlusion is more common when the iliac limb of the stent graft is extended in to the external iliac artery. Occlusion may occur any time after implantation in up to 5% of patients.[8]

A special group of iatrogenic occlusion of external iliac and femoral vessels is related to the maldeployment or failure of arterial closure devices. These achieve closure of arteries after endovascular intervention using percutaneously delivered sutures or plugs. Inadvertently they can cause arrest of flow through direct closure or stenosis of the artery, or by dissection of the

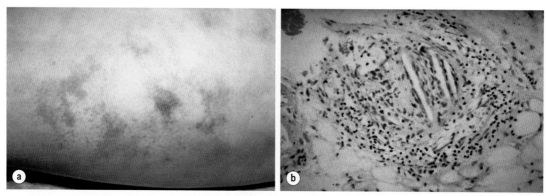

Figure 8.3 • Livedo reticularis **(a)** caused by cholesterol embolism **(b)**.

vessel. Presentation is usually in the early post-intervention period but may be delayed.

Spontaneous native arterial thrombosis occasionally occurs without an underlying flow-limiting stenosis and these patients should be investigated for an intrinsic clotting abnormality/thrombophilia, e.g. antiphospholipid syndrome, activated protein C deficiency or malignancy.

Occasionally, acute arterial occlusion may be due to arterial dissection, trauma, extrinsic compression or illicit drug use (cocaine and 'crack' cocaine). In a young patient with acute popliteal artery occlusion, either popliteal entrapment or cystic adventitial disease should be considered (see Chapter 2 on chronic limb ischaemia).

Recent changes

A number of factors may have changed the presentation of ALI. For example, many patients are now treated with risk factor-modifying drugs such as antiplatelet therapy and statins. Antiplatelet therapy probably reduces the risk of limb deterioration and the need for limb revascularisation in those patients with established PAD.[9] It is not yet clear whether this has had an effect on the incidence of ALI. Similarly, patients with atrial fibrillation are now assessed using the CHA2DS2-VASc risk score to establish their future risk of stroke. Patients with non-valvular AF with a score of ≥2 should be anticoagulated using warfarin or a novel oral anticoagulant (NOAC) to reduce their future risk of stroke. The CHA2DS2-VASc is better at identifying truly low-risk patients with AF who do not require anticoagulation and is at least as good as the previously used CHAD2 score in identifying patients who develop strokes and thromboembolism.[10] The long-term effect of more patients being formally anticoagulated on the incidence and presentation of acute limb ischaemia has yet to be demonstrated.

A randomised double-blind placebo-controlled trial evaluating Vorapaxar used acute limb ischaemia as one of the endpoints. They found that in selected patients with symptomatic PAD without atrial fibrillation Vorapaxar reduced the incidence of acute limb ischaemia regardless of the cause. With further research this protease-activated receptor 1 antagonist could be used to reduce the risk of acute limb ischaemia in patients with known PAD.[11]

Clinical features

The severity of ischaemia at presentation is the most important factor affecting outcome of the leg.[12,13] Complete occlusion of a proximal artery in the absence of preformed collateral vessels (as in cardiac embolism) results in the classical clinical presentation of pain, paralysis, paraesthesia, pallor, pulselessness and a perishingly cold leg. The pain is severe and frequently resistant to analgesia. Calf pain and tenderness with a tense muscle compartment indicates severe muscle ischaemia or necrosis and often irreversible ischaemia. Sensorimotor deficit including muscle paralysis and paraesthesia is indicative of muscle and nerve ischaemia with the potential for salvage if treated promptly. Initially the leg is white with empty veins but after 6–12 hours vasodilatation occurs, probably caused by hypoxia of the smooth muscle. The capillaries then fill with stagnant deoxygenated blood, resulting in a mottled appearance that blanches on digital pressure (**Fig. 8.4**). If flow is not restored rapidly, the arteries distal to the occlusion fill with propagated thrombus and the capillaries rupture, resulting in a fixed blue staining of the skin that is a sign of irreversible ischaemia. These features are typical of an acute arterial occlusion in the absence of existing collaterals and suggest an embolic cause. When arterial occlusion occurs as part of a chronic process where collaterals have developed (in patients with pre-existing PAD), typically the leg is less severely

Figure 8.4 • Clinical outcome after acute leg ischaemia.

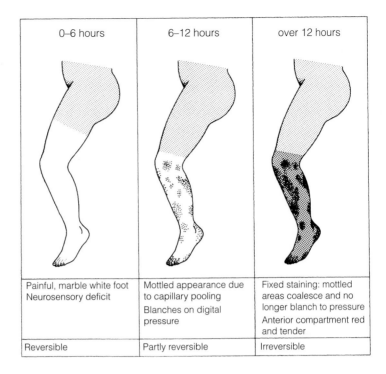

0–6 hours	6–12 hours	over 12 hours
Painful, marble white foot Neurosensory deficit	Mottled appearance due to capillary pooling Blanches on digital pressure	Fixed staining: mottled areas coalesce and no longer blanch to pressure Anterior compartment red and tender
Reversible	Partly reversible	Irreversible

ischaemic. Patients with peripheral atherosclerosis deteriorate in a stepwise fashion as thrombosis supervenes on an existing arterial plaque. Patients often report a sudden change in symptoms, which progress over a few days: the foot often has a dusky hue with slow capillary return. Previous claudication or absent pulses in the contralateral foot help make a clinical diagnosis of in situ thrombosis. Palpation of a mass in either popliteal fossa suggests thrombosis of a popliteal aneurysm. Young patients (<50 years), those with an atypical history (e.g. severe back pain associated with aortic dissection) or recent endovascular intervention raise the possibility of non-atherosclerotic/embolic ALI.

Initial management

Patients presenting with ALI are often in poor general health, which contributes to the observed high mortality rate from associated cardiovascular disease. Dehydration, cardiac failure, hypoxia and pain should all be managed in the standard way. An intravenous infusion is required for rehydration and is also often the best means of providing analgesia with an infusion pump. If thrombolysis is an option, intramuscular analgesia should be avoided because of the risk of bleeding. Intravenous calcium heparin (5000 units) should be given immediately, followed by systemic heparinisation, principally to restrict propagation of thrombus, although there is also evidence that it improves the prognosis.[14] In many units low-molecular-weight heparins have

replaced calcium heparin because of their more reliable effect on anticoagulation. Anticoagulation should be delayed if the patient is likely to need epidural anaesthesia. The short half-life of the latter, however, is helpful in this situation. In order to improve oxygenation, 24% oxygen should be given by face mask.

Venous blood should be taken for full blood count, urea, electrolytes and glucose. An electrocardiogram (ECG) and chest radiograph may be of value in diagnosing and managing cardiac arrhythmias and heart failure. If a primary thrombotic tendency is suspected, investigation of this should be delayed as the diagnostic tests are inaccurate in the face of fresh thrombus.

Revascularisation

The clinical assessment of the severity of limb ischaemia will largely dictate the most appropriate form of therapy (**Fig. 8.5**).

Irreversible (category III) leg ischaemia

A small number of patients will present in a moribund state or with irreversible leg ischaemia (muscle paralysis, tense swollen fascial compartments, fixed skin staining) and terminal care should be considered. For the irreversibly ischaemic leg,

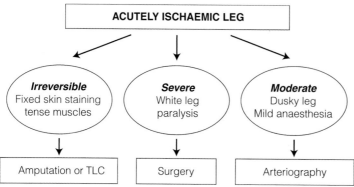

Figure 8.5 • Clinical approach to the management of the acutely ischaemic leg.

revascularisation is, by definition, inappropriate and may be dangerous. This includes the patient who develops ALI while being treated for another condition, usually as an inpatient on an elderly care ward. Prognosis is particularly dismal in this group.[15] Surviving patients should be resuscitated and stabilised before considering amputation.

Immediately threatened (category IIb ischaemia)

The acute white leg with sensorimotor deficit requires urgent intervention to prevent limb loss. Although the differentiation between thrombosis and embolus is often difficult, it is in this group of patients that embolism is more likely. An acute white leg with no prior history of claudication, normal contralateral pulses and a probable embolic source, such as atrial fibrillation, would indicate that embolisation is the likely cause. Urgent surgery is indicated in these patients, after resuscitation. Thrombolysis is often inappropriate, given the potential delay in revascularisation; however, Byrne et al. found that patients with an immediately threatened limb did not fare worse when treated with thrombolysis, suggesting that thrombolysis may have a role in treating patients who are at high risk from operative intervention.[16] Imaging may help guide revascularisation but should not be allowed to delay revascularisation. Many vascular and trauma centres now have rapid access to computed tomography (CT) angiography, which is a useful investigation, especially when the femoral pulse is absent and alternative diagnoses such as aortic dissection are possible. An alternative approach is to perform on-table angiography at the same time as groin exploration. Duplex ultrasound imaging is often unhelpful because of the low-flow state in the limb arteries and the need for expert interpretation in the emergency setting.

Both groins and lower limbs should be prepared in theatre. If inflow cannot be re-established into the groin then a femoral crossover graft can be inserted (or aortic dissection managed according to Chapter 9).

Threatened (category IIa ischaemia)/viable (category I ischaemia)

The majority of patients presenting with ALI have acute onset of rest pain but no paralysis and no, or only mild, sensory loss. The cause is often acute thrombosis of either an atherosclerotic artery or graft. Because the leg is not immediately threatened, time is available to plan appropriate intervention after investigation. Conventionally, acute leg ischaemia was investigated using catheter angiography (**Fig. 8.6**). The advantage was that imaging could be followed by therapeutic thrombolysis at the same sitting. There are now, however, non-invasive alternatives such as duplex imaging CT and MR angiography, both of which can provide enough information on which to plan intervention. The method of investigation will depend on the time of presentation and the available facilities. The two main alternatives in these patients are intervention with surgery or percutaneous thrombolysis. Thromboembolectomy is unlikely to reopen an artery occluded by thrombus and atherosclerotic plaque; formal arterial bypass is more likely to be needed. Nationwide registries suggest that surgical revascularisation is used three to five times more frequently than thrombolysis in everyday clinical practice for patients with ALI.[17] Logistics (multiple angiographies) and experience may account in part for this distribution.

Thrombolysis is arguably less invasive than revascularisation surgery. It has the capacity to open small as well as large arteries. It may also uncover the cause of the in situ thrombosis, such as an arterial stenosis, which can be treated by angioplasty to produce a lasting outcome.

Figure 8.6 • Treatment pathways following arteriography.

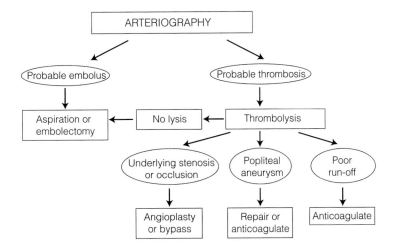

Some patients are admitted to hospital with acute thrombosis of a peripheral artery (usually the superficial femoral) but have only claudication and no ischaemic pain at rest. Thrombolysis might appear an attractive option to treat the claudication, but the risks are as high as in patients with limb-threatening ischaemia.[18] Initial anticoagulation followed by expectant management, depending on the progression of ischaemia, reduces the risk to both life and limb.[15] Some patients' symptoms improve and never require revascularisation. In others (especially those with short-distance claudication) it may be more appropriate to angioplasty the occluded arterial segment 6–12 weeks after the acute event, when the thrombus has organised and embolic risk is reduced.

Choice between surgery and thrombolysis: the evidence

There remains considerable controversy about the individual roles of surgery and thrombolysis for ALI. A summary of the available evidence in 2016 critically evaluated 26 studies, 4 of which were randomised prospective clinical trials. The authors concluded that thrombolysis was effective for limb salvage and safer in the short term than urgent open revascularisation.[19]

✔✔ Between 1994 and 1996 three randomised studies compared the effectiveness of thrombolysis with operative intervention.[20–25] The New York study was the first to show that thrombolysis improves survival in patients with limb-threatening ischaemia of less than 14 days.[20] This study was small and the advantage was due to the high incidence of cardiorespiratory deaths following emergency surgery. The STILE study was much larger and

included patients with ischaemia for longer than 14 days.[20] This study has been much criticised because of the failure to insert a catheter successfully for peripheral thrombolysis in one-third of cases. The study introduced the concept of amputation-free survival but failed to show any significant improvement in this primary endpoint between the treatment groups. In the subgroup of patients with ischaemia for fewer than 14 days, thrombolysis reduced the rate of amputation. Subsequent analysis of patients from this study up to 1 year revealed that thrombolysis was a better initial treatment for graft occlusions, whereas surgery was more effective and durable for native vessel occlusions.[22,23] However, few of the patients in the STILE study had critical ischaemia. The TOPAS trial was designed, using lessons learned from the above studies, to try to settle this debate. In the first phase, an optimal dose of thrombolytic therapy was selected (urokinase 4000 IU/hour)[24] and in phase II this was compared with urgent surgery in 544 patients.[25] Amputation-free survival was similar in both groups at 6 months and 1 year (72% and 65% for urokinase vs 75% and 70% for surgery, respectively), though thrombolysis reduced the need for open surgical procedures.

Since these trials a number of retrospective studies have compared the effectiveness of contemporary thrombolysis with surgery. Taha et al. concluded that operative intervention as an initial treatment had improved technical success in Rutherford II ischaemia, especially when caused by a failed stent or bypass.[26] This was at the expense of a higher mortality rate compared with endovascular treatment without any added advantage in patency or limb salvage at 30 days and 1 year. The decision between surgery and thrombolysis should therefore be made on an individual basis, taking into account the class of ischaemia, aetiology and the patient's comorbidities.[26]

Peripheral artery thrombolysis

Thrombus dissolution is achieved by stimulating the conversion of fibrin-bound plasminogen into the active enzyme plasmin. Plasmin is a non-specific protease capable of degrading fibrin and producing thrombus dissolution.

In contrast to the thrombolytic treatment of acute myocardial infarction, systemic infusion of thrombolytic agents for ALI results in a poor success rate and unacceptable complications. By selectively placing a catheter within the thrombus via the percutaneous route and delivering the thrombolytic agent locally, the concentration of agent is maximised and plasmin is less likely to be neutralised by circulating antiplasmins. The dose of thrombolytic agent can be optimised to the minimum level that results in a local effect without producing systemic thrombolysis and the attendant complications.

Contraindications (Box 8.2)

Perhaps the only absolute contraindication to lysis is active internal bleeding. Most other contraindications are relative, where the risk of complications from thrombolysis must be weighed against the potential benefits of limb salvage. The elderly (>80 years) are at particularly high risk of bleeding complications. It is unwise to consider thrombolysis within 2 weeks of surgery or within 2 months of a stroke. Dacron grafts may take 3 months to seal, and if they do not become fully incorporated they may become porous if thrombolytic therapy is employed. Care should be exercised when using thrombolysis to open Dacron grafts within the abdomen where manual compression is not possible should bleeding occur. The presence of cardiac thrombus theoretically increases the likelihood of systemic embolisation during thrombolysis, but there is no evidence

that patient selection based on echocardiography affects management or outcome. Patients with end-stage renal disease fare significantly worse with catheter-directed thrombolysis when considering amputation risk, primary, primary assisted and secondary patency rates, suggesting that patients with CKD stage 5 are poor candidates for thrombolysis.[16]

Technique

All patients should have adequate analgesia and a cannula inserted for venous access, analgesia and hydration. Patients should be managed in units where nursing and medical staff are experienced in thrombolysis and clear protocols exist to manage complications. A critical care environment is desirable for close monitoring during thrombolysis. The extent of occlusive disease needs to be defined by arteriography or duplex imaging before intervention. The number of arterial punctures should be kept to a minimum to reduce the risk of puncture-site bleeding during treatment. The initial diagnostic approach is tailored to the distribution of disease. If there is an absent femoral pulse in the affected leg but a palpable femoral pulse on the contralateral side, then it is reasonable to anticipate an iliac artery occlusion. In this situation, a contralateral femoral puncture will provide access for the diagnostic arteriogram and subsequently the iliac thrombosis can be approached from the same puncture site using a crossover technique (**Fig. 8.7**). If there is a normal femoral pulse on the side of acute ischaemia, then initial diagnostic information may be provided by CT angiography or duplex imaging. As long as adequate inflow can be confirmed using one of these methods, an antegrade puncture should be attempted to treat occlusions below the femoral bifurcation so that adjuvant procedures such as angioplasty or thrombus aspiration can be performed from the same side (Fig. 8.7). An occluded arterial bypass graft is optimally accessed from the native artery proximal to the graft so that any stenoses can be treated via the same puncture site. However, this is not always possible for technical reasons, although direct puncture of the most proximal accessible part of the graft results in a high success rate from thrombolysis. Once access has been achieved, a guidewire should be passed through the occlusion; indeed, the ability to do this implies the presence of soft thrombus and is a good predictor of success (guidewire traversal test). The catheter used to deliver the lytic agent is then placed within the thrombus.

Several techniques are described for delivering thrombolysis. The low-dose infusion method involves running the thrombolytic drug through the catheter over several hours. This may be combined with an initial high-dose bolus.

Box 8.2 • Contraindications to thrombolysis

- Active internal bleeding
- Pregnancy
- Stroke within 2 months
- Transient ischaemic attack within 2 months
- Known intracerebral tumour, aneurysm or arteriovenous malformation
- Severe bleeding tendency
- Craniotomy within 2 months
- Vascular surgery within 2 weeks
- Abdominal surgery within 2 weeks
- Puncture of a non-compressible vessel or biopsy within 10 days
- Previous gastrointestinal haemorrhage
- Trauma within 10 days

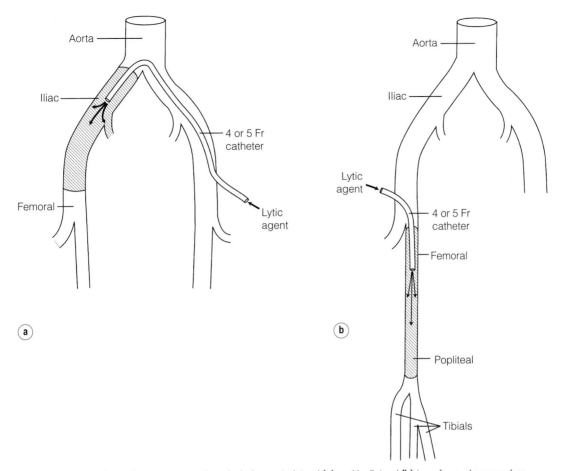

Figure 8.7 • Technique of percutaneous thrombolysis: contralateral **(a)** and ipsilateral **(b)** transfemoral approaches.

☑☑ More recently, high-dose techniques have been described that accelerate the rate of thrombus dissolution.[27] This may be achieved by administering a number of high-dose boluses sequentially or by using the 'pulse spray' technique.[23] The latter involves high-pressure injection of tiny pulses of lytic agent through a catheter with multiple side-holes, and thus it combines enzymatic thrombolysis with mechanical disruption. The high-dose techniques accelerate thrombolysis and allow patients to be treated within the normal working hours of a radiology department.

Several randomised trials comparing low-dose and accelerated methods of thrombolysis have found that limb salvage rate and complication rates appear similar, though accelerated methods are quicker.[27–30]

Streptokinase and urokinase were the agents initially used for peripheral thrombolysis. Urokinase was used in the STILE and TOPAS trials discussed above; however, it is no longer available in North America. Tissue plasminogen activator (t-PA) is the most common lytic agent used in current practice.[16] A number of recombinant t-PAs have subsequently been developed using molecular cloning and bioengineering techniques with the aim of lengthening the duration of bioavailability and avoiding the need for continuous infusion.

☑☑ There are very few high-quality trials to determine which drug is most effective, but most agree that t-PA and urokinase are superior to streptokinase.[31] Recombinant t-PAs have been found to be as effective and safe as urokinase[32] and are the agent of choice in the UK.

The STILE trial suggested that urokinase and t-PA had equivalent activity,[21] and this was confirmed in unpublished manufacturers' data. A number of new agents such as staphylokinase and alfimeprase are under investigation, but as yet they have not been shown to be better than existing agents.

Heparin is often administered systemically before and after thrombolysis to counteract the associated prothrombotic tendency, although some data from trials of the thrombolytic treatment of acute stroke suggest that heparin may increase haemorrhagic complications. An alternative is concurrent administration of low-dose heparin (200 units/hour) via the proximal arterial sheath while delivering the thrombolytic agent via an end-hole catheter to an occlusion below the inguinal ligament. Heparin should be given routinely for 48 hours after completion of thrombolysis. Consideration will then be needed to determine whether individual patients need lifelong anticoagulation with warfarin. No data exist to guide appropriate therapy. Thrombolysis should be considered a diagnostic process aimed at exposing the underlying flow-limiting lesion (**Fig. 8.8**). This should be found in the majority of patients using duplex ultrasonography of the suspect arterial segment. The majority of lesions can be managed by angioplasty or stent placement. Where the disease appears too extensive, surgical reconstruction may be required, particularly when an anastomotic stenosis results in graft occlusion.

ALI due to a popliteal aneurysm remains a difficult clinical problem. The bulk of thrombus within the aneurysm restricts the use of thrombolysis because of the high risk of massive distal embolisation, the slow clearance and large amount of residual thrombus after recanalisation. If thrombolysis does have a role to play, then it is to open run-off vessels for distal bypass grafting. This is achieved by placing a catheter through the popliteal artery into a tibial vessel and then lysing it until a distal vessel becomes patent for bypass. Alternatively, urgent surgery may be performed with on-table angiography and thrombolysis to clear the run-off (see later).

Percutaneous thrombectomy devices

Percutaneous mechanical thrombectomy (PMT) devices have been developed to hasten thrombus removal and either replace the need for thrombolytic drugs or reduce the dose required.[33] The devices may be classified according to their mode of action. The most basic technique involves simply aspirating the thrombus by applying suction to a wide-bore catheter (e.g. Pat-Rat aspiration catheter ™, Angiomed Bard, Karlsruhe, Germany). Some devices simply macerate thrombus into particles so small that they are removed by natural fibrinolysis (e.g. Amplatz Thrombectomy™ Device, Microvena, White Bear Lake, MN, USA).

Mechanical Rotational Catheter systems (e.g. Rotarex™, Straub Medical, Wangs, Switzerland) use the principle of the 'Archimedes screw' to break up the clot up and aspirate it. Other mechanisms include a clot aspiration system based on the Bernoulii or Venturi principle to remove fragments of thrombus and prevent distal embolisation (e.g. Angiojet™, Possis Medical Inc., Minneapolis, MN, USA). Ultrasound catheters use ultrasound energy

to lyse thrombus (e.g. the Acolysis™ catheter, Angiosonics, Morrisville, NC, USA). Thrombolysis is often required as a supplement to mechanical thrombectomy: in the Trellis Thrombectomy System™ (Covidien, Mansfield, MA, USA), the occluded segment of the artery is isolated by proximal and distal balloons. An oscillating wire fragments the thrombus while a thrombolytic infusion helps to dissolve it before the liquefied material is aspirated from the isolated segment.

The most comprehensive data for percutaneous mechanical thrombectomy are for the Rotarex™ device. Current studies report a greater than 90% technical success rate of primary reopening of infra-aortic vessels using either the Rotarex™ or Angiojet™ devices[34]. The amputation rate using the Angiojet™ device is between 4% and 11%. By contrast the amputation-free survival rate at 12 months for the Rotarex™ catheter is 95–100%.[34] The results available for these devices need to be interpreted with caution as they are predominantly from small retrospective studies with heterogeneous groups.

Thrombosuction has only been used sporadically for ALI, with 12 studies published from 1984 to 2015. Technical success is reported in 70–97% of cases, but it has predominantly been used in Rutherford class I ischaemia. There may be a role for this device in patients who are too high risk to undergo operative thromboembolectomy. The 30-day mortality rate was 4.6% in a study examining a single centre's experience over 5 years, which is in line with previous studies.[35] Only a few case reports have been published evaluating the performance of the Trellis system; however, these have reported promising results.

The current evidence for these devices is predominantly retrospective in nature. Multicentre prospective studies would provide more robust data for the efficacy and safety of pharmacomechanical thrombolysis in treating acute limb ischaemia.

Complications

There are significant risks associated with percutaneous thrombolytic therapy, most of which can be attributed to severe comorbidity of the patients and their advanced systemic atherosclerosis. Myocardial infarction and stroke are the commonest causes of death. The rate of reported adverse outcomes is variable, depending on the condition of the patients treated. A recent review of the mortality after thrombolysis was 2–8%.[19]

The National Audit of Thrombolysis for Acute Limb Ischaemia (NATALI) database, which includes over 1100 episodes of thrombolysis (mostly for limb-threatening ischaemia), records a 12.4% mortality rate at 30 days.[36] Other large series report intermediate results.[37,38] Major haemorrhage occurs

Figure 8.8 • (a) Arteriography demonstrates an occlusion of the popliteal artery extending into the tibial vessels. **(b)** Thrombolysis reveals a popliteal stenosis but persistent occlusion of the tibial trifurcation. **(c)** The stenosis was treated by balloon angioplasty and the thrombus aspirated from the tibial vessels using an aspiration catheter.

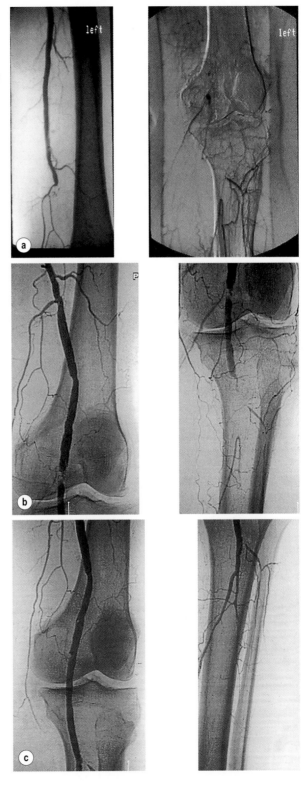

in approximately 9% of patients, usually at a groin puncture site but occasionally retroperitoneal or intra-abdominal. If major haemorrhage occurs during thrombolysis, aprotinin is an effective plasmin inhibitor and the administration of whole blood, fresh-frozen plasma and, in particular, fibrinogen concentrate will replenish the clotting factors. Stroke is seen in approximately 3% of patients (2.3% in the TSG database); this must be interpreted in the context of other risk factors for stroke in this population. Most occur after thrombolysis, during therapeutic anticoagulation. About half are thrombotic rather than haemorrhagic. If a stroke occurs, cerebral haemorrhage should be excluded by urgent CT. If haemorrhage is not the cause, then a clinical decision needs to be made whether to persist with thrombolysis to salvage the affected limb, with possible additional benefits to the intracerebral circulation.

Minor haemorrhage is common (approximately 40% of infusions) and usually occurs at the groin puncture site. It can be managed by direct compression or by exchanging the catheter system for a larger catheter or sheath. Distal embolisation during thrombolysis is a nuisance, occurring in 4% of patients, and is usually managed by either aspiration thromboembolectomy or continued lysis. Reperfusion damage has been reported in 2% and pericatheter thrombosis in 1%.

Outcome

Diffin and Kandarpa[39] report successful thrombolysis in 70% of treatments, with limb salvage in 93%, although many patients in the collected review did not have limb-threatening ischaemia. The British Thrombolysis Study Group (TSG) database records complete lysis in 45.5% and clinically useful lysis in a further 27.9% of infusions, leading to a limb salvage rate of 75.2%; 12.4% of patients required an amputation and 12.4% died.[40] Thrombolysis was similarly effective in bypass grafts and native vessels. The outcome seems dependent on the nature of the lesion treated and the clinical state of the patient. Patients with subcritical ischaemia appear less likely to need amputation than patients with critical ischaemia including a neurosensory deficit. In addition, the following are more likely to predict failure of thrombolysis: inability to traverse the occlusion with a guidewire or place a catheter within the thrombus, diabetes, multilevel disease, vein graft occlusion, advancing age and female sex.[37] In the long term, approximately 75% of successfully opened native vessels remain patent at 1 year and 55% at 2 years.[38,41] When an identifiable lesion is found after graft thrombolysis, the 2-year patency is approximately 85%. Long-term patency is less good where no underlying lesion is found in native vessels or grafts. In addition, successfully treated iliac occlusions and emboli have a better long-term outlook.[42,43]

The results of thrombolysis for vein graft occlusion have proved disappointing.[44] It is assumed that ischaemia of the vein graft reduces the chances of success. In contrast, the results of prosthetic graft thrombolysis are better. Where an underlying lesion is responsible for occlusion of a prosthetic graft, patency rates at 1 year are encouraging (86% vs 37%).[45]

There is currently great interest in trying to improve the results of peripheral thrombolysis. It is unlikely that advances in techniques will make a significant difference as no one method can be shown to be superior.

Other scoring systems may be used to try to identify patients unlikely to survive after thrombolysis.[46] Detailed analysis of available data and large databases may help identify patients at greater risk of a poor outcome from thrombolysis. A detailed statistical analysis of the TSG database has shown that the following factors were associated with reduced amputation-free survival: increasing patient age, increasing severity of ischaemia (Rutherford Classification and presence of a sensorimotor deficit), shorter duration of ischaemia and diabetes.[36] Being on warfarin at the time of the occlusion improved the chance of amputation-free survival. The risk of death after thrombolysis was highest in patients with an embolic occlusion, women, older patients and those with ischaemic heart disease. Amputation risk was highest in younger men, legs with a sensorimotor deficit, and graft and thrombotic occlusions.

Surgical management

With the increasing age of the population, underlying atherosclerosis often complicates ischaemia even if the cause is primarily embolic. Consequently, complex secondary procedures may well be necessary if initial balloon catheter embolectomy fails (**Fig. 8.9**). It is therefore advisable that an experienced vascular surgeon performs or supervises the operation. Local anaesthesia may be considered in frail patients where a straightforward femoral embolectomy is considered likely, but an epidural is a better option. An anaesthetist should always be present to monitor the ECG and oxygen saturation, administer sedation or analgesia and convert to general anaesthesia if required.

Balloon catheter embolectomy

Both groins and the entire leg should be prepared to permit surgical access and arteriography. The foot should be placed in a sterile transparent bag for easy inspection. The common femoral artery bifurcation is exposed via a groin incision and the vessels controlled with Silastic slings. Clamps should be avoided initially because they fragment thrombus

Figure 8.9 • Possible treatment pathway required when exploring the femoral artery.

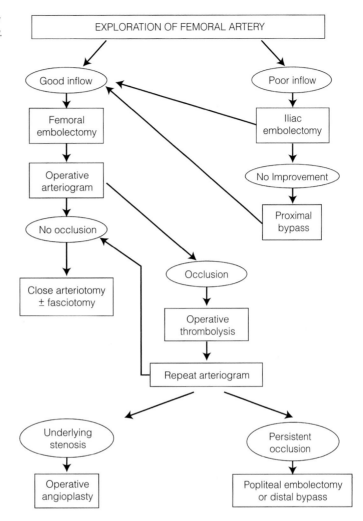

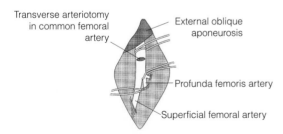

Transverse arteriotomy in common femoral artery

External oblique aponeurosis

Profunda femoris artery

Superficial femoral artery

Figure 8.10 • Exploration of the femoral artery using Silastic slings to control the vessels and a transverse arteriotomy proximal to the common femoral bifurcation.

that may otherwise be removed intact. A transverse arteriotomy is made in the common femoral artery proximal to the bifurcation, avoiding any obvious plaque (**Fig. 8.10**). A transverse arteriotomy is easier to close without narrowing and it can be converted to a diamond shape for proximal anastomosis if a bypass is required. Any thrombus at the bifurcation can be removed by gentle suction or forceps and

momentary release of the sling or clamp. Some surgeons send the embolic material for histological and microbiological assessment, although there is little evidence to support this routinely.

If pulsatile inflow is not present, then a 4-Fr or 5-Fr balloon catheter is passed proximally up into the aorta, inflated and withdrawn. Pressure should be applied to the contralateral femoral artery during this procedure to prevent contralateral embolisation. If good inflow cannot be achieved, then a femorofemoral or axillofemoral bypass will be required. A saddle embolus can usually be retrieved by bilateral femoral embolectomy. Next, a 3-Fr or 4-Fr balloon catheter is passed as far distally as possible down both the profunda and superficial femoral arteries. Force should not be used if resistance is met as dissection or perforation may result. The balloon is inflated only as the catheter is withdrawn and the amount of inflation adjusted to avoid excessive intimal friction. The procedure is repeated until no more thromboembolic material can be retrieved. Conventional embolectomy is performed blind and the surgeon has no control over the direction of the catheter past the popliteal trifurcation. Use of an 'over-the-wire' embolectomy catheter permits selective catheterisation of the tibial arteries under fluoroscopic control, which is preferable to performing an additional popliteal trifurcation exposure (**Fig. 8.11**).

Completion angiography

✅ A completion arteriogram should always be performed because persistent thrombus may be present even if the catheter passes to the foot;[47] back-bleeding is of no prognostic value as it may arise from established proximal collaterals. Modern vascular operating theatres now have excellent fluoroscopic facilities capable of high-quality arteriography. Routine angiography results in a higher rate of extension of the procedure for a residual lesion and a lower re-occlusion rate at 24 months.[48] The procedure involves flushing the distal arteries with heparin saline and if no thrombus is present on the arteriogram, the arteriotomy is repaired with 5/0 prolene. On removing the clamps the foot should become pink with palpable pulses.

Failed embolectomy

If the arteriogram shows persistent occlusion, then 15 mg t-PA in 100 mL heparin saline can be infused via an umbilical catheter over 30 minutes and the arteriogram repeated (**Fig. 8.12**). This often results in complete lysis and reduces the need for popliteal

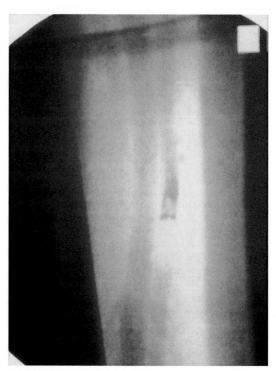

Figure 8.11 • Angiographically controlled balloon catheter embolectomy. The balloon occluding the lumen and the thrombus above it can be seen as negative images against the contrast-filled artery.

exploration.[49] The technique may also be used to lyse residual thrombus in the tibial arteries during bypass of a popliteal aneurysm.[50] If an underlying stenosis of the superficial femoral artery is revealed, then on-table angioplasty may be attempted.

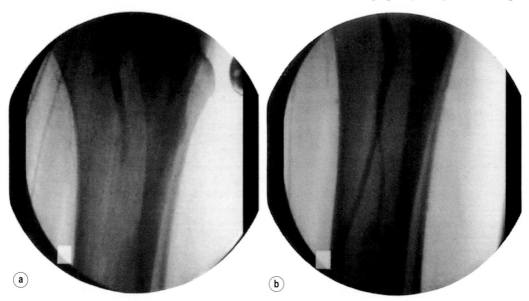

(a) (b)

Figure 8.12 • Completion angiogram after embolectomy showing persistent occlusion of the popliteal trifurcation **(a)** and complete lysis after intraoperative thrombolysis **(b)**.

Persistent distal occlusion requires exploration of the below-knee popliteal artery and either popliteal embolectomy or distal bypass. The origins of the anterior tibial artery and tibioperoneal trunk should be controlled with slings and selective embolectomy performed via a longitudinal arteriotomy. The popliteal arteriotomy requires repair with a vein patch to prevent stenosis.

Further management

Revascularisation of an ischaemic leg results in a sudden venous return of blood with anaerobic metabolites, low pH and a high potassium concentration. Even if these procedures are performed under local anaesthetic it is important to have an anaesthetist present to correct electrolyte abnormalities, hypotension and arrhythmias when they occur. The importance of a specialist vascular anaesthetist is recognised in 'The Provision of Services for Patients with Vascular Disease 2015' executive statement.[51] Reperfusion of a large mass of ischaemic tissue results in a systemic inflammatory response. This may lead to multiple inflammatory responses. This may lead to multiple organ dysfunction and failure. Renal function may be further impaired by myoglobinuria, which is helped by maintaining a good diuresis.

✅ Revascularisation of ischaemic muscle can result in considerable swelling within the fascial compartments of the leg. This swelling leads to increased compartment pressures causing venous compression, worsening oedema and, if not treated promptly, permanent neurological insult. Patients with prolonged ischaemia or ischaemia from an embolic source are at highest risk of compartment syndrome.[52]

In patients with a severely ischaemic limb or where the compartments are tense it is wise to perform a fasciotomy at the time of the initial revascularisation procedure. Diagnosis of compartment syndrome is a clinical one. Measurement of compartment pressures may be unreliable. All four muscle compartments should be decompressed via full-length skin and fascial incisions from knee to ankle if any muscle tenseness is present at the time of embolectomy or subsequently.[53] The anterior fasciotomy should be made about two finger-breadths lateral to the anterior border of the tibia, which avoids the peroneal nerve. The posterior fasciotomy incision is done in a line about two finger-breadths posterior to the medial condyle of the femur and the medial malleolus, which avoids the long saphenous vein. The defect can be closed later with sutures or a split-skin graft.

After embolectomy, anticoagulation with heparin and then warfarin is continued as this reduces the risk of recurrent embolism, especially if atrial fibrillation is present.[54–56] There is little guidance about the role of anticoagulation in patients who are not fibrillating and have no other obvious cause. Results of a search for proximal sources of emboli using echocardiography and CT angiography may indicate the need for lifelong anticoagulation, but in many patients an individual decision will need to be made based on the risks of warfarinisation and the state of the distal circulation.

Overall prognosis

There has been little change in overall outcome from ALI because the improvements in radiological and surgical techniques have been balanced by increasing atherosclerotic arterial disease in ever older patients. Ten per cent of patients presenting with ALI will have an unsalvageable lower limb. A Swedish population study demonstrated that between 1965 and 1983 there was an increasing incidence of ALI, without any improvement in amputation rates or survival,[57] although outcome after treatment in a university hospital was better than in a district hospital.[58] A prospective survey by the Vascular Surgical Society of Great Britain and Ireland that included 539 episodes in 474 patients recorded a limb salvage rate of 70% and an overall mortality rate of 22%.[59] An analysis of the Medicare population in the USA recorded an in-hospital mortality rate of 9% and an amputation rate of 11% at 1 year.[3] Patients with embolism have a higher mortality rate due to their underlying cardiac disease. In contrast, those with thrombosis are at increased risk of amputation. Patients with a high mortality rate after embolectomy are characterised by:[55]

- poor cardiac function;
- associated peripheral vascular disease;
- short duration of symptoms;
- the need for amputation.

The amputation risk appears higher in patients with a longer duration of ischaemia and poor preoperative and postoperative cardiac function.[60] Recently, an analysis of preoperative cardiac troponin T has suggested it can be used to predict outcome after embolectomy.[61] Patients with ALI are often elderly and within this group there is a cohort of individuals whose leg problem heralds the end of life. Patients with concomitant malignancy represent a very high-risk population and most studies have found that these patients have a very poor prognosis. It is important to recognise this group and to offer appropriate palliative care rather than aggressive intervention.[62]

Conclusions

Although there have been huge changes in the therapeutic options for patients with ALI, there remains debate over the optimal management. Clinical trials in this area are difficult to organise and are often flawed by the great variation in the condition of the patients and their lower limbs. However, further stratification of existing data could help define which occlusions are most suitable for thrombolysis or surgery. A clear comparison between the different drugs available and delivery techniques would help. New drugs will undoubtedly become available with improved safety profiles. Thrombolysis combined with percutaneous mechanical thrombectomy seems to enhance its effectiveness in certain clinical situations.

Key points

- Patients with ALI have high morbidity and mortality rates.
- Optimal management is based on the severity of the ischaemia at presentation.
- Randomised trials have failed to show superiority of thrombolysis or surgery as primary management for all cases.
- The best results are achieved when management is agreed jointly by a team consisting of vascular surgeon and interventional radiologist using available expertise and local guidelines.
- Further research is required to identify which patients with salvageable legs at presentation may be better managed by primary amputation rather than futile attempts at revascularisation.
- For some patients ALI heralds end of life and palliative care should be instituted.

🌐 Full references available at **http://expertconsult.inkling.com**

Key references

1. Norgeren L, Hiatt WR, Dormandy JA, et al. Inter-Society Consensus for the management of peripheral arterial disease. Eur J Vasc Endovasc Surg 2007;33:S1–75. PMID: 17140820.
   The Trans-Atlantic Inter-Society Consensus document on the management of peripheral arterial disease (TASC). This updated document discusses the diagnosis and management of artery disease.

20. Ouriel K, Shortell CK, DeWeese JA, et al. A comparison of thrombolytic therapy with operative revascularisation in the initial treatment of acute peripheral arterial ischaemia. J Vasc Surg 1994;19:1021–30. PMID: 8201703.
    This randomised controlled trial involved 114 patients who were randomised to thrombolytic therapy or operative management. It concluded that thrombolysis provided a safe alternative treatment for patients with acute limb ischaemia.

21. The STILE Investigators. Results of a prospective randomized trial evaluating surgery versus thrombolysis for ischaemia of the lower extremity. Ann Surg 1994;220:1–68. PMID: 8092895.
    This multicentre study compared open revascularisation with catheter-directed thrombolysis (either urokinase or recombinant tissue plasminogen activator) for non-embolic leg ischaemia.

22. Comerota AJ, Weaver FA, Hosking JD, et al. Results of a prospective randomized trial of surgery versus thrombolysis for occluded lower extremity bypass grafts. Am J Surg 1996;172:105–12. PMID: 8795509.
    This randomised controlled trial of 134 patients compared surgery with catheter-directed thrombolysis for occluded lower limb bypass grafts. It showed that those with chronic ischaemia (>14 days) had better outcomes with surgery. In acute limb ischaemia successful thrombolysis improved limb salvage.

23. Weaver FA, Comerota AJ, Youngblood M, et al. Surgical revascularisation versus thrombolysis for nonembolic lower extremity native artery occlusions: results of a prospective randomized trial. J Vasc Surg 1996;24:513–23. PMID: 8911400.
    This randomised controlled trial involved 237 patients who were randomised to surgery or catheter-directed thrombolysis. It showed that at 1 year the incidence of recurrent ischaemia and major amputation was higher in the thrombolysis group.

24. Ouriel K, Veith FJ, Sasahara AA, for the TOPAS investigators. Thrombolysis or peripheral arterial surgery: phase I results. J Vasc Surg 1996;23:64–75. PMID: 8558744.
    This multicentre randomised controlled trial involved 213 patients who were treated with surgery or recombinant urokinase at one of three dose regimes. It found that 4000 IU/min was safe and effective in the treatment of acute lower limb ischaemia.

25. Ouriel K, Veith FJ, Sasahara AA, for the TOPAS investigators. A comparison of recombinant

urokinase with vascular surgery as initial treatment for acute arterial occlusion of the legs. N Engl J Med 1998;338:1105–11. PMID: 9545358.

This multicentre randomised controlled trial compared surgery and thrombolysis in the treatment of acute limb ischaemia; 272 patients were randomised to surgery and 272 patients to thrombolysis. It found that thrombolysis with urokinase reduced the need for open surgery with no significant increase in the risk of amputation or death.

27. Braithwaite BD, Buckenham TM, Galland RB, et al. on behalf of the Thrombolysis Study Group. Prospective randomized trial of high-dose bolus versus low-dose tissue plasminogen activator infusion in the management of acute limb ischaemia. Br J Surg 1997;84:646–50. PMID: 9171752.

This randomised trial involved 100 patients treated with either a high-dose bolus or conventional low-dose tissue plasminogen activator thrombolysis to treat acute lower limb ischaemia. It found that the high-dose bolus regime significantly accelerated thrombolysis without compromising outcome.

28. Yusuf SW, Whitaker SC, Gregson RHS, et al. Prospective randomised comparative study of pulse spray and conventional local thrombolysis. Eur J Vasc Endovasc Surg 1995;10:136–41. PMID: 7655964.

This randomised study involved 18 patients and compared pulse spray with conventional thrombolysis. It found that significantly shorter time was required to achieve lysis in the pulse spray group.

29. Kandarpa K, Chopra PS, Arung JE. Intra-arterial thrombolysis of lower extremity occlusion: prospective randomized comparison of forced periodic infusion and conventional slow continuous infusion. Radiology 1993;188:861–7. PMID: 8351363.

This randomised controlled trial involved 25 patients and compared forced infusion of urokinase with conventional slow infusion. If found no significant difference between the two groups in the speed of lysis, initial success rates, complications rates or 30-day clinical outcome.

30. Plate G, Jansson L, Forssell C, et al. Thrombolysis for acute lower limb ischaemia – a prospective, randomised multicenter study comparing two strategies. Eur J Vasc Endovasc Surg 2006;31:651–60. PMID: 16427339.

This prospective randomised study involved 121 patients who were randomised to receive pulse spray or standard low-dose thrombolysis. It found that there was no obvious advantage with pulse spray thrombolysis.

31. Berridge DC, Gregson RHS, Hopkinson BR, et al. Randomized trial of intra-arterial recombinant tissue plasminogen activator, intravenous recombinant tissue plasminogen activator and intra-arterial streptokinase in peripheral thrombolysis. Br J Surg 1991;78:988–95. PMID: 1913123.

This randomised trial involved 60 patients and compared three different thrombolysis agents. It found that intra-arterial recombinant tissue plasminogen activator is a more effective, safer thrombolysis agent than intra-arterial streptokinase.

32. Cina CS, Goh RH, Chan J, et al. Intraarterial catheter-directed thrombolysis urokinase versus tissue plasminogen activator. Ann Vasc Surg 1999;13:571–5. PMID: 10541608.

This prospective study compared two thrombolysis agents, urokinase and tissue plasminogen activator. There was no significant difference in efficacy between the two agents. t-PA acted faster but also had a higher incidence of bleeding complications.

9

Vascular trauma

Jacobus van Marle
Dirk A. le Roux

Introduction

Fewer than 10% of patients with polytrauma have associated vascular injuries, but these injuries can cause significant morbidity and mortality.[1] In most European countries the majority of vascular trauma is caused by blunt (traffic accidents) and iatrogenic injuries.[2] In South Africa, injuries are mostly penetrating and have also changed from predominantly stab wounds to injuries caused by firearms.[3]

Complex vascular injuries have a high morbidity and mortality, and a clear understanding of the pathophysiology of vascular trauma and a logical approach to the management of those injuries are essential for a favourable outcome.

Mechanism of injury

Vascular injuries are classified according to the mechanism of the injury.

Blunt trauma

Direct trauma to the artery accounts for the majority of blunt vascular injuries. Indirect trauma is usually the result of shearing and distraction forces following dislocation of major joints, displaced long-bone fractures and acceleration/deceleration injuries as seen with high-speed motor vehicle accidents and falls from a height. Blunt trauma causes contusion of the arterial wall with disruption of the intima. This intimal tear may cause immediate obstruction due to an intimal flap or may predispose to thrombosis and delayed occlusion (**Fig. 9.1a–d**). As the vessel is stretched

further, progressive layers of the media are disrupted until the continuity of the vessel is maintained only by the elastic adventitia or there is complete disruption.

Penetrating trauma

Penetrating trauma may result in partial or complete transection of a vessel. Bleeding is often brisk and distal flow may be interrupted. Stab and low-velocity missile injuries cause localised damage confined to the injury tract. High-velocity missiles cause total tissue destruction around the missile tract, surrounded by an area of doubtful tissue viability, causing extensive associated soft-tissue trauma. The shock wave of a high-velocity missile can also cause intimal injury.[4] The vessel may be macroscopically intact with minimal bruising, but on opening the vessel there is an intimal tear with superimposed thrombosis. Shotgun injuries cause extensive local tissue destruction with often multiple sites of perforation (**Fig. 9.2**). Bomb blasts cause complex injuries due to the combination of extensive local tissue trauma, high-velocity fragments and thermal injury.

Iatrogenic injuries are becoming increasingly important and account for more than 40% of vascular trauma in many European countries.[2]

Sequelae of vascular injuries

Vascular injuries have significant sequelae (Box 9.1, **Figs 9.3** and **9.4**). A contused artery may be patent initially but thrombose later. Subsequent propagation of thrombus may cause progressive

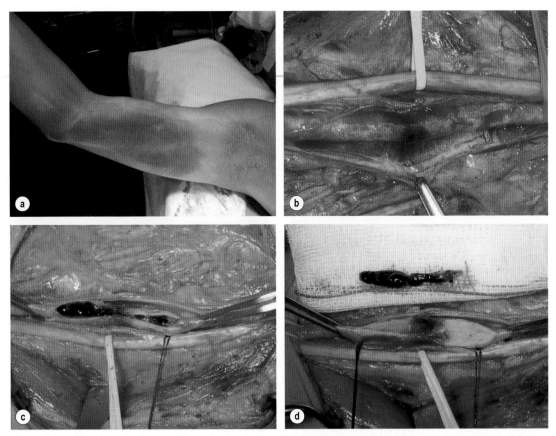

Figure 9.1 • Blunt injury to the arm **(a)** causing contusion of the brachial artery, **(b)** predisposing to thrombosis, **(c)** due to underlying intimal damage **(d)**.

ischaemia by obstructing essential collaterals. Acute ischaemia leads to degeneration and necrosis of muscle cells and Wallerian degeneration in nerves. Findings from large-animal studies indicate that early restoration of flow within 3 hours is associated with near-complete recovery, whereas delayed revascularisation at 6 hours was associated with significant muscle necrosis and nerve degeneration.[5]

Concomitant fractures, dislocations, injuries to accompanying veins and nerves, soft-tissue trauma and contamination of the wound with foreign material serve to compound vascular injury. Other determinants of the final outcome are the level of vascular injury, the quality of the collateral circulation and pre-existing occlusive arterial disease.

Clinical assessment

History

Information regarding the mechanism of the trauma, blood loss prior to hospital admission and underlying vascular disease should be obtained.

Examination

Initial assessment should be carried out according to advanced trauma life support (ATLS) principles and life-threatening conditions managed. Vascular injury may present with any of the sequelae listed in Box 9.1. Clinical signs of vascular injuries can be divided into hard and soft signs.

Hard signs of vascular injury:

- Active pulsatile bleeding.
- Shock with ongoing bleeding.
- Absent distal pulses.
- Symptoms and signs of acute ischaemia.
- Expanding or pulsating haematoma.
- Bruits or thrill over the area of injury.

Soft signs of vascular injury:

- History of severe bleeding.
- Diminished distal pulse.
- Injury of anatomically related structures.
- Small non-expanding haematoma.
- Multiple fractures and extensive soft-tissue injury.
- Injury in anatomical area of major blood vessel.

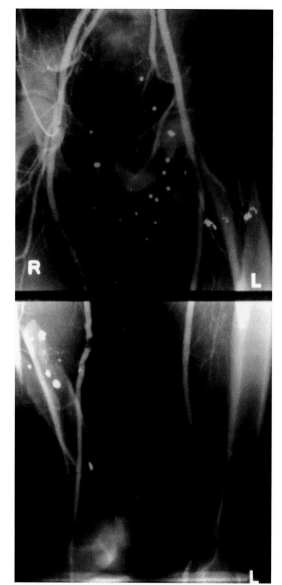

Figure 9.2 • Arteriogram of the pelvis and thighs to demonstrate multiple arterial perforations together with extensive local trauma to bone and soft tissue caused by shotgun injury.

Distal pulses may be difficult to evaluate in patients with extensive soft-tissue trauma, swelling and multiple wounds. A diminished or absent pulse is due to arterial occlusion until proven otherwise and should not be attributed to vascular spasm, external compression or any other ill-defined factor.

Signs of acute arterial insufficiency (ischaemia) include pulse deficit (absent/diminished pulse), pain, pallor, paraesthesia and paralysis. Neurological deficit must be evaluated carefully in order to distinguish between ischaemic neuropathy and direct injury to the nerve.

Box 9.1 Sequelae of vascular injuries

Acute haemorrhage
- Overt external bleeding
- Contained bleeding (e.g. in muscle compartment)
- Concealed bleeding (e.g. pleural cavity)

Hypovolaemia, shock
Haematoma with or without secondary infection
Delayed bleeding and rebleeding
Thrombosis: acute or delayed
Ischaemia: acute or delayed
Arteriovenous fistula (see **Fig. 9.3**)
Pseudoaneurysm formation (see **Fig. 9.4**)

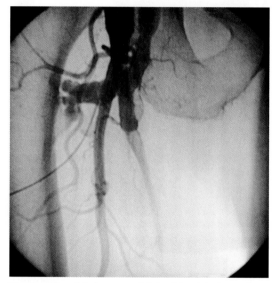

Figure 9.3 • Arteriovenous fistula of the right femoral vessels following iatrogenic injury after diagnostic cardiac catheterisation.

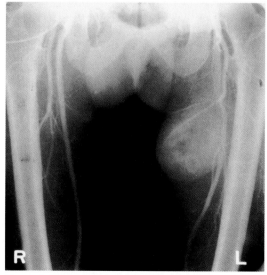

Figure 9.4 • False aneurysm of the left thigh after gunshot wound.

Diagnosis

✔✔ The value and accuracy of a thorough clinical examination in predicting significant vascular injury has been reported in various series.[6]

Arterial Doppler pressure measurement is a useful supplement to the clinical examination. An arterial pressure index (API) above 0.9 reliably excludes significant occult arterial injury.[7]

Special investigations should only be performed in patients who have been adequately resuscitated and who are haemodynamically stable. Haemodynamic instability, active bleeding and an expanding haematoma are indications for immediate surgery.

Resuscitation and initial management

ATLS guidelines are followed, keeping in mind that the resuscitation of the unstable patient in urgent need of surgery may be best conducted in the operating room.

✔✔ The amount, type and timing of fluid resuscitation is important. In uncontrolled haemorrhagic shock where bleeding has been temporarily stopped due to hypotension, vasoconstriction and thrombus formation, aggressive fluid resuscitation may lead to increased intravascular pressure, decreased blood viscosity and loss of the haemostatic plug, with resultant increased bleeding and mortality.[8] *Hypotensive resuscitation* (permissive hypotension) aims at a systolic blood pressure of between 70 and 90 mmHg to maintain cerebral and renal perfusion until operative control of bleeding has been achieved. *Haemostatic resuscitation* is indicated in patients with massive bleeding/blood loss. Immediate administration of plasma, platelets and red blood cells as part of the resuscitation protocol has resulted in improved survival.[9]

Active bleeding is an indication for urgent exploration, but can usually be temporarily controlled by direct pressure. Blind clamping of vessels in the depth of a wound is discouraged, because of the danger of injuring adjacent nerves and vessels. Tourniquets should be used in cases of massive bleeding that cannot be controlled with direct pressure.

Fractures must be stabilised during the period of resuscitation and diagnostic investigation in order to protect blood vessels and other soft tissue from further trauma. Preliminary reduction of a displaced fracture or dislocation may improve distal circulation.

Special investigations

Plain radiography

Plain radiographs are usually taken for associated skeletal injuries. A high index of suspicion for vascular trauma should exist with dislocations and displaced fractures (**Fig. 9.5**). Chest radiography is valuable in patients with chest trauma.

Angiography

✔✔ Computed tomographic angiography (CTA) is valuable in diagnosing blunt and penetrating vascular injuries in the neck, thorax, abdomen and extremities and should be the first-line investigation for all patients with suspected vascular trauma who do not require immediate surgical intervention.[10]

Digital subtraction angiography (DSA) may still be indicated for selected conditions in haemodynamically stable patients, and where endovascular management of the injury is considered. The use of magnetic resonance angiography (MRA) in trauma is limited due to time constraints and inaccessibility to the patient during the examination.

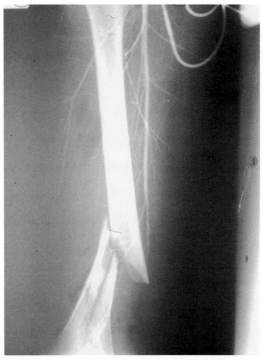

Figure 9.5 • Displaced fracture of the femur with injury to the superficial femoral artery.

Surgical intervention should not be delayed for special investigations where vascular injury is evident and the patient is unstable or the limb is at ischaemic risk. On-table arteriography can be performed in the operating room for vascular injuries where surgery cannot be delayed and the additional information is considered valuable.

Ultrasound

Duplex Doppler examination is mostly used as a screening test in the absence of hard signs, in zone 2 neck injuries, in extremity vascular trauma and for follow-up evaluation in patients managed expectantly.

General principles of management of vascular injury

Procedures are performed under general anaesthesia in a suitably equipped theatre. Blood products should be available and arrangements for intraoperative autotransfusion should be made where further bleeding is expected. The value of prophylactic antibiotics in vascular surgery is established.

Adequate exposure is vital for obtaining proximal and distal control of injured vessels. This often requires inclusion of adjacent anatomical areas in the operative field, e.g. preparing the neck in thoracic injuries (and vice versa) and the abdomen in groin injuries. An uninjured leg is prepared for possible vein harvesting should bypass be required. Vascular control must be achieved proximally and distally before directly approaching the area of injury. Bleeding may be temporarily arrested by digital compression or by endovascular means until clamps have been applied.

In blunt and high-velocity trauma there is often extensive intimal damage, and careful debridement of the vessel is necessary until normal-appearing intima is found (**Fig. 9.6**). Antegrade and retrograde flow should be evaluated. Arteries are cleared of thrombus by careful passage of embolectomy catheters followed by irrigation with heparin-saline solution.

Simple laceration of the vessel wall is repaired by lateral suture, provided it does not lead to stenosis, when patch graft angioplasty is indicated. Where more than 50% of the circumference of a vessel wall is damaged, this area should be excised followed by

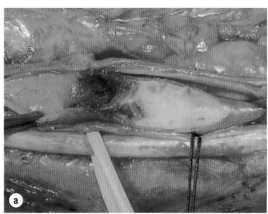

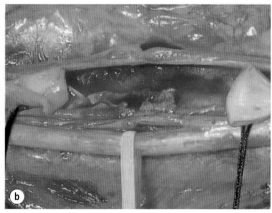

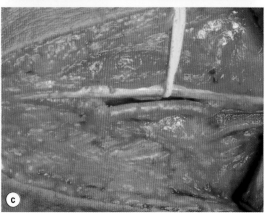

Figure 9.6 • Blunt injury of the intima **(a)**, resected **(b)** and replaced with a venous interposition graft **(c)**.

end-to-end anastomosis. This requires mobilisation of the proximal and distal arterial stumps to achieve approximation without tension. Failing this, an interposition graft is indicated. Autologous vein is the preferred conduit for reconstruction. Where there is a mismatch in diameter between the vessel that needs to be repaired and the available autologous vein, either a panelled or spiral vein graft should be used. Prosthetic material may be used in the absence of available autologous vein or as part of a damage control strategy.[11]

✔✔ Where complex arterial repair will result in delay in revascularisation, intraluminal shunts should be used to maintain antegrade flow during repair, thereby reducing ischaemic time.[12]

Completion angiography should be performed to document a technically perfect repair and to assess the distal arterial tree. Associated injuries are addressed once vascular repair has been completed. Wound debridement should be performed with removal of all devitalised and contaminated tissue. Contaminated wounds are left open, but the vascular repair must be covered by soft tissue. Repeated wound inspections are performed, with delayed primary suture when the wound is clean.

Venous injuries

Venous injuries found during exploration for associated arterial injury should be repaired, if the repair itself can be done simply (e.g. lateral suture repair) and only if it will not significantly delay treatment of associated injuries or destabilise the patient's condition. Complex venous repair or bypass should only be attempted if the patient is haemodynamically stable. All veins, including the inferior vena cava (IVC), can be tied off in cases of haemodynamic instability.

Endovascular management of vascular trauma

The application of endovascular techniques in the injured patient has many potential advantages. General anaesthesia is not required. Surgical trauma, with further blood loss, hypothermia, etc., as well as cross-clamping of major vessels, distal ischaemia and subsequent reperfusion injury, is avoided. The main advantage is the option of approaching complex arterial lesions in anatomically challenging locations from a remote site. A difficult exploration in an injured area is avoided, with less potential damage to surrounding structures, and preventing fresh bleeding.

Endovascular techniques are increasingly applied in vascular trauma, but still have certain limitations. These techniques are usually not applicable, mainly due to time constraints, in patients with active bleeding, in unstable patients or where there is end-organ ischaemia. Endovascular techniques are contraindicated where there are compression symptoms, infected wounds or where concomitant injuries require open exploration. Technical restrictions include inability to traverse the lesion by guidewire, where intraluminal thrombus prevents the safe passage of a guidewire due to the danger of distal embolisation or where luminal discrepancy exists between the proximal and distal involved segments.

Endovascular techniques are used to manage vascular trauma in three ways:

1. **To obtain haemostasis.** Damaged vessels are embolised using a variety of substances including haemostatic agents (gel foam), coils and balloons.

✔✔ Embolotherapy has become the standard treatment for managing significant bleeding following pelvic fractures[13] and also to control bleeding due to penetrating and blunt trauma of the liver, kidneys and spleen.[14]

Embolotherapy is also the preferred option for treating vertebral artery lesions[15] and lesions of non-essential, inaccessible vessels in other regions.

2. **To obtain vascular control.** Temporary balloon occlusion of a damaged vessel at the time of diagnostic angiography can prevent exsanguinating bleeding until surgical control is achieved. It is especially valuable in relatively inaccessible regions and allows limiting the extent of the exposure to obtain surgical control.[16] This technique is valuable in injuries in zones 1 and 3 of the neck, the abdominal aorta, proximal subclavian and iliac arteries.

3. **For vascular repair.** Covered stent grafts are used for repairing vessels in anatomically challenging locations and to avoid major surgical exposures, e.g. the thoracic aorta, thoracic outlet vessels, internal carotid and vertebral arteries (**Fig. 9.7**).[17–19] This will be discussed in more detail in the relevant sections. Covered stent grafts may also be used as a temporary measure to allow stabilisation of the patient until definitive open repair later.

In-stent stenosis, graft migration, stent breakage and endoleaks are well-known complications of

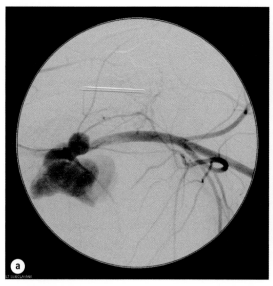
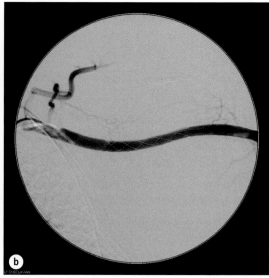

Figure 9.7 • False aneurysm of left subclavian artery after infraclavicular stab wound **(a)** repaired by means of a covered stent graft **(b)**.

stent graft repair. Durability is therefore of concern in the younger population, who are the main victims of trauma. However, good long-term results have been published for endograft repair of carotid, subclavian and thoracic aortic injuries (see later).

Cervical vascular injuries

Carotid artery injuries

The cervical vessels are involved in 25% of patients with neck trauma. Carotid artery injury constitutes 5–10% of all arterial injuries.[20] The mortality for carotid injuries ranges from 10% to 31%, with permanent neurological deficit ranging from 16% to 60%.[21]

Mechanism

More than 90% of carotid injuries are caused by penetrating trauma. Blunt trauma is caused by a direct blow to the artery, hyperextension, hyper-rotation, or contusion by bone fragments associated with fractures of the mandible, temporal bone or cervical spine.

Penetrating injury may cause partial or complete transection of the vessel, pseudoaneurysm or arteriovenous fistula (**Fig. 9.8**). Pseudoaneurysm may have an acute or delayed onset, with progressive enlargement causing compression of the aerodigestive tract or brachial plexus. Blunt trauma may cause intimal flaps, intramural haematomas, dissection,

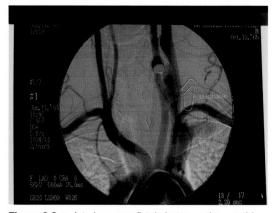

Figure 9.8 • Arteriovenous fistula between the carotid artery and internal jugular vein caused by gunshot wound.

complete disruption of the arterial wall with pseudoaneurysms, arteriovenous fistulas and total occlusion (**Fig. 9.9**).

Neurological sequelae are caused by hypoperfusion (transected or thrombosed vessels) or embolisation from thrombus, pseudoaneurysm or arteriovenous fistula.

Clinical signs

Active external bleeding, rapidly expanding cervical haematoma, absent carotid pulse and a bruit or thrill are indicative of vascular injury. Signs that may indicate an associated vascular injury warranting further investigation include bleeding

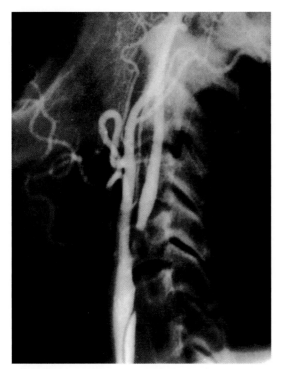

Figure 9.9 • Dissection of the common carotid artery with blunt trauma to the neck following a motor vehicle accident.

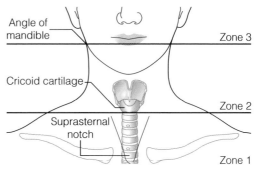

Figure 9.10 • Zones of the neck.

from wounds of the neck or the pharynx, a deficit of the superficial temporal artery pulse, ipsilateral Horner's sign, dysfunction of cranial nerves IX–XII, a widened mediastinum, fractures of the skull base and temporal bone, and fractures and dislocation of the cervical spine. Neurological deficit may be present, but obscured due to concomitant head injury, shock or the use of alcohol or drugs. About 50% of patients with established blunt injury to the carotid and vertebral arteries could initially be asymptomatic, but 43–58% of these will eventually develop neurological signs after hospital admission.[22]

Diagnosis

Only patients who are haemodynamically stable and have a patent airway should undergo further appropriate investigations.

The neck has been divided into three anatomical zones in order to standardise diagnosis and management of cervical vascular injuries (**Fig. 9.10**).

Anteroposterior chest radiography can provide valuable information regarding associated haemothorax or pneumothorax, widening of the mediastinum, surgical emphysema of the neck with concomitant aerodigestive tract injuries, etc.

CTA is accurate in detecting blunt and penetrating cervical vascular injuries and provides important information regarding associated bony and aerodigestive tract injuries.[23,24]

Duplex Doppler examination is useful for investigating zone 2 vascular injuries and is now the preferred diagnostic modality in experienced hands.[25]

DSA is used in equivocal CTA findings and as part of the endovascular management.

Computed tomography (CT) of the brain should be used to investigate patients with associated head trauma, bone injuries of the spine and skull, and neurological deficit. It is a good predictor of outcome: patients who have an infarct on initial CT on admission have a high mortality with poor chance of neurological recovery compared with those who have a normal CT on admission. MRA may be valuable in carotid artery and vertebral artery dissection.[26]

Management

Active external bleeding can be controlled in the emergency room by direct digital compression or a Foley catheter inflated in the wound tract to obtain balloon tamponade.[27]

✅✅ Mandatory exploration of all penetrating neck injuries has been replaced by a selective approach.[28]

Active pulsatile haemorrhage, expanding cervical haematoma and airway compromise are indications for urgent surgical exploration. Some low-velocity penetrating injuries may be managed expectantly with careful observation, provided there is no active bleeding and the distal circulation is normal.[29,30] These injuries include intimal defects, small pseudoaneurysms (<5 mm) and non-obstructive intimal flaps. The majority of penetrating carotid artery injuries, however, are best managed by primary arterial repair or endovascular stent grafting.

Neurological deficit is only a contraindication to surgical repair in a deeply comatose patient with a dense neurological deficit, arterial occlusion and a huge infarct on cerebral CT.[31] All other patients with associated neurological deficit would benefit from arterial repair, with improved mortality and final neurological status.

Most blunt injuries of the carotid and vertebral arteries result in intimal disruption, with dissection and/or thrombosis, and the immediate goal of management is to restore cerebral perfusion and to prevent embolisation. Systemic anticoagulation is therefore the treatment of choice, because it limits the formation, propagation and/or embolisation of the thrombus. Intravenous heparin is administered in the acute phase, followed by oral anticoagulation for at least 3 months.[32]

Operative technique

Detailed description of operative technique falls outside the scope of this chapter and the reader is referred to the standard textbooks on operative surgery.[33] The general principles of management include the following:

- The patient should be in a supine position with a bolster between the scapulae and with the neck extended and the head rotated to the contralateral side. The patient must be draped to allow access from the base of the skull to the xiphisternum.
- Zone 2 injuries are explored by the standard carotid incision overlying the anterior border of the sternocleidomastoid muscle.
- Zone 1 injuries may require a median sternotomy.
- Various techniques have been described to improve exposure of the distal internal carotid artery in zone 3 injuries, including subluxation of the mandible, mandibular osteotomy, excision of the styloid process, etc.
- Some authors recommend routine shunting to maintain antegrade flow.
- Where simple repair is not feasible, a bypass should be performed. Saphenous vein should preferably be used in the internal carotid artery whereas polytetrafluoroethylene (PTFE) is used to repair the common carotid artery.
- The external carotid artery can be safely ligated if the internal carotid artery is patent. Internal carotid artery ligation is only recommended when the distal vessel is thrombosed with no back-bleeding following extraction of thrombus.

- Minor venous injuries can be managed by lateral suture repair, but complex venous repair is not indicated as there is a high occlusion rate and it increases the magnitude of the operative procedure. Ligation of the jugular vein can be performed without significant sequelae.[34]
- In the presence of associated injuries to the trachea and oesophagus, the vascular repair should be protected by soft-tissue interposition (sternocleidomastoid muscle).

Vertebral artery injuries

The occurrence of vertebral artery injury is low, with the reported incidence in penetrating neck trauma ranging from 1% to 7.4%. Gunshot wounds are the most common mechanism of injury.[35] Blunt injury of the vertebral artery is even less common and is caused by fractures of the lateral mass of the cervical vertebrae involving the foramen transversarium, vertebral fractures, ligamentous cervical spine injury, or severe and sudden rotation and/or hyperextension of the head. These injuries are seen with motor vehicle accidents, near-hanging injuries and after extreme chiropractic manipulation.[36]

The majority of patients with vertebral artery injuries have associated injuries of the cervical spine, spinal cord and other vascular structures in the neck or aerodigestive tract.[37]

Angiographic embolisation is the treatment of choice in the majority of patients with vertebral artery injuries.[15,38] Operative management is only indicated for severe active bleeding or when embolisation has failed. Haemodynamically stable patients with a thrombosed vertebral artery do not need any intervention.

A detailed description of surgical approaches to, and management of, vertebral artery injuries is given by Hatzitheofilou et al.[39]

Subclavian and axillary vascular injuries

All patients with periclavicular trauma should be evaluated for possible vascular injury. Most of these injuries are caused by penetrating trauma. The presence of a peripheral pulse does not reliably exclude significant proximal arterial injury. A difference in blood pressure of more than 20 mmHg between the upper limbs warrants further investigation. The brachial plexus is injured in about one-third of patients with subclavian or axillary artery injuries. A thorough neurological assessment should be performed.

Duplex ultrasound reliably assesses arterial and venous injuries but has certain limitations, for example visualising the origin of the subclavian artery.[40] CTA is the preferred diagnostic modality in cervico-mediastinal injuries. DSA has a therapeutic role in embolisation of injured vessels and for stent graft repair.

Where surgical repair is required, the neck and chest should be included in the operative field. The patient is placed supine and the arm is draped free and abducted to 30°. The head is turned to the other side. The standard incision starts at the sternoclavicular joint and extends over the medial half of the clavicle, curving over the deltopectoral groove. For proximal subclavian artery injuries this incision can be combined with a median sternotomy, which gives excellent exposure of both proximal subclavian arteries.[33] The so-called 'trapdoor' incision (supraclavicular incision, upper third median sternotomy and left anterior thoracotomy) is not recommended due to significant postoperative morbidity.

The axillary artery is exposed through an infraclavicular incision between the clavicular and sternal parts of the pectoralis major muscle. Dividing the clavicle should be avoided whenever possible due to postoperative morbidity.

Promising results have been obtained with endovascular repair of pseudoaneurysms and arteriovenous fistulas in selected patients (**Figs 9.7** and **9.11**). Most studies report a significant incidence of brachial plexus injury associated with surgical repair of subclavian artery injuries; this may be avoided with endovascular repair.

Endovascular management of cervical vascular injuries

An important advantage of endovascular repair of cervico-mediastinal trauma is the avoidance of general anaesthesia and the ability to monitor neurological status during the procedure. Endovascular therapies are used in three ways in the management of cervical vascular trauma:

1. **Angiographic embolisation.** This is indicated for (a) injury to the vertebral artery in the osseus vertebral canal and (b) persistent bleeding from external carotid artery branches (face, oro- and nasopharynx).[15,41]

2. **Temporary balloon occlusion.** This is used as an adjunct to support standard open vascular repair in neck zone 1 and 3 injuries. An occlusion balloon is placed via the femoral artery to provide proximal endoluminal control of the injured vessel, allowing surgical exposure in a more controlled fashion, and possibly avoiding sternotomy for proximal control.

3. **Covered stent grafts.** These are indicated for penetrating wounds, arteriovenous fistulae and pseudoaneurysms in (a) surgically inaccessible regions, and (b) in patients where extensive surgical exploration is to be avoided due to multiple trauma, local aggravating factors or high surgical risk due to medical comorbidities.

✓✓ Endovascular stentgrafting should be considered in all patients with penetrating injuries of the brachiocephalic trunk, proximal common carotid, distal internal carotid and subclavian arteries[42–44] (Fig. 9.12).

Thoracic vascular injuries

The majority of thoracic vascular injuries are caused by penetrating trauma, with a mortality rate as high as 90%.[45] Blunt aortic injury is considered as the second most common cause of death in trauma

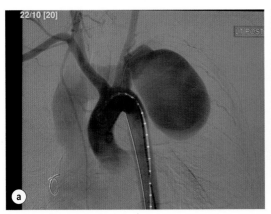
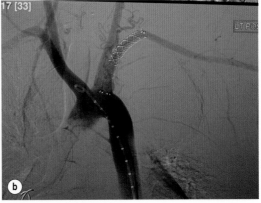

Figure 9.11 • Arteriovenous fistula of the subclavian artery **(a)** repaired by stent graft **(b)**.

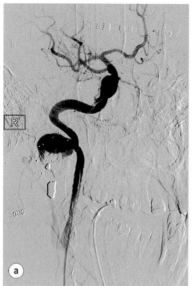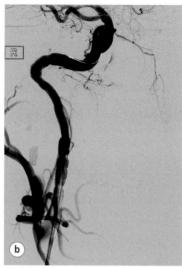

Figure 9.12 • Stent graft repair of a pseudoaneurysm in the R-internal carotid artery, pre-stent **(a)** and post-stent **(b)**.

patients; 70–90% of patients sustaining these injuries will die before reaching a hospital and, if left untreated, 90% will die within 4 months.[46] The site of insertion of the ligamentum arteriosum, just distal to the origin of the left subclavian artery, is the typical point of injury. Deceleration or compression injury may also involve the brachiocephalic trunk, the pulmonary veins and the vena cava.

Clinical presentation and initial management

Patients with penetrating thoracic vascular trauma are usually haemodynamically unstable, often with continuing haemorrhage into the pleural cavity or the mediastinum and should be taken for urgent thoracotomy. Patients with blunt thoracic trauma may initially be haemodynamically stable and the injury may not be immediately apparent due to the high incidence of concomitant trauma. The following clinical findings may be associated with underlying thoracic great vessel injury:

- shock/hypotension;
- difference in blood pressure or pulses between the two upper extremities;
- difference in blood pressure between upper and lower extremities (pseudocoarctation syndrome);
- expanding haematoma at the thoracic outlet;
- left flail chest;
- infrascapular murmur;
- palpable fracture of the sternum;
- palpable fracture of the thoracic spine;

- external evidence of major chest trauma;
- history indicating deceleration or compression injury to the chest.

Diagnostic studies

The number and type of diagnostic studies performed will be determined by the patient's haemodynamic stability and general status, as well as the type of aortic lesion and concomitant injuries.

Chest radiography

A frontal chest radiograph is an important screening tool and should be obtained in all patients with penetrating and suspected blunt thoracic trauma. Radio-opaque markers are useful for identifying entrance and exit sites.

A widened mediastinum on chest radiography is associated with more than 90% of thoracic aortic injuries, with a 90% sensitivity and 95% negative predictive value.[47] Other radiographic findings associated with blunt injuries of the descending aorta include the following:

1. Mediastinal findings:
   a. widening of the mediastinum greater than 8 cm;
   b. obliteration of the aortic knob contour;
   c. depression of the left main stem bronchus greater than 140°;
   d. loss of the paravertebral pleural line;
   e. lateral displacement of the trachea;
   f. deviation of a nasogastric tube;
   g. calcium layering of the aortic knob.

2. Fractures of sternum, first and second ribs and thoracic spine. Scapular and clavicular fractures in a polytrauma patient.

3. Other findings on (a) anteroposterior chest radiograph: apical pleural haematoma (apical cap), massive left haemothorax/effusion, ruptured diaphragm; (b) lateral chest radiograph: anterior displacement of trachea, loss of the aortopulmonary window.

Positive findings on chest radiography are indications for CTA.

Angiography

> ✅ CTA is recommended as the primary diagnostic modality in patients with suspected blunt thoracic aortic injury.[48]

CTA is also preferred to conventional arteriography for penetrating trauma in haemodynamically stable patients with suspected injury to the innominate, carotid and subclavian arteries. CTA is less invasive, faster to obtain and more readily available than catheter angiography, and also provides important information regarding associated lesions. However, the relative inaccessibility to the patient during examination limits its use in unstable patients.

The proximity of a missile trajectory to the brachiocephalic vessels may in itself be an indication for CTA even without any physical findings of vascular injury. DSA is used as part of the endovascular management of the injured vessel.

Other imaging modalities

Intravascular ultrasound is valuable for sizing and accurate placement of thoracic endografts during endovascular repair.[49]

Treatment

Indications for urgent surgery are haemodynamic instability, increasing haemorrhage from chest tubes and radiographic evidence of an expanding haematoma. An initial large volume of blood drained from a chest tube (>1500 mL) or ongoing haemorrhage of more than 200–300 mL/hour may indicate great vessel injury that requires thoracotomy.

The Vancouver classification of thoracic aortic injuries is useful in terms of staging the extent of injury and guiding intervention. Minimal aortic lesions, i.e. Vancouver grade I (intimal flap/intramural haematoma/thrombus <10 mm) or grade II (intimal flap/intramural haematoma/thrombus >20 mm) are managed non-operatively with close observation, whilst grade III lesions (pseudoaneurysm, simple or complex but no extravasation) and grade IV

lesions (active contrast extravasation) will require intervention.[50]

Patients selected for initial non-operative management should be closely monitored, with systolic blood pressure kept below 120 mmHg or mean arterial pressure below 80 mmHg. Intravenous beta-blockade, titrated to heart rate, was shown to be beneficial in patients with a blunt aortic injury.

Endovascular repair

Injuries to the arch outflow vessels can be successfully managed with endovascular stent grafting.[42–44]

> ✅✅ Endovascular stent grafting is currently the preferred method for treating traumatic rupture of the descending thoracic aorta. Mortality is significantly lower compared to open surgery (9% vs 19%) with a decreased risk of spinal cord ischaemia, renal injury, graft and systemic infection (**Fig. 9.13**).[51]

Numerous recent studies have reported on the durability of thoracic stent grafts up to 10 years with low complication and re-intervention rates.[52]

Surgical repair

Open surgery is reserved for unstable, hypotensive patients, for injuries of the ascending aorta and arch, and where endovascular treatment is not readily available. The basic surgical approaches are: median sternotomy, left anterolateral thoracotomy and left posterolateral thoracotomy. The reader is referred to the standard textbooks on thoracic surgery for a detailed description of these procedures.

Abdominal vascular injuries

Penetrating trauma accounts for 90–95% of abdominal vascular injuries (**Fig. 9.14**), with a high mortality due to the nature of these injuries as well as associated injuries to other intra-abdominal organs. It is important to consider intra-abdominal injury with all penetrating injuries from the fourth intercostal space anteriorly (level of T8 posterior) to the upper thighs.

Diagnosis

The unstable patient with a possible abdominal vascular injury requires immediate surgery. The

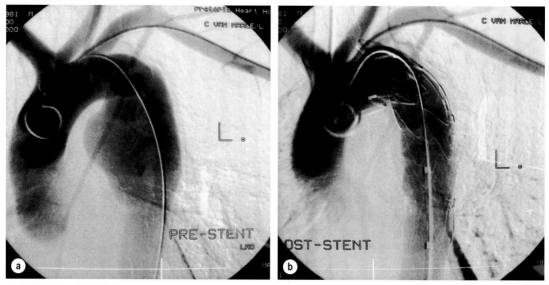

Figure 9.13 • Thoracic aneurysm after blunt injury to the chest **(a)** treated with a covered aortic stent graft **(b)**.

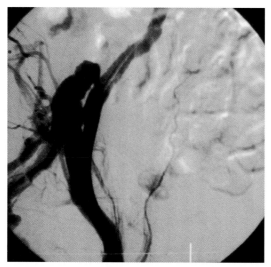

Figure 9.14 • A-V fistula between the left common iliac artery and vein after a gunshot wound to the lower abdomen.

stable patient should be investigated according to the injuries. Plain abdominal radiography using radio-opaque markers (paperclips) placed on the entrance and exit wounds is of value in establishing the trajectory of missiles in penetrating injuries. DSA and CTA have little, if any, role in the diagnosis of abdominal vascular injury when the patient is unstable. CTA is the investigation of choice in stable patients with penetrating or blunt abdominal trauma.[10,53]

Management

Abdominal vascular injuries are usually associated with haemodynamic instability or concomitant bowel injuries requiring a laparotomy. The abdominal cavity should be entered rapidly as tamponade and haemodynamic stability may be lost with relaxation of the abdominal musculature at the induction of anaesthesia. A generous laparotomy incision is required from xiphisternum to suprapubis. Four-quadrant packing of the abdomen is performed immediately and the proximal aorta is controlled at the diaphragmatic crus. Once the vascular injury is controlled, resuscitation with blood products is started. Bowel injuries are temporarily controlled until vascular repair is effected.

The retroperitoneum is divided into three anatomical zones for purposes of treatment. Central retroperitoneal haematomas (zone 1) are formally explored due to the high incidence of associated major vascular, pancreatic or duodenal injuries, and the high morbidity and mortality if these are overlooked. Flank/perinephric haematomas (zone 2) caused by penetrating injuries should routinely be explored, whilst haematomas caused by blunt trauma can be left alone if they are not expanding and the urogram on contrast-enhanced CT scan is normal. Zone 3 injuries, which are confined to or originate from the pelvis, are most often associated with pelvic fractures; exploration in these cases can be hazardous and is usually avoided. Retroperitoneal haematomas following penetrating injuries are usually explored to exclude major vascular injuries.

Different surgical exposures are used for specific injuries:

- Medial visceral rotation of the left-sided viscera (Mattox manoeuvre), i.e. spleen, tail of the pancreas, left colon and kidney allows access to the supracoeliac aorta, coeliac axis with its branches to the left, superior mesenteric artery (SMA), inferior mesenteric artery, left renal artery and left iliac vessels.
- The Cattell–Braasch or extended Kocher manoeuvre (right-sided medial visceral rotation) allows access to infrahepatic inferior vena cava, right renal vein, portal system and right iliac vessels.
- The infrarenal aorta and IVC are exposed by reflecting the transverse colon superiorly and the small intestine to the right and then dividing the midline retroperitoneum.
- The iliac arteries are exposed via separate incisions lateral to the caecum and sigmoid, respectively, avoiding injury to the ureters as they cross the common iliac arteries. The iliac veins may be accessible only after dividing the arteries that lie anterior to them.

Aortic injury

Direct repair is used for simple lacerations; this should be done transversely to avoid narrowing. An interposition polyester or PTFE graft may be necessary where there is extensive destruction, but should be avoided in a contaminated field.

In the 'damage control' scenario, a temporary shunt using a sterile intercostal drain can be placed in the aorta. Definitive repair is performed once the patient is stable and all physiological parameters are normal.[54]

In the absence of contamination, in situ graft replacement with either a PTFE or polyester (Dacron) graft soaked in rifampicin, can be used. In cases with contamination the aorta is ligated and an extra-anatomic bypass (axillo-bifemoral bypass) is performed.[55] Autologous veins using the superficial femoral–popliteal veins have been used to replace infected aortic prosthesis, but this procedure is invasive, time-consuming and is associated with significant blood loss. It is therefore not indicated in the unstable patient.[56] Abdominal aortic dissection after blunt trauma ('seat-belt aorta') is relatively uncommon, but endovascular repair has been described in such cases.[57]

Visceral artery injury

Injuries to the coeliac trunk and its branches are usually dealt with by primary ligation.[55] The superior mesenteric artery is divided into four zones.[58] Injuries to the first two zones (i.e. SMA trunk to the origin of the middle colic artery) should be repaired. Where primary repair is not possible due to extreme damage, bypass with saphenous vein or PTFE should be performed to maintain midgut viability. Injuries to the inferior mesenteric artery can usually be ligated.

Renal artery injury

Blunt injury, usually caused by acceleration/deceleration, results in intimal disruption with subsequent thrombosis of the vessels. These injuries should be repaired within 12 hours, since renal viability beyond this period is very slim. Proximal injuries are approached from the midline through the base of the mesentery, while distal injuries are approached laterally. Repair is performed by either primary repair or interposition grafting using saphenous vein.

Traumatic renal artery dissection can be managed endovascularly with either bare metal or covered stent grafts.[59]

Inferior vena cava injury

The IVC consists of four parts: infrarenal, suprarenal, retrohepatic and intrapericardial. The retrohepatic and intrapericardial portions are usually affected by blunt trauma. Approximately 50% of patients die before reaching hospital and the in-hospital mortality ranges between 20% and 57%.[60]

Wounds in the infrahepatic IVC can be temporarily controlled by means of digital pressure or intraluminal balloon catheters. When clamps are applied, one should be aware of the abundant lumbar collateral circulation. Repair is effected by means of lateral suture or, when there are large defects, even prosthetic material. The anterior laceration in a through-and-through lesion may need to be extended so that the posterior defect can be repaired first. In dire attempts to save an exsanguinating patient this part of the IVC may be ligated. The retrohepatic IVC should be approached with extreme caution. If haemorrhage can be controlled with packing this should be the method of treatment. Various strategies to repair these injuries have been described but the prognosis is still dismal, with a reported mortality of 70–90%.[61] The Shrock shunt, which is inserted through the right atrium, can be used to control these injuries temporarily. We use a modified technique by inserting an endotracheal tube through the infrahepatic IVC and inflating the balloon in the right atrium. Total hepatic isolation (Heany manoeuvre) is associated with a high mortality, especially in an exsanguinated patient.

Emergency endovascular stent graft repair for traumatic injury of the inferior vena cava was described by Castelli et al.[62]

Pelvic vascular injury

Haemorrhage is the primary cause of death in patients with pelvic fractures. The major sources of bleeding are branches of the internal iliac artery and vein, bone and soft tissues. These injuries are managed by embolising the relevant bleeding branches.[13] The common iliac, external iliac and common femoral arteries and corresponding veins are the source of catastrophic blood loss in about only 1% of pelvic fractures. Penetrating and blunt injuries to the common and external iliac arteries can be repaired by primary suturing or interposition grafting. In the case of severe contamination, ligation and femorofemoral bypass is an accepted technique.[55] The internal iliac artery may be ligated. Reports support a role for the endovascular management of iliac artery injuries.[63]

Extremity vascular trauma

The incidence of peripheral vascular injury depends on the extent and type of trauma, ranging from 0.6–3.6% for isolated extremity fractures to 25–30% for all penetrating injuries of the extremities.[1] The risk of limb loss is greatest following blunt trauma and injuries from high-velocity missiles or close-range shotgun wounds.

Diagnosis

Any extremity injury warrants a complete physical examination of the injured extremity and distal vessels. The absence of hard signs of vascular injury reliably excludes surgically significant arterial injury.[64]

✅✅ CTA has proven excellent sensitivity and specificity for diagnosing extremity vascular injury and can replace DSA as a diagnostic modality.[65]

The occurrence of delayed thrombosis stresses the importance of regular reassessment of the peripheral circulation for at least 24 hours after orthopaedic injury. There is a role for duplex Doppler studies in patients with soft signs of vascular injury or with proximity injuries.[66]

General principles of management

- Restoration of perfusion to an ischaemic extremity should be performed as quickly as possible. Contemporary studies emphasise the importance of restoration of perfusion within 3–4 hours to optimise neuromuscular recovery of the injured limb.[5] Adjunctive therapies such as hypertonic saline resuscitation, temporary intravascular shunts, fasciotomy, limb cooling and ischaemic reconditioning may reduce the severity of ischaemic injury.[5,67]

- Non-operative observation of asymptomatic non-occlusive arterial injuries is acceptable. These injuries can be defined as small pseudoaneurysms, intimal flaps or irregularities, small arteriovenous fistulas and haemodynamically insignificant narrowing of the vessels. Should subsequent repair of these injuries be required, it can be done without significant increase in morbidity.[6]

- Extremity arterial trauma is usually addressed by conventional open surgical techniques. Endovascular treatment usually consists of embolisation of non-essential vessels after penetrating trauma.

- Simple arterial repairs do better than grafts. If complex repair is required, vein grafts appear to be the best choice.[68] PTFE is an acceptable conduit when no vein is available and may even be used in a contaminated field.[11] Effort should be made to cover the graft with soft tissue.

- Temporary shunting is valuable for maintaining antegrade flow in order to allow stabilisation of unstable fractures and/or dislocations prior to definitive arterial repair (**Fig. 9.15**).[12]

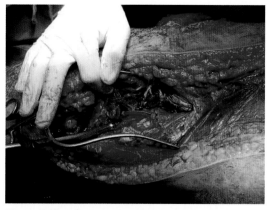

Figure 9.15 • Temporary shunt in right superficial femoral artery, allowing distal perfusion while external fixator is applied to the femur.

- Early four-compartment lower leg fasciotomy should be applied liberally. Indications for fasciotomy include: (i) ischaemic time greater than 4–6 hours; (ii) signs of acute ischaemia; (iii) extensive soft-tissue injuries; (iv) combined arterial and venous injuries; (v) intra-compartmental bleeding; and (vi) increased compartmental pressure. Measurement of compartment pressures is an important adjunct, and must be done in all compartments. Pressures should be interpreted in the context of each individual patient, because tissue perfusion is a balance between compartment pressure and blood pressure. Acceptable compartment pressures have been defined as absolute compartment pressures of less than 20 mmHg and at least 30 mmHg less than mean arterial pressure.[69]
- Completion arteriogram should be performed after arterial repair to assess patency and technical perfection of the repair.
- Although amputation rates increase with longer ischaemia times, quantifying the relationship is difficult, because amputation rates also depend on other factors such as extent of soft-tissue damage, the capacity of collaterals, pre-existing arterial disease and the vessels injured.[70]
- In certain cases primary amputation may be considered. Scoring systems such as the mangled extremity severity score (MESS) have been developed to help predict the outcome of limb salvage procedures.[71] A MESS score of 7 or more has a predicted amputation rate of 100%. Several MESS score calculators are available online. Given the significance of amputation, delaying the procedure even by a day or two is preferred as it allows careful examination of the limb and discussion with the patient and family.
- Measures should be taken to protect against the systemic effects of reperfusion injury and subsequent renal damage. A diuresis of at least 2–3 mL/kg per hour is maintained with the administration of adequate volumes of normal saline. This should be started during the operation and is continued postoperatively for as long as the serum myoglobin and creatine kinase remain elevated. Measures to treat hyperkalaemia may be required.

Vascular injuries to the upper limb (Fig. 9.16)

Brachial artery injuries

The most common injuries to the brachial artery are associated with either a supracondylar fracture or an elbow dislocation followed by penetrating vascular trauma.[72] Upper extremity vascular injuries are usually not life-threatening, but significant morbidity

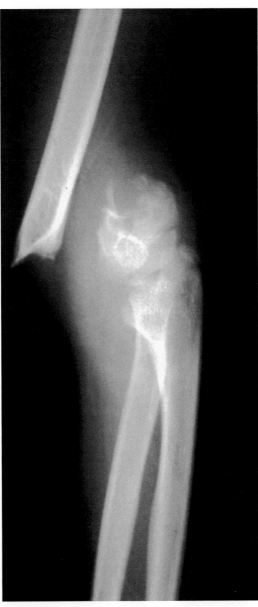

Figure 9.16 • Fractures of the supracondylar humerus are often associated with vascular injuries and should alert the physician to the possibility of a vascular injury.

may occur. Return of function is often related to associated nerve injury. In the case of blunt injury the fracture or dislocation should be reduced. If the distal pulse returns the patient should be treated expectantly with regular, i.e. 2-hourly, evaluation of the circulation. If the limb remains ischaemic or even if the hand is pink with no pulses, it is mandatory to explore and repair the arterial injury in order to avoid complications like an ischaemic contracture.[73] With penetrating trauma the injury should be repaired by open surgical repair.

Distal arterial injuries to the upper limb

Most of the injuries to the forearm circulation are due to a penetrating mechanism. When only one vessel in the forearm is injured it may usually be ligated without any adverse effects. If both the radial and ulnar arteries are injured at least one should be repaired – preferably the ulnar artery as this vessel is in most cases the dominant supply to the hand. These injuries are often accompanied by injuries to the accompanying nerve and will require repair of the nerve.[72]

Venous injuries to the arm rarely require repair and even injuries to the brachial and axillary veins may be ligated because the collateral venous network is extensive.

Vascular injuries to the lower limb

These injuries are often associated with skeletal injuries, especially posterior dislocation of the knee, proximal tibial fractures and supracondylar femur fractures. Immediate arterial repair should be performed when the skeletal injury is stable and not significantly displaced. When there is instability,

severe displacement and where extreme orthopaedic manipulation is anticipated, a temporary shunt should be placed to restore blood flow while the orthopaedic repair is completed, after which definite arterial repair is performed. Patients may have significant bleeding from extremity vascular injuries and a tourniquet should be used if the bleeding cannot be controlled with direct pressure.[74]

Femoral vascular injuries

Bleeding from the femoral triangle can be difficult to control, particularly if both artery and vein are injured. The suprainguinal region should be entered through a separate incision above the inguinal ligament to obtain proximal control of the vessels.

> ✔✔ Common femoral artery injuries should always be repaired as ligation has a 50% amputation rate.[70]

Effort should be made to also repair the common femoral vein.

Iatrogenic injuries (pseudoaneurysms and arteriovenous fistula) secondary to attempted femoral access are fairly common. Primary treatment of femoral pseudoaneurysms consists of ultrasound-guided compression and thrombin injection.[75]

Popliteal vascular injury

The lower leg is almost totally dependent on the popliteal artery. Popliteal artery injury has an amputation rate of up to 16%.[70] The association between posterior knee dislocation and popliteal artery disruption is well known (**Fig. 9.17**). All patients with posterior knee dislocations should have a complete neurovascular examination of the

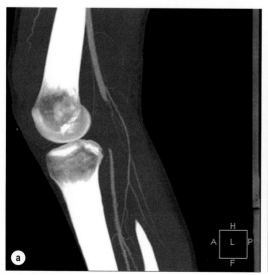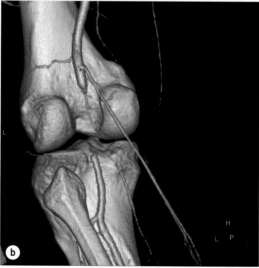

Figure 9.17 • Popliteal artery injury after posterior dislocation of the left knee, angiogram **(a)**, and 3D reconstruction **(b)**.

affected limb. Most popliteal artery injuries present with hard signs of arterial injury. The absence of hard signs is usually sufficient to rule out injuries to the popliteal artery.[76]

✅✅ Selective angiography (CTA or DSA) following knee dislocation is safe as there is a strong correlation between results of serial physical examinations and the need for arteriography. Patients who are managed expectantly should be closely observed, with regular reassessment of the peripheral circulation.[77,78]

Injury to popliteal veins should be repaired in order to minimise postoperative swelling and compartment syndrome and to improve the patency of arterial repairs.

Compartment syndrome is a major risk factor for amputation following popliteal artery injury.[79] There is evidence that fasciotomy performed at the time of arterial repair, but before the development of compartment syndrome (prophylactic fasciotomy),

may lower amputation rates, particularly in patients with long preoperative delays, extensive injuries, injuries of the artery and vein, and venous injuries treated with ligation.[80]

Single tibial vessels may be ligated if there is documented collateral flow distally.

Resuscitative endovascular balloon occlusion of the aorta (REBOA)

Temporary occlusion of the aorta with a percutaneously placed balloon has been used as an adjunct to resuscitation and haemorrhage control in thoracic, abdominal and pelvic trauma.[81–83] A detailed description of the technique has been published in the *Journal of Trauma*.[84] High quality evidence in support of this technique is, however, lacking. A recent systematic review of REBOA concluded that the evidence is weak, with no clear reduction of haemorrhage-associated mortality.[85] A study from Japan found an association between the use of REBOA and an excess mortality in patients with haemodynamically unstable torso trauma.[86]

Key points

- A high index of suspicion should be maintained regarding possible vascular injuries in the trauma patient.
- A thorough clinical examination is accurate in predicting significant vascular injury.
- Special investigations should only be performed in adequately resuscitated and haemodynamically stable patients.
- Haemodynamic instability, active bleeding and an expanding haematoma are indications for immediate surgery.
- The absence of hard signs of arterial injury justifies an expectant non-operative approach with careful observation.
- Restoration of arterial blood supply should be achieved as soon as possible; temporary intra-arterial shunts are valuable in this regard.
- Adequate surgical exposure is vital for proper management of vascular injuries.
- Fasciotomy should be applied liberally in lower-extremity vascular trauma.
- Endovascular treatment is useful in managing arterial lesions in anatomically challenging locations and is currently indicated for injuries of the descending thoracic aorta, proximal aortic arch branches, and distal internal carotid and vertebral arteries.

🌐 Full references available at **http://expertconsult.inkling.com**

Key references

6. Dennis JW, Frykberg ER, Veldenz HC, et al. Validation of non-operative management of occult vascular injuries and accuracy of physical examination alone in penetrating extremity trauma: 5–10 year follow up. J Trauma 1998;44:243–53. PMID: 9498494.

   A prospective study with 10-year follow-up proving the accuracy of clinical assessment and conservative management of occult vascular trauma.

7. Johansen K, Lynch K. Non-invasive vascular tests reliably exclude occult arterial trauma in injured extremities. J Trauma 1991;31:515–22. PMID: 2020038.

In this prospective study it was shown that an API of more than 0.9 has a negative predictive value of 99% for excluding significant arterial trauma. Reserving arteriography for limbs with an API of less than 0.9 is safe, accurate and cost-effective.

8. Bickell WH, Wall MJ, Pepe PE, et al. Immediate vs delayed fluid resuscitation for hypotensive patients with penetrating torso injuries. N Engl J Med 1994; 331:1105–9. PMID: 7935634.
   In a randomised controlled trial of patients with penetrating torso injuries, reduced mortality and complications were seen when fluid resuscitation was delayed until haemorrhage was controlled.

9. Johansson PI, Stensballe J, Oliveri R, et al. How I treat patients with massive haemorrhage. Blood 2014;124:3052–8. PMID: 25293771.
   Comprehensive literature review on haemostatitc resuscitation with recommendations regarding the monitoring of haemostasis and targeted administration of blood products.

10. Patterson BO, Holt PJ, Cleanthis M, et al on behalf of the London Vascular Injuries Working Group. Imaging vascular trauma. Br J Surg 2012;99:494–505. PMID: 22190106.
    A systematic review of the literature on the radiological diagnosis of vascular trauma. CTA was found to have acceptable sensitivity and specificity for diagnosing blunt and penetrating vascular injuries and is recommended as the primary investigation for vascular trauma.

12. Inaba K, Aksoy H, Seamon MJ, et al. Multicentre evaluation of temporary intravascular shunt use in vascular trauma. J Trauma 2016;80:359–64. PMID: 26713968.
    This multicentre report represents the largest civilian experience of temporary intravascular shunts used for damage control, staged procedures and for referral due to insufficient surgeon skill. Description of the indication, technique and outcome in a range of vascular injuries.

13. Velmahos GC, Toutouzas KG, Sarkisyan G, et al. A prospective study on the safety and efficacy of angiographic embolisation for pelvic and visceral injuries. J Trauma 2002;53:303–8. PMID: 12169938.
    100 consecutive patients were evaluated by angiography for bleeding from major pelvic fractures (n=65) or solid visceral organ injuries (n=35). Angiographic embolisation was found to be highly effective in controlling bleeding in patients with selected injuries of the pelvis and abdominal visceral organs.

14. Stratil PG, Burdick TR. Visceral trauma: principles of management and role of embolo therapy. Semin Intervent Radiol 2008;25:271–80. PMID: 21326517.
    This article reviews the general management of visceral injuries with special reference to embolising lesions of the liver, kidneys and spleen.

28. Feliciano DV. Penetrating cervical trauma. World J Surg 2015;39:1363–72. PMID: 25561188.
    Detailed discussion on the management of patients with penetrating cervical trauma.

42. Du Toit DF, Odendaal W, Lampbrechts A, et al. Surgical and endovascular management of penetrating innominate artery injuries. Eur J Vasc Endovasc Surg 2008;36:56–62. PMID: 18356085.
    The authors discuss the diagnosis and management of patients with penetrating innominate artery injuries with special reference to surgical and endovascular technique.

43. Du Toit DF, Coolen D, Lampbrechts A, et al. The endovascular management of penetrating carotid artery injuries: long-term follow up. Eur J Vasc Endovasc Surg 2009;38:267–70. PMID: 19570690.
    This article discusses the indications and technique of carotid artery stenting and reports on the long-term follow-up.

44. Du Toit DF, Lampbrechts A, Stark H, et al. Long-term results of stentgraft treatment of subclavian artery injuries: management of choice for stable patients? J Vasc Surg 2008;47:739–43. PMID: 18242938.
    The authors report their extensive experience with endovascular management of subclavian artery injuries discussing their technique, with immediate results and long-term follow-up (mean 49 months, range 5–104 months).

48. Fox N, Schwartz D, Salazar JH, et al. Evaluation and management of blunt traumatic aortic injury: a practice management guideline from the Eastern Association for the Surgery of Trauma. J Trauma Acute Care Surg 2015;78:136–46. PMID: 25539215.
    These guidelines represent a comprehensive overview of the literature regarding the evaluation and management of blunt thoracic aortic injury (BTAI). Three important and evidence-based recommendations regarding BTAI are made: (1) CTA is strongly recommended for the identification of clinical significant BTAI. (2) The use of endovascular repair is strongly recommended in patients with BTAI who do not have contraindications to endovascular repair. (3) The use of delayed repair in patients with BTAI is suggested with strict blood pressure control.

51. Lee WA, Matsumura MD, Mitchell RS, et al. Endovascular repair of traumatic thoracic aortic injury: clinical practice guidelines for the Society for Vascular Surgery. J Vasc Surg 2011;53:187–92. PMID: 20974523.
    A systematic review and meta-analysis of the literature including 7768 patients from 139 studies. The mortality was significantly lower in patients who underwent endovascular repair compared with open repair (9% vs 19%). Endovascular repair also had decreased risk of spinal chord ischaemia, renal impairment, graft and systemic infections.

54. Aucar JA, Hirshberg A. Damage control for vascular injuries. Surg Clin North Am 1997;77:853–62. PMID: 9291986.

A good review of the different techniques in vascular damage control.

65. Jens S, Kerstens MK, Legemate DA, et al. Diagnostic performance of computed tomography angiography in peripheral arterial injuries due to trauma: a systematic review and meta-analysis. Eur J Vasc Endovasc Surg 2013;46:329–37. PMID: 23726770.

A systematic review and meta-analysis of literature comparing CTA with surgery, DSA or follow-up in extremity vascular trauma. Excellent sensitivity and specificity was found with CTA and it is recommended that CTA replaces DSA as diagnostic modality.

70. Hafez HM, Woolgar J, Robbs JV. Lower extremity arterial injury: results of 550 cases and review of risk factors associated with limb loss. J Vasc Surg 2001;33:1212–9. PMID: 11389420.

The authors review their experience with 641 lower limb arterial injuries in 550 patients with reference to diagnosis, management, results and risk factors for amputation.

77. Stannard JP, Shiels TM, Lopez-Ben RR, et al. Vascular injuries in knee dislocations: the role of physical examination in determining the need for arteriography. J Bone Joint Surg 2004; 86:910–4. PMID: 15118031.

In a prospective study of 138 consecutive patients with acute multiligamentous knee injury, a strong correlation was found between the results of physical examination and the need for arteriography. It was concluded that selective arteriography, based on serial physical examination, is a safe and prudent policy following knee dislocation.

78. Holtis JD, Daley BJ. 10-year review of knee dislocations: is arteriography always necessary? J Trauma 2005;59:672–6. PMID: 16361911.

In this retrospective review of patients with knee dislocation, the result of routine arteriography was compared to that of physical examination. It was concluded that routine arteriography was unnecessary in patients with a normal physical examination after reduction of the knee.

10

Extracranial cerebrovascular disease

A. Ross Naylor
Jos C. van den Berg

Introduction

Stroke is the third commonest cause of death and a major cause of neurological disability. It is defined as acute loss of focal cerebral function with symptoms exceeding 24 hours (or leading to death), with no apparent cause other than of vascular origin. A transient ischaemic attack (TIA) has the same definition, but lasts <24 hours. In the UK, the annual incidence of stroke is 2:1000 and 150 000 patients will suffer their first stroke each year.[1] Although mortality has diminished by about 20%, attributed to improved survival rather than a declining incidence, overall stroke incidence could increase by 30% by 2033 because of the ageing population.[1] About 36 000 patients will suffer a TIA each year, giving an annual UK incidence of 0.5:1000. TIA incidence increases with age from 0.9:1000 (55–64 years) to 2.6:1000 (75–84 years).[2]

Aetiology and risk factors

About 80% of strokes are ischaemic and 20% haemorrhagic (intracerebral/subarachnoid). Approximately 80% of ischaemic strokes affect the carotid territory. Risk factors include increasing age, smoking, hypertension, ischaemic heart disease, cardioembolic source, previous TIA, diabetes, peripheral artery disease (PAD), high plasma fibrinogen and hypercholesterolaemia. The main causes of ischaemic, carotid territory stroke include thromboembolism of the internal carotid artery (ICA) or middle cerebral artery (MCA) (50%); small vessel disease (25%); cardiac embolism (15%); haematological disorders (5%); and non-atheromatous disease (5%).[2]

Large-vessel thromboembolism

Commonest cause is thromboembolism from a stenosis at the origin of the ICA (**Fig. 10.1**). Haemodynamic failure accounts for <2% of strokes. Stenoses develop at the ICA origin because of a region of low shear stress, flow stasis and flow separation that predisposes towards atherosclerotic plaque formation. If the plaque undergoes acute disruption (rupture, ulceration, haemorrhage), the core of subendothelial collagen is exposed, triggering thrombus formation and secondary embolism.

Small-vessel disease

Occlusion of penetrating end-arterioles causes lacunar infarcts. The occlusive process follows fibrinoid necrosis (hypertensive encephalopathy), lipohyalinosis, micro-atheroma (chronic hypertension) or microcalcinosis (diabetes). The commonest sites for lacunar infarction include the basal ganglia, thalamus and internal capsule.

Cardiogenic brain embolism

Sources include ventricular mural thrombus (post-myocardial infarction [MI], cardiomyopathy), left atrial thrombus (atrial fibrillation) and valvular lesions (vegetations, prostheses, calcified annulus, endocarditis).

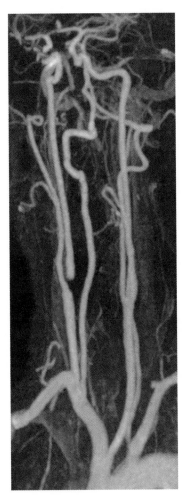

fibroplasia, perimedial fibroplasia, medial hyperplasia) and (iii) adventitial (periarterial) fibroplasia. The commonest is medial fibroplasia (75–80% of cases), characterised by alternating stenotic webs and dilatation/aneurysm formation (**Fig. 10.2**). In up to 60%, FMD is bilateral. Patients with carotid FMD may be asymptomatic or symptomatic (TIA/stroke, dissection, false aneurysm). Management is conservative in asymptomatic individuals, but surveillance is recommended. Once symptomatic, patients should be treated as for symptomatic atherosclerotic disease.

Figure 10.1 • CEMRA in the right anterior oblique orientation providing overview anatomical imaging, i.e. from the arch origin to the circle of Willis. There is an extremely tight stenosis (>95%) at the right carotid bulb/proximal internal carotid artery.

Haematological disorders

Myeloma, sickle-cell disease, polycythaemia, the oral contraceptive pill and related prothrombotic disorders predispose towards stroke.

Non-atheromatous carotid diseases

Fibromuscular dysplasia (FMD)

FMD is a rare disorder of unknown aetiology affecting the renal (60–75%) and carotid arteries (25–30%) in young to middle-aged women. The commonest presentation is hypertension. FMD is classified as: (i) intimal fibroplasia, (ii) medial dysplasia (medial

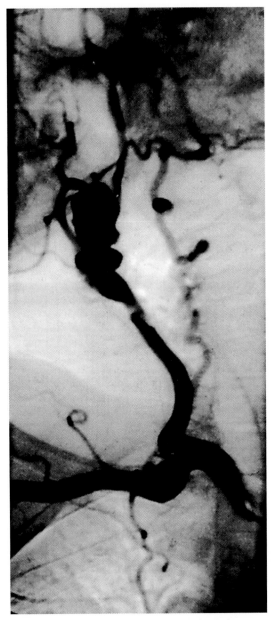

Figure 10.2 • Example of fibromuscular dysplasia causing early aneurysm formation in the carotid artery.

Options include resection and interposition bypass, open graduated internal dilatation or (more commonly) percutaneous angioplasty.

Arteritis

Takayasu's arteritis (TA) is a transmural, granulomatous inflammatory condition, ultimately causing occlusion through fibrosis. TA predominantly affects younger females (female:male ratio 7:1) and presentation may be a relatively innocuous illness comprising malaise, fever and arthralgia/myalgia. In the acute phase, there is a granulomatous vasculitis with medial disruption, followed by transmural fibrosis. Occasionally, focal aneurysms form after disruption of the internal elastic lamina and media. Neurological symptoms follow vessel occlusion or via renovascular hypertension. Type I TA (arch branches) and Type IIa (ascending aorta, aortic arch, arch branches) presents with cerebral vascular/ocular symptoms or asymptomatic stenoses. Type III TA (arch vessels plus abdominal aorta and its branches) accounts for 65% of cases and is associated with stroke, renovascular hypertension and mesenteric ischaemia.

The mainstay of treatment is immunosuppression (steroid/cyclophosphamide/methotrexate). Surgery should be avoided in the acute phase where possible. Neither endarterectomy nor angioplasty/stenting is really an option with involvement of the carotid vessels because of the long segments of fibrotic disease. If surgery becomes necessary, bypass is the preferred option and the inflow should be taken from the ascending aorta (as opposed to the subclavian artery) as the latter may be involved in the disease process.

Giant-cell arteritis (GCA) is the most common vasculitis in adults and primarily affects older females (female:male ratio 4:1). There are three recognised subtypes (systemic inflammatory syndrome; cranial arteritis and large vessel arteritis). The intracranial vessels are unaffected. The commonest presentation is malaise, headache and myalgic pain. Jaw claudication occurs in 50%, while 50% will develop pain over the temporal artery. Stroke is rare, the commonest presentation being transient/permanent blindness. Ocular symptoms (blindness, corneal ulcers/cataracts) can occur up to 6 months after initial presentation. Treatment is corticosteroid therapy.

Carotid aneurysm

Carotid aneurysms are rare (<2% of peripheral aneurysms, 0.2% of all carotid interventions). The accepted definition is a diameter >150% of the common carotid artery (CCA) or twice the diameter of the distal ICA. The aetiology is unknown, but may be 'atherosclerotic' or follow trauma/infection. Presentations include pulsatile swelling (with/without pain), Horner's syndrome, thrombosis, dissection, rupture or embolisation (TIA/stroke). Treatment involves exclusion and primary re-anastomosis or interposition bypass. Endovascular exclusion is the preferred option in patients with distal ICA aneurysms.

Carotid dissection

Acute carotid dissection causes 2% of strokes, increasing to 20% in young adults (**Fig. 10.3**). One-fifth of trauma patients with an unexplained neurological deficit will have a dissection and 25% will be bilateral. Dissection can be spontaneous (fibromuscular dysplasia), iatrogenic (angioplasty/stenting), be part of a type A dissection or follow blunt trauma (forced hyperextension or forced rotation with compression of the ICA between the mastoid process and the transverse process of C2). Type I dissections involve irregularity, but no significant stenosis (**Fig. 10.3a**); type II involves a 70–99% stenosis and/or >50% dilatation, while type III dissections present with a characteristic 'flame'-shaped occlusion about 2–3 cm distal to the bifurcation (**Fig. 10.3b**). The latter is due to compression of the true lumen by thrombus in the false channel.

The commonest presentation is ipsilateral head/neck pain (70%), but 50–75% of patients will present with TIA/stroke (usually embolic), pulsatile tinnitus, syncope, ocular signs or cranial nerve palsies (III, IV, VI, VII, IX, X, XII). Cranial nerve signs probably follow mechanical compression from mural haematoma or stretching. Up to 60% with spontaneous dissection will have ocular signs (oculo-sympathetic paresis, amaurosis fugax, aggravated by sitting/standing), hemianopia, ischaemic optic neuropathy and painful Horner's syndrome). The latter follows segmental ischaemia of the postganglionic fibres distal to the superior cervical ganglion and may persist in 50%.

> ✔ Recognition of ocular symptoms in patients with suspected dissection is important as up to 25% will suffer a stroke within 7 days.

Patients suspected of having a dissection should undergo ultrasound and computed tomographic/magnetic resonance (CT/MR) angiography (to include axial T2 fat-saturated images). This typically shows the dissection to start 2–3 cm beyond the origin of the ICA (**Fig. 10.3b**). The distal limit is variable (occasionally the petrous segment) with varying combinations of stenosis, dilatation, intimal flaps and occlusion in the intervening segment. The majority of dissections are managed conservatively. The aim is to reduce the risk of thrombosis and embolism.

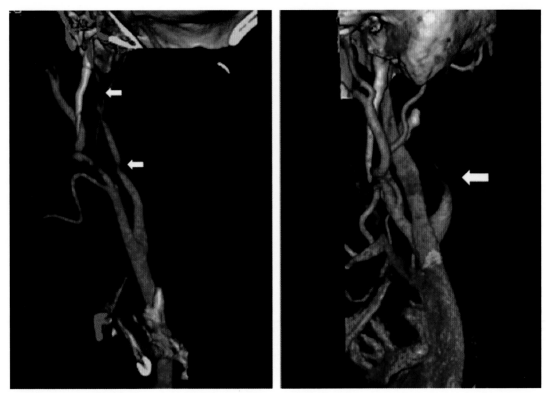

Figure 10.3 • 3-D CTA reconstruction showing bilateral carotid dissections in the same patient. Left panel shows asymptomatic, spontaneous internal carotid artery (ICA) dissection (type 1 lesion) with entry and exit tears (*small arrows*), causing no significant stenosis. Right panel: symptomatic 'flame'-shaped type 3 dissection with subocclusion of the ICA, 2–3 cm beyond the bifurcation.

> ✔ Most acute carotid dissections are treated with anticoagulation (heparin then warfarin), but systematic reviews suggest that there is no evidence that this is preferable/safer to antiplatelet therapy.[3]

Surgery (or endovascular intervention) is reserved for complex symptomatic trauma cases (usually type II), but may be indicated in patients with recurrent cerebral events despite medical therapy. Overall, dissection carries a 20% mortality and a 30% rate of disability. About 10–40% of patients suffering a carotid dissection will develop a false aneurysm, usually in the distal ICA. A recent systematic review of 166 non-operated distal ICA false aneurysms revealed that in 95% of cases the false aneurysm either stayed the same size or regressed, while <3% became symptomatic.[4]

> ✔ Most distal false aneurysms following carotid dissection do not increase in size or cause symptoms. The majority should, therefore, be managed conservatively. Interventions are only warranted if the aneurysm increases in size or causes symptoms.

Carotid body tumour

The carotid body is located within the adventitia of the posterior aspect of the carotid bifurcation and is responsible for monitoring blood gases/pH. A carotid body tumour (CBT) is derived from cells originating from the neural crest ectoderm (chemoreceptor cells). It is typically located in the space between the ICA and external carotid arteries (ECA), and consists of nests of neoplastic epithelioid chief cells. As it enlarges, the bifurcation splays (**Fig. 10.4**) and the patient becomes aware of a neck swelling. Other presentations include pain, invasion/compression causing hoarseness, cranial nerve palsies and Horner's syndrome. CBTs rarely cause cerebral ischaemia, but can present as a hormonally mediated syndrome comprising flushing, dizziness, arrhythmias and hypertension.

Diagnosis requires awareness, supplemented by ultrasound, MR/CT angiography. Overall, 5% are bilateral and 5% are malignant. Treatment involves excision, although a conservative approach may be preferable in elderly patients with small asymptomatic tumours. Preoperative embolisation or insertion of a covered stent into the proximal

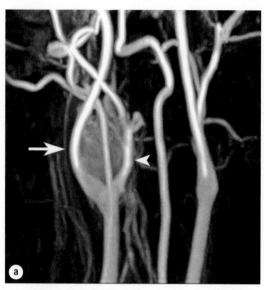 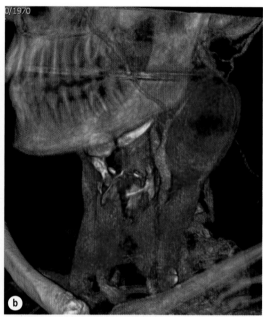

Figure 10.4 • (a) Maximum intensity projection reconstruction of MRA of a highly vascular right carotid body tumour causing splaying of the bifurcation (right internal carotid, *arrow*; right external carotid artery, *arrowhead*). **(b)** 3-D CT angiogram of a probable glomus vagale tumour. Note that the tumour does not splay the bifurcation, but it pushes between the external and internal carotid arteries from a posterior location higher up in the neck.

ECA may reduce intraoperative bleeding, but this is probably only necessary in large tumours. Patients with bilateral CBTs or a family history of CBTs should be referred for testing for mutations of the succinyl dehydrogenase gene as they may be associated with worse disease-free survival after resection in patients with carotid body paragangliomas and may therefore benefit from resection at an earlier stage.[5]

Differential diagnoses include glomus vagale/glomus jugulare tumours. A glomus vagale tumour arises from chemoreceptor cells within the vagus nerve and can be differentiated from a CBT because the bifurcation is not splayed. Instead, the tumour causes deviation of the ICA above the bifurcation (**Fig. 10.4b**). It is important to consider a glomus vagale tumour preoperatively as resection leads to swallowing problems (injury to motor fibres) and hoarseness (recurrent laryngeal nerve) and the patient has to be warned of this.

Presentation of carotid disease

Asymptomatic cerebrovascular disease

Four per cent of the population aged over 45 years will have a bruit, increasing to 12% in those older than 60 years.[6] One-third of patients with a 70–99% ICA stenosis will not have a bruit, increasing to 60% for those with 90–99% stenoses. Up to 30% of patients with ICA occlusion will still have a bruit. The commonest reasons for a false-positive bruit are systolic cardiac murmurs, haemodynamic causes and bruits arising from the vertebrals or ECA.

> ✅ The presence/absence/quality of a bruit does not correlate with degree of stenosis.

Symptomatic cerebrovascular disease

Carotid territory

'Classical' carotid territory symptoms include: (1) hemimotor/sensory signs, (2) transient monocular blindness (TMB) and (3) higher cortical dysfunction (Box 10.1). TMB usually develops over a few seconds and clears within a few minutes. Failure to resolve within 24 hours is analogous to a stroke.

> ✅ A history of TMB in the absence of a source of embolisation should prompt referral to an ophthalmologist to exclude anterior ischaemic optic neuropathy (microvascular disease of the posterior ciliary arteries), which causes acute ischaemia of the optic nerve head.

Differential diagnoses for carotid territory events include epilepsy, tumour, giant aneurysm, hypoglycaemia and migraine (i.e. stroke mimics). Where TIAs are precipitated by a heavy meal, hot bath, exercise or where there is a 'limb shaking' TIA, a haemodynamically critical ICA stenosis should be suspected.

Conventional teaching advises that the risk of stroke after a TIA/minor stroke is 1–2% at 7 days and 2–4% at 30 days. This, in conjunction with a reluctance to perform carotid surgery within the hyperacute period (because of concerns about increased procedural risks), has led to little urgency regarding referral, investigation and management. However, there is now compelling evidence that the incidence of recurrent stroke after the index TIA in patients with 50–99% ICA stenoses ranges from 5–8% at 48 hours, 4–17% at 72 hours, 8–22% at 7 days and 11–25% at 14 days.[7] Interestingly, pooled data from patients randomised to 'best medical therapy' (BMT) in the ECST (European Carotid Surgery Trial), NASCET (North American Symptomatic Carotid Endarterectomy Trial) and Veterans Affairs trials observed only a 21% risk of ipsilateral stroke at 5 years.[8] This would suggest that most patients who were previously destined to suffer an early recurrent stroke after their TIA were rarely randomised within these trials. The decision to refer should never be influenced by the presence/absence of a carotid bruit.

Vertebrobasilar

Vertebrobasilar (VB) symptoms (Box 10.1) include bilateral blindness, problems with gait/stance, hemilateral/bilateral motor or sensory impairment (10% will have hemisensory/motor signs), dysarthria, homonymous hemianopia, nystagmus, dizziness, diplopia and vertigo (provided the latter three are not isolated).

> ✔ VB TIAs carry early stroke risks comparable to carotid territory events, especially if they have an ipsilateral 50–99% stenosis (20–30% stroke risk within 90 days[9]). Patients reporting VB symptoms need to be treated more urgently in future.

Non-hemispheric

The term 'non-hemispheric' is applied to patients with isolated syncope (blackout, drop attack), presyncope (faintness), isolated dizziness, isolated double vision (diplopia) and isolated vertigo.

> ✔ 'Non-hemispheric' symptoms should never be considered to be carotid or VB in origin unless other 'classical' symptoms are present. It is very important to exclude a cardiac or inner ear pathology.

Box 10.1 • 'Classical' carotid and vertebrobasilar features

Carotid territory
Hemimotor/hemisensory signs
Monocular visual loss (amaurosis fugax)
Higher cortical dysfunction (dysphasia, visuospatial neglect etc.)

Vertebrobasilar
Bilateral blindness
Problems with gait and stance
Hemi- or bilateral motor/sensory signs
Dysarthria
Homonymous hemianopia
Diplopia, vertigo and nystagmus (provided it is not the only symptom)

Investigation of carotid disease severity

> ✔✔ The 2016 Intercollegiate Stroke Working Party recommends that any patient with a suspected acute TIA should be assessed and imaged <24 hours by a specialist physician in a single-visit neurovascular clinic or an acute stroke unit.[10]
>
> The 2016 Intercollegiate Stroke Working Party recommends that any patient with a suspected TIA that occurred more than 7 days prior should be assessed and imaged within 7 days by a specialist physician in a single-visit neurovascular clinic.[10]
>
> Every centre should know which carotid stenosis measurement method is being used in their unit (i.e. ECST or NASCET).[10]

There are three methods for measuring stenosis severity, each using the luminal diameter at the point of maximum stenosis as the numerator (**Fig. 10.5**). Stenoses measured using the ECST method generate higher grades of stenosis than those using the NASCET method. In reality, a 50% NASCET stenosis is broadly equivalent to a 70% ECST, while a 70% NASCET stenosis equates to a 85% ECST stenosis. However, while the CCA method may be the most reproducible, most guidelines of practice now recommend using the NASCET measurement method.

Duplex ultrasound

Stenosis severity is usually evaluated using duplex ultrasound (DUS), which combines B-mode (real-time) imaging with waveform analysis using pulsed-wave Doppler. Advantages include: (i) low cost, (ii) accessibility within 'single-visit' clinics and (iii) being non-invasive. There are recognised limitations, mostly relating to the expertise of the operator. With highly experienced sonographers, however, DUS can

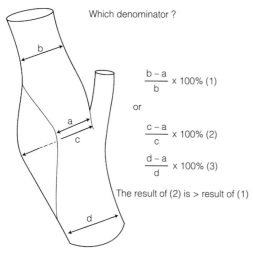

Which denominator ?

$$\frac{b - a}{b} \times 100\% \quad (1)$$

or

$$\frac{c - a}{c} \times 100\% \quad (2)$$

$$\frac{d - a}{d} \times 100\% \quad (3)$$

The result of (2) is > result of (1)

Figure 10.5 • Measurement of carotid stenosis by the ECST, NASCET and common carotid methods.

identify up to 95% of lesions responsible for carotid territory symptoms and there is no evidence that operating on the basis of DUS (alone) compromises patient safety.[11] A joint working group of the Vascular Society of Great Britain and Ireland and the Society of Vascular Technologists[12] developed consensus criteria for diagnosing the severity of carotid disease based on the NASCET measurement method (Table 10.1).

In most UK centres, carotid endarterectomy (CEA) procedures are planned on the basis of DUS alone. DUS can only insonate the cervical portion of the extracranial ICA and is therefore relatively unreliable at excluding disease elsewhere and cannot be used for planning carotid artery stenting (CAS). Any suspicion of additional lesions (damped proximal CCA waveform, unable to image above

the stenosis) requires alternative imaging (MR/CT angiography). Because the benefit conferred by CEA in patients with 50–69% stenoses falls significantly with delays to surgery (see later), it has been recommended that if 4 weeks or more have elapsed after the index event, corroborative imaging with either contrast-enhanced MR angiography (CEMRA) or multi-detector CT angiography (MDCTA) should be performed in order to confirm stenosis severity. If, however, DUS was performed within 4 weeks of the index event, a 2006 Health Technology Assessment (HTA) felt it reasonable to proceed to CEA on the basis of DUS alone, as the number of strokes prevented through rapidly performed surgery exceeded the potential risk to patients with <50% stenoses undergoing inappropriate surgery.[13]

The Gray–Weale classification[14] classifies plaques according to whether they are echolucent (type 1), predominantly echolucent (type 2), predominantly echogenic (type 3) or echogenic (type 4). Unfortunately, correlation with histology and clinical risk is variable. The Grey Scale Median (GSM) is a computerised measurement of plaque echogenicity that was developed to differentiate echogenic carotid plaques (that have a fibro-calcified content that is thought to be associated with a stable plaque) and echolucent plaques (with a thin fibrous cap and a higher lipid or haemorrhagic content that are supposedly unstable). The presence of a low GSM is associated with a higher incidence of neurologic events after CAS.[15] Several studies have indicated that plaque echogenicity on high-resolution B-mode ultrasound is related to the histological components of carotid plaques, and low echogenicity (or echolucency) is associated with the development of neurological events, especially in asymptomatic patients.[16]

Table 10.1 • Diagnostic duplex ultrasound criteria for NASCET-based carotid stenosis measurement

% stenosis NASCET	ICA$_{PSV}$ cm/s	ICA$_{PSV}$/CCA$_{PSV}$ ratio	St Mary's ratio ICA$_{PSV}$/CCA$_{EDV}$
<50%	<125	<2	<8
50-69%	>125	2–4	8–10
60-69%			11–13
70-79%	>230	>4	14–21
80-89%			22–29
>90 but no near occlusion	>400	>5	>30
Near occlusion	High, low – string flow	Variable	Variable
Occlusion	No flow	Not applicable	Not applicable

CCA, common carotid artery; EDV, end diastolic velocity; ICA, internal carotid artery; NASCET, North American Symptomatic Carotid Endarterectomy Trial; PSV, peak systolic velocity.

Reproduced with permission from Oates C, Naylor AR, Hartshorne T, et al. Reporting carotid ultrasound investigations in the United Kingdom. Eur J Vasc Endovasc Surg 2009;37:251–61.

Catheter angiography

Digital subtraction angiography (DSA) was previously the gold standard in carotid imaging. It is, however, associated with a small risk of perioperative stroke. In patients with symptomatic ischaemic cerebrovascular disease, the risk for disabling stroke and death can be as high as 4% and 1%, respectively.[17] Awareness of local angiographic complication rates is important in the selection process of diagnostic tests to be performed. Minor adverse reactions, including TIA, groin haematoma, unstable angina, need for blood transfusion, leg ischaemia and iliac artery dissection, can occur in up to 10% of procedures.[17] The morbidity and mortality of angiography can be significantly reduced by performing non-selective angiography in multiple projections, with contrast being injected into the aortic arch.[18] The main advantages of angiography are its high resolution and ability to demonstrate flow dynamics within the diseased artery and of the collateral circulation (circle of Willis and external carotid artery). In the era of high-quality non-invasive imaging, no centre would currently advocate any role for routine DSA, because of the risk of angiographic stroke and arterial access site complications.

> ✔✔ In the Asymptomatic Carotid Atherosclerosis Study (ACAS), selective catheter angiography incurred a stroke/death risk of 1.5% (>50% of the overall surgical risk[19]). It is no longer part of the routine work-up of a TIA patient.

Magnetic resonance angiography

CEMRA uses the paramagnetic agent gadolinium and (compared to non-enhanced TOF-MRA), images are obtained more rapidly. CEMRA incurs fewer flow-related artefacts and provides a much greater field of view that enables high-resolution imaging from the aortic arch up to the circle of Willis (**Fig. 10.1**), whilst retaining the ability to evaluate flow directionality. CEMRA is, however, limited by availability, accessibility, and occasionally patient incompatibility (e.g. pacemaker) or claustrophobia. Whilst MRA is non-invasive and avoids ionising radiation, gadolinium has recently been identified as the cause of nephrogenic systemic fibrosis (NSF).

MRI can also be used to characterise atherosclerotic plaque. MRI indicators of vulnerable plaque (signal intensity ratio [SIR] and plaque volume) correlate with new cerebral lesions following CAS. Plaque bleeding or the presence of a lipid-rich necrotic core may lead to an increase in symptoms and therefore it can be anticipated that crossing these lesions may lead to a higher burden of cerebral emboli detected using transcranial Doppler (TCD).[20] SIR and plaque volume are independent predictors of DWI (diffusion weighted imaging) lesions following protected CAS.

> ✔ NSF is a systemic scleroderma-like condition, which affects 3–5% of patients with pre-existing renal impairment exposed to gadolinium-based compounds. Five per cent of affected individuals exhibit a rapidly progressive course.

Computed tomographic angiography (CTA)

Multidetector CTA permits rapid acquisition of large amounts of cross-sectional data that can be reformatted into any plane. The advantages of CTA include: (i) being minimally invasive, (ii) overview anatomical imaging with short scan times, while thinner 'slices' mean less artifact, (iii) CTA is more accessible than MRA and (iv) CTA is generally well tolerated. Disadvantages include: (i) requirement for iodinated contrast, (ii) radiation burden, (iii) inability to impart dynamic information, i.e. 'trickle flow' not reliably identified and (iv) heavy calcification can increase the difficulty of reliable estimates of stenosis severity.

Comparison of methods

A 2006 Health Technology Assessment (HTA) performed a meta-analysis of the accuracy of non-invasive imaging for all carotid stenosis subgroups and imaging modalities (Table 10.2).[13] CEMRA had the highest sensitivity (94%; 95%CI 0.88–0.97), specificity and least heterogeneity, followed by DUS (89%; 95%CI 0.85–0.92).

Management of cerebrovascular disease

'Best medical therapy'

All patients benefit from optimisation of risk factors, antiplatelet/statin therapy and exclusion of important comorbidities. Everyone should undergo an ECG to exclude occult cardiac pathology. Baseline blood tests will exclude diabetes, arteritis, polycythaemia, anaemia, thrombocytosis, sickle-cell disease and hyperlipidaemia.

> ✔✔ Table 10.3 summarises recommendations from the American Heart Association regarding levels of evidence for what should constitute 'best medical therapy' in patients with symptomatic and asymptomatic carotid disease.

Table 10.2 • Meta-analysis of the accuracy of non-invasive imaging for all carotid stenosis subgroups and imaging modalities

Stenosis group	Imaging	Sensitivity % (95% CI)	Specificity % (95% CI)
70–99%	DUS	89% (0.85–0.92)	84% (0.77–0.89)
	CTA	77% (0.68–0.84)	95% (0.91–0.97)
	MRA	88% (0.82–0.92)	84% (0.76–0.90)
	CEMRA	94% (0.88–0.97)	93% (0.89–0.96)
50–69%	DUS	36% (0.25–0.49)	91% (0.87–0.94)
	CTA	67% (0.30–0.90)	79% (0.63–0.89)
	MRA	37% (0.26–0.49)	91% (0.78–0.97)
	CEMRA	77% (0.59–0.89)	97% (0.93–0.99)
<49%, 100%	DUS	83% (0.73–0.90)	84% (0.62–0.95)
	CTA	81% (0.70–0.88)	91% (0.74–0.98)
	MRA	81% (0.70–0.88)	88% (0.76–0.95)
	CEMRA	96% (0.90–0.99)	96% (0.90–0.99)

CEMRA, contrast-enhanced MRA; CTA, computed tomographic angiography; DUS, duplex ultrasound; MRA, magnetic resonance angiography.
Adapted from Wardlaw JM, Chappell FM, Stevenson M, et al. Accurate, practical and cost-effective assessment of carotid stenosis in the UK. Health Technol Assess 2006;10:iii–iv, ix–x,1–182.

Table 10.3 • Summary of American Heart Association recommendations for 'best medical therapy' and interventions in patients with symptomatic and asymptomatic carotid disease

	Symptomatic*	Asymptomatic[†]
Blood pressure <140/90 mmHg	Class I, Level B	Class I, Level A
Statin therapy	Class I, Level A	Class I, Level C
Antiplatelet therapy	Class I, Level A	Class I, Level C
Aspirin 50–325 mg daily	Class I, Level B	
Aspirin 25 mg + dipyridamole 200 mg b.d.	Class IIa, Level B	
Clopidogrel 75 mg	Class IIb, Level B	
Aspirin + clopidogrel <24 h of TIA onset		
Smoking cessation	Class I, Level C	Class I, Level B
Obesity advice	Class I, Level C	Class I, Level A
Physical exercise	Class IIa, Level C	Class I, Level B
Reduce alcohol consumption	Class I, Level C	Class I, Level A
70–99% stenosis: CEA	Class I, Level A	Class IIa, Level A
50–69% stenosis: CEA	Class I, Level B	
70–99% stenosis: CAS	Class IIa, Level B	Class IIb, Level B

*Levels of evidence adapted from Kernan et al.[21]
[†]Levels of evidence adapted from Meschia et al.[22]
CAS, carotid artery stenting; CEA, carotid endarterectomy; TIA, transient ischaemic attack.

Angina therapy should be optimised as the principal cause of late death is cardiac. Blood pressure (BP) should be maintained <140/90 mmHg. Systematic reviews suggest that reducing diastolic BP by 5 mmHg lowers the relative risk of stroke by 35%, while the relative risk of MI falls by 25%.[23] However, evidence suggests that only 60% with known hypertension will receive treatment prior to suffering their first stroke and only half will have a documented diastolic BP <90 mmHg.[24]

✅✅ The Heart Protection Study showed that patients randomised to statin had a 25% relative risk reduction (RRR) in: (i) any major coronary event, (ii) any stroke and (iii) the need for revascularisation at 5 years. This benefit was irrespective of age, gender or presenting cholesterol level.[25]

No randomised controlled trial (RCT) has evaluated the role of antiplatelet agents in asymptomatic patients. However, most guidelines recommend low-dose aspirin in order to minimise the risk of late cardiovascular events.[22] There are, however, discrepancies amongst practice guidelines regarding antiplatelet strategies in symptomatic patients. The 2014 American Heart Association (AHA) guidelines (Table 10.3) recommend either aspirin monotherapy (50–325 mg) or aspirin (25 mg) plus slow-release dipyridamole (200 mg b.d.) in patients with a recent ischaemic stroke/TIA. The AHA advised that clopidogrel (75 mg daily) was an alternative antiplatelet strategy in recently symptomatic patients. The AHA also advised that it was reasonable to consider dual antiplatelet therapy (DAPT) using aspirin and clopidogrel in TIA patients, provided this was started <24 hours of TIA onset.[21] This is because there is evidence that DAPT may reduce the risks of early recurrent events.[26,27]

By contrast, the 2016 Intercollegiate Working Party for Stroke Prevention (ICWPSP) guidelines advise that clopidogrel monotherapy (75 mg daily) is now the preferred antithrombotic treatment in patients with an ischaemic TIA or minor stroke, with aspirin (75 mg daily) plus modified-release dipyridamole (200 mg twice daily) for those who are unable to tolerate clopidogrel. Aspirin (75 mg daily) should be used if both clopidogrel and modified-release dipyridamole are contraindicated or not tolerated. The ICWPSP, however, did not recommend DAPT unless there was another indication, such as an acute coronary syndrome or recent coronary stent.[10]

One possible reason for discrepancies between guidelines regarding choice (and dose) of antiplatelet therapy in patients scheduled to undergo CEA is surgeon concerns regarding perioperative bleeding. Most guidelines advocate low-dose aspirin (75–325 mg) in CEA patients, although studies have demonstrated that DAPT can reduce recurrent stroke immediately prior to CEA, without increasing perioperative bleeding complications.[27] There has also been controversy regarding the optimal aspirin dose during CEA. NASCET reported that patients receiving high-dose aspirin (650–1300 mg) had a lower perioperative risk than patients taking 0–325 mg aspirin daily.[28] This was an unplanned analysis and an RCT subsequently showed that the risk of stroke, MI or death within 30 and 90 days of CEA was significantly lower in patients receiving

80–325 mg as opposed to 650–1300 mg.[29] This suggests greater evidence for prescribing low-dose aspirin (75–325 mg).

The early risk of stroke after suffering a TIA is higher than previously thought. This has led to a review of practice regarding the timing of surgery (see later), but also regarding the benefit of very early implementation of BMT. The EXPRESS study evaluated early stroke rates in two cohorts of TIA patients. In the first (2002–2004), patients were seen in a daily TIA clinic (appointment based, usual referral delays, etc.) with treatment recommendations faxed to the referring doctor. The patient then contacted their doctor to obtain their prescription, but an average of 19 days elapsed before medications were started. In the second cohort (2004–2007), there was a daily 'walk-in' service, but statin and antiplatelet therapy were started in the outpatient clinic.[30] The 90-day stroke risk fell from 10% in the first cohort to 2% in the second. The reduction in risk was independent of age and gender, with no increase in rates of haemorrhagic stroke.

✅✅ Rapid institution of 'best medical therapy' significantly reduces the risk of early stroke and should be started in the TIA clinic.

Management of carotid disease

Symptomatic carotid artery disease

The Carotid Endarterectomy Trialists Collaboration (CETC) combined data from ECST, NASCET and the Veterans Affairs trials, having re-measured pre-randomisation angiograms using the NASCET measurement method. This database[8,31,32] now provides 5-year outcome data in >6000 patients (Table 10.4). Notwithstanding concerns regarding the 'historical' nature of the RCTs, the 5-year CETC data should now be quoted in preference to the constituent RCTs.

✅✅ CEA is not indicated in symptomatic patients with <50% NASCET stenoses. CEA confers modest (but significant) benefit in recently symptomatic (<6 months) with a 50–69% NASCET stenosis (ECST 70–85%). CEA confers maximum benefit in recently symptomatic (<6 months) with a 70–99% NASCET stenosis, excluding those with the 'string sign'.

✅ Surgeons must know and also quote their own operative risks rather than justifying practice on the basis of the RCTs.

Table 10.4 • Carotid Endarterectomy Trialists Collaboration (CETC): 5-year risk of any stroke (including 30-day stroke/ death) from a pooled individual patient meta-analysis from the VA, ECST and NASCET trials*

NASCET stenosis	n	30 days death/stroke after CEA	5-year risk		ARR in stroke at 5 years	RRR in stroke at 5 years	NNT	Strokes prevented per 1000 CEAs at 5 years
			CEA	BMT				
<30%	1746	No data	18.4%	15.7%	−2.7%	NB	NB	None at 5 yrs
30–49%	1429	6.7%	22.8%	25.5%	+2.7%	10%	37	27 at 5 yrs
50–69%	1549	8.4%	20.0%	27.8%	+7.8%	28%	13	78 at 5 yrs
70–99%	1095	6.2%	17.1%	32.7%	+15.6%	48%	6	156 at 5 yrs
Near occlusion	262	5.4%	22.4%	22.3%	−0.1%	NB	NB	None at 5 yrs

*Data derived from the CETC[8,31,32] with all pre-randomisation angiograms re-measured using NASCET method. ECST, European Carotid Surgery Trial; NASCET, North American Symptomatic Carotid Endarterectomy Trial; VA, Veterans Affairs.
ARR, absolute risk reduction; BMT, 'best medical therapy'; CEA, carotid endarterectomy; NB, no benefit conferred by CEA; NNT number needed to treat; RRR, relative risk reduction.

ECST/NASCET have published over 50 papers since 1991, most being secondary analyses that have increased knowledge about the role of CEA in patients with symptomatic cerebral vascular disease.[33] These should not be used to *exclude* patients from intervention, but rather to identify clinical and/or imaging predictors of increased risk of stroke on BMT (Box 10.2).

One of the most important issues facing CEA and CAS practitioners is the effect of 'delay to intervention'. Previously, there was no impetus for expediting carotid interventions, other than recommending that CEA be performed 'as soon as reasonably possible'. This approach has, however, been challenged because of increasing evidence that the most vulnerable patients are suffering recurrent strokes before they can undergo CEA. A recent review suggested that the incidence of recurrent stroke after the index TIA in patients with 50–99% ICA stenoses ranged from 5–8% at

48 hours, 4–17% at 72 hours, 8–22% at 7 days and 11–25% at 14 days.[7] Second, the CETC has published evidence that 'delay to surgery' significantly reduces the benefit conferred by CEA.[8,31,32] By implication, the same will apply to CAS. Table 10.5 presents a reanalysis of CETC data showing long-term stroke prevention conferred by CEA in male and female patients with NASCET 50–99% stenoses (i.e. ECST 70–99%), stratified for delay from randomisation to surgery. In practice, the median delay from symptom onset to randomisation was about 7 days (P. Rothwell, personal communication). Note that the benefit conferred in males with 70–99% stenoses persisted with increasing delay, but rapidly diminished in males with 50–69% stenoses. By contrast, the benefit conferred in females appeared to disappear after 4 weeks had elapsed, even in those with 70–99% stenoses.[8,31,32]

Box 10.2 • Which patients with symptomatic 50–99% stenoses are at higher risk of suffering a stroke on 'best medical therapy'?*

Clinical features

Male versus female gender
Increasing age (especially >75 years)
Hemispheric versus ocular symptoms
Cortical versus lacunar stroke
Recurrent symptoms for >6 months
Increasing medical comorbidity
Symptoms within 2 weeks

Imaging features

Irregular versus smooth plaques
Increasing stenosis but not near occlusion
Contralateral occlusion
Tandem intracranial disease

✅✅ Maximum benefit, regarding late stroke prevention, was observed when surgery was performed within 2 weeks. If surgery was delayed beyond 12 weeks, only eight ipsilateral strokes were prevented at 5 years by performing 1000 CEAs.[8,31,32]

✅ Symptomatic women gain less benefit from CEA than men and maximum benefit was only conferred if CEA was performed as soon as possible. Excessive delays to treatment could mean that female patients face all the risks of intervention with little prospect of gaining any benefit.[8,31,32]

However, there have been concerns that expedited CEA may be associated with increased 30-day risks of death/stroke, which may negate any benefit from intervening early. In a review of 1046 symptomatic patients undergoing CEA in New York, the 30-day death/stroke rate was three times higher (5.1%) if CEA was performed within 4 weeks, as compared with 1.6% if surgery was deferred for >4 weeks.[34] Data like these have been used as a reason to delay interventions in order to achieve the 'lowest' procedural risks. However, three national registries have now published 30-day death/stroke rates after CEA stratified for delays to surgery (Table 10.6). Only one (SwedVasc[35]) observed a very high procedural risk (11.5%) when CEA was performed within 48 hours of symptom onset; the German and UK registries did not.[36,37] After 48 hours, all three national registries reported acceptably low procedural risks when CEA was performed in the first 7–14 days after symptom onset.[35–37]

> ✅ Evidence suggests that more strokes will be prevented in the long term through rapid intervention, even if the procedural risk is increased. Future guidelines must consider whether it is reasonable to accept a slightly higher procedural risk if the operation is carried out early.

CAS is now an alternative to CEA (see later). However, the Carotid Stent Trialists Collaboration (CSTC) undertook a meta-analysis of outcomes from EVA-3S, SPACE and ICSS (for abbreviations see Table 10.7), stratified for delay from index symptom

Table 10.5 • Absolute risk reduction conferred by CEA in the 5-year risk of ipsilateral carotid territory ischaemic stroke (including the perioperative risk) in patients with a NASCET 50–69% and 70–99% stenosis, stratified for delay from index event to randomisation and gender*

	50–69% stenosis			70–99% stenosis		
	ARR	NNT	CVA/1000	ARR	NNT	CVA/1000
(1) All patients						
<2 weeks	14.8%	7	148	23.0%	4	230
2–4 weeks	3.3%	30	33	15.9%	6	159
4–12 weeks	4.0%	25	40	7.9%	13	79
>12 weeks	−2.9%	NB	NB	7.4%	14	74
(2) Males						
<2 weeks	15.2%	7	152	23.3%	4	233
2–4 weeks	6.8%	15	68	23.8%	4	238
4–12 weeks	5.0%	20	50	18.3%	5	183
>12 weeks	6.3%	16	63	20.4%	5	204
(3) Females						
<2 weeks	13.8%	7	138	41.7%	2	417
2–4 weeks	−5.7%	NB	NB	6.6%	15	66
4–12 weeks	−2.2%	NB	NB	−2.2%	NB	NB
>12 weeks	−21.7%	NB	NB	−2.4%	NB	NB

*Data derived from the CETC[8,31,32] with all pre-randomisation angiograms re-measured using the NASCET method.
CVA/1000 = number of ipsilateral strokes prevented at 5 years by performing 1000 CEAs.
ARR, absolute risk reduction; CEA, carotid endarterectomy; CETC, Carotid Endarterectomy Trialists Collaboration; NASCET, North American Symptomatic Carotid Endarterectomy Trial; NB, no benefit; NNT, number needed to treat.

Table 10.6 • 30-day death/stroke after CEA, stratified for delay from index symptom onset to undergoing CEA, in national audits of practice

National audit	0–2 days	3–7 days	8–14 days	>15 days
Sweden [35]	17/148	29/804	27/677	52/967
n = 2596	(11.5%)	(3.6%)	(4.0%)	(5.4%)
UK[36]	29/780	128/5126	132/6292	254/11037
n = 23 235	(3.7%)	(2.5%)	(2.1%)	(2.3%)
Germany [37]	157/5198	480/19117	427/16205	370/15759
n = 56 279	(3.0%)	(2.5%)	(2.6%)	(2.3%)

CEA, carotid endarterectomy.

Table 10.7 • 30-day outcomes following CEA and CAS in trials that randomised >500 recently symptomatic patients into EVA-3S, SPACE, ICSS and CREST*

30-day risks	EVA-3S[43]		SPACE[40]		ICSS[42]		CREST[41]	
	CEA $n=262$	CAS $n=261$	CEA $n=589$	CAS $n=607$	CEA $n=857$	CAS $n=853$	CEA $n=653$	CAS $n=668$
Death	1.2%	0.8%	0.9%	1.0%	0.8%	2.3%		
Any stroke	3.5%	9.2%	6.2%	7.2%	4.1%	7.7%	3.2%	5.5%
Death/any stroke	3.9%	9.6%	6.5%	7.4%	4.7%	8.5%	3.2%	6.0%
Disabling stroke/death	1.5%	3.4%	3.8%	5.1%	3.2%	4%		
Death/stroke/MI					5.2%	8.5%	5.4%	6.7%
Cranial nerve injury	7.7%	1.1%			5.3%	0.1%	5.1%	0.5%

Trials: CREST, Carotid Revascularization Endarterectomy versus Stenting Trial; EVA-3S, Endarterectomy Versus Angioplasty in Patients with Symptomatic Severe Carotid Stenosis; ICSS, International Carotid Stenting Study; SPACE, Stent-Protected Angioplasty versus Carotid Endarterectomy.
CAS, carotid artery stenting; CEA, carotid endarterectomy; MI, myocardial infarction.

to intervention.[38] Patients undergoing CEA within the first 7 days after the index TIA/stroke had a 30-day death/stroke rate of 2.8%, compared with 9.4% in patients undergoing CAS during the same time period (HR 3.4; [95% CI 1.01–11.8]; $P=0.03$) after adjusting for age, sex and type of qualifying event. Patients treated between 8 and 14 days had a periprocedural death/stroke rate of 3.4% after CEA, versus 8.1% following CAS (HR 2.42; 95% CI, 1.0–5.7; $P=0.04$).[38] These data would therefore suggest that CEA is probably preferable to CAS in the first 7–14 days after symptom onset, especially as a recent systematic review of procedural risks following CAS in symptomatic patients in large administrative datasets showed that 70% of registries reported death/stroke rates that exceeded the accepted 6% procedural risk.[39] Twenty per cent of registries reported death/stroke rates in excess of 10% after CAS.[39]

Randomised trials comparing CEA with CAS in symptomatic patients

Table 10.7 summarises the 30-day risks of death/ stroke after CEA and CAS in the four largest contemporary RCTs involving recently symptomatic patients.[40–43] Overall, CAS was associated with a significantly higher rate of procedural death/ stroke (HR 1.80 [95%CI 1.40–2.31]). However, the available evidence suggests that once the 30-day perioperative period has elapsed, the long-term risks of ipsilateral stroke were very similar, suggesting that CAS appears to be as durable as CEA.[40–43] Accordingly, the key issue as to whether CEA or CAS is preferable (safer) in recently symptomatic patients will be the predicted 30-day risk in individual patients. As described (above), CAS was associated with significantly higher rates of death/stroke (than CEA) when performed in the first 7–14 days after

onset of symptoms.[38] A pooled meta-analysis of RCT data has also shown that while increasing age had no effect on operative risks after CEA, it was associated with significantly higher rates of 30-day death/stroke after CAS in patients aged 70–74 years (HR 4.01 [95%CI 2.19–7.32]), 75–79 years (HR 3.94 [95%CI2.14–7.28]) and >80 years (HR 4.15 [95%CI 2.2–7.84]). Below 65 years of age, CAS had the same procedural risks as CEA.[44] A further subgroup analysis from CREST showed that CAS was associated with significantly lower risks of clinical/biomarker MI in the perioperative period compared to CEA, which was associated with poorer long-term survival.[45] However, CREST observed that perioperative stroke (which was significantly higher following CAS) was also associated with poorer long-term survival as well.[46] CAS was associated with better health-related quality of life (HRQoL) during the early recovery period (compared with CEA), especially for physical limitations and pain $(P=0.01)$. These differences were significant at 4 weeks, but at 1 year there was no difference in any HRQoL measure. Perhaps most importantly, periprocedural stroke was associated with poorer 1-year HRQoL scores across all domains, while periprocedural MI and CNI were not.[47]

✔✔ After the perioperative period has elapsed, CAS appears to be as durable as CEA with similar rates of long-term ipsilateral stroke.[40–43]

The key to determining whether CEA or CAS is preferable (in individual patients) will be largely governed by factors that increase the 30-day risk of death/stroke.

Performing CAS in the first 7–14 days after symptom onset is associated with significantly higher rates of death/stroke, compared to CEA.[38]

CEA appears to be safer (than CAS) in recently symptomatic patients aged >70 years.[44]

CAS had similar procedural risks to CEA in patients aged <65 years.[44]

Perioperative stroke and MI (clinical and/or biomarker) were both associated with poorer long-term survival.[45,46]

New ischaemic lesions on MR imaging

In a meta-analysis of two RCTs and 18 non-randomised studies (CAS = 989; CEA = 1115), the incidence of new DWI cerebral lesions was significantly greater after CAS than CEA (40% vs 12%; OR 5.17 [95% CI 3.31–8.06]; $P <0.00001$).[48] In ICSS,[49] CAS was associated with a fivefold increase in new ischaemic lesions in the immediate postoperative period, which persisted at 30 days (compared with CEA). There were more (smaller) lesions following CAS and fewer (larger) lesions following CEA, such that the median affected brain volume was similar for CEA and CAS. To date, there is no evidence that these lesions predispose towards cognitive impairment. However, ICSS has reported that the 5-year incidence of recurrent stroke/TIA was 22.8% in CAS patients with new DWI lesions postoperatively, compared with 8.8% in CAS patients with no new DWI–MRI lesions (HR 2.85 [95% CI 1.05–7.72]; $P = 0.04$). ICSS concluded that new ischaemic brain lesions may be a marker for an increased risk of recurrent cerebrovascular events and that DWI-positive patients might benefit from more prolonged DAPT.[50]

Asymptomatic carotid artery disease

Five randomised trials have compared CEA + 'best medical therapy' (BMT) with BMT alone, but only two (ACAS and the Asymptomatic Carotid Surgery Trial [ACST]) have really influenced practice.[19,51,52] The 5- and 10-year outcomes from ACAS/ACST are summarised in Table 10.8.

✗ ✓ The 2014 AHA guidelines continue to retain the recommendation that intervention should only be considered in 'highly selected' average-risk patients with an asymptomatic 60–99% stenosis.[22]

The AHA is highly influential in determining guidelines of practice. However, the management of asymptomatic disease remains controversial. Those who feel it is time to rethink management strategies cite the following observations: (i) the overall benefit conferred by CEA (CAS) is small – at 10 years, only 45 strokes are prevented per 1000 operations; (ii) in a recent audit, 50% of clinicians around the world would not offer CEA/CAS to patients fulfilling AHA criteria;[53] (iii) the AHA recommends treating 'highly selected' patients, but never defined what this meant; (iv) the majority of patients were never destined to suffer a stroke. At 5 years, 88% treated medically were stroke-free, with 82% stroke-free at 10 years; (v) up to 94% of interventions in asymptomatic patients are ultimately unnecessary, costing US Health providers $2 billion annually;[54] and (vi) there is accumulating evidence that the stroke risk on medical therapy has declined over the last 20 years.[54]

Conversely, those who believe that guidelines should remain unchanged cite the following reasons for adopting this position: (i) the AHA guidelines are based on level I, RCT evidence and should not be changed until guided by further RCTs; (ii) the procedural risks associated with CEA and CAS have reduced significantly and will further increase the benefit accrued to the patient.; (iii) CEA/CAS offers the only chance of preventing stroke in the 80% of

Table 10.8 • Perioperative and late outcomes following carotid endarterectomy and 'best medical therapy' in, ACAS and ACST

RCT	30-day death/ stroke after CEA	Ipsilateral stroke plus perioperative death or stroke		Any stroke plus perioperative death or stroke	
		CEA	BMT	CEA	BMT
ACAS[19]	2.3%	5.1% at 5 years	11.0% at 5 years	17.8% at 5 years	12.4% at 5 years
ACST-1[51]	2.8%			6.4% at 5 years	11.8% at 5 years
ACST-1[52]	2.8%			13.4% at 10 years	17.9% at 10 years

ACAS, Asymptomatic Carotid Atherosclerosis Study; ACST, Asymptomatic Carotid Surgery Trial; BMT, 'best medical therapy'; CEA, carotid endarterectomy.

stroke victims who do not have a prior TIA; and (iv) the alleged decline in stroke risk is based on flawed data because some studies included patients with subsurgical (50–60%) stenoses.

The most controversial issue is the apparent decline in stroke risk over the last decade. This has been consistent across all stenosis severities and was also evident in ACAS and ACST.[54] In 1995, the 5-year risk of 'any' stroke in ACAS was 17.5% (3.5% p.a.) in patients randomised to BMT. When ACST reported in 2004, the first 5-year risk of 'any' stroke had fallen to 11.8% (2.4% p.a.). When ACST reported its 10-year data, the second 5-year risk of 'any' stroke was now only 7.2% (1.4% p.a.). In effect, the 5-year risk of 'any' stroke has declined by 60% since 1995. There is an identical trend for 'ipsilateral' stroke. In 1995, ACAS reported 5-year rates of 'ipsilateral' stroke in medically treated patients of 11.0% (2.2% p.a.). By 2004, ACST reported 5-year risks of ipsilateral stroke of 5.3% (1.1% p.a.), while in years 6–10, the 5-year risk of 'ipsilateral stroke' had fallen to 3.6% (0.7% p.a.). This represents a 70% decline in the 5-year risk of ipsilateral stroke since 1995.[54] It is hoped that future randomised studies in asymptomatic patients will include a third arm for 'best medical therapy' so as to determine whether the observed decline in stroke risk in non-randomised studies is a real phenomenon or not.

☑ It is inevitable that a small cohort of asymptomatic patients will benefit from intervention. It is essential that more research is undertaken to identify a 'higher or lower risk for stroke' cohort in whom to either target or avoid CEA/CAS. Until then, most surgeons/ interventionists will continue to adhere to the 2014 AHA Guidelines (if only for medico-legal protection) as the AHA never defined what being 'highly selected' meant.

☑ An overview suggests that a number of clinical and/or imaging modalities could be used to develop algorithms for identifying 'high-risk for stroke' patients, including; spontaneous embolisation on transcranial Doppler, computerised plaque analysis (Gray Scale Median, juxta-luminal black area, plaque area), silent infarction on CT/MRA, stenosis progression, multiple plaque microulcers, impaired cerebral vascular reserve, contralateral TIA/stroke and MRI evidence of intra-plaque haemorrhage.[55]

Comparison of CEA and CAS in randomised trials

Five RCTs have compared CEA with CAS in 'average-risk for CEA' asymptomatic patients.[56–60] Table 10.9 details 30-day outcome data from these RCTs, one of which was stopped early after poor recruitment.[59] A meta-analysis involving data from four of five RCTs in Table 10.9 (Lexington was excluded as there were no complications), observed a 30-day death/stroke of 1.6% after CEA (95%CI 1.02–2.45) and 2.7% (95%CI 2.1–3.6%) after CAS (OR 1.71 [95%CI 0.98–2.94]; $P = 0.0553$).[57–60]

As was observed with the symptomatic RCTs, CAS appeared to be as durable as CEA once the 30-day perioperative period had elapsed. In CREST, the 4-year rate of ipsilateral stroke (including the perioperative risk) was 8% following CAS, versus 6.7% after CEA.[57] In ACT-1, the 5-year rate of ipsilateral stroke (excluding perioperative events) was 2.2% (CAS) versus 2.7% after CEA ($P = 0.51$).[58] In Mannheim's study, there were no late strokes at a mean follow-up of 26 months.[60]

CEA/CAS and coronary bypass

Recently symptomatic patients who are unable to undergo CEA/CAS because of unstable cardiac disease should undergo staged or synchronous CEA + coronary bypass (CABG) as soon as

Table 10.9 • 30-day morbidity and mortality in randomised trials comparing CEA and CAS in asymptomatic patients

30-day outcomes	Brooks[56] CEA $n=42$	CAS $n=43$	CREST[57] CEA $n=587$	CAS $n=364$	ACT-1[58] CEA $n=364$	CAS $n=1089$	SPACE-2[59] CEA $n=203$	CAS $n=197$	BMT $n=113$	Mannheim[60] CEA $n=68$	CAS $n=68$
Death/stroke	0%	0%	1.4%	2.5%	1.7%	2.9%	2.0%	2.5%	0.0%	1.5%	2.9%
Death/disabling stroke	0%	0%	0.3%	0.5%	0.6%	0.6%					
Death/stroke/ MI	0%	0%	3.6%	3.5%	2.6%	3.3%				1.5%	2.9%

Trials: ACT, Asymptomatic Carotid Trial; CREST, Carotid Revascularization Endarterectomy versus Stenting Trial; SPACE, Stent-Protected Angioplasty versus Carotid Endarterectomy.
CAS, carotid artery stenting; CEA, carotid endarterectomy; MI, myocardial infarction.

possible. This is because the risk of stroke is highest in the early period after onset of symptoms. In reality, this only applies to <5% of all cardiac surgery patients.[61] A recent meta-analysis suggested that CAS + CABG carried a much higher risk of perioperative stroke (15%) compared with CEA + CABG in patients with a prior history of stroke/TIA.[62]

The role of prophylactic CEA/CAS in CABG patients with an asymptomatic carotid stenosis remains enduringly controversial. In the USA, about 96% of staged/synchronous interventions are undertaken in patients with asymptomatic carotid disease, the majority with unilateral stenosis.[61] So what is the evidence supporting prophylactic CEA/CAS in these patients? In a pooled series of 23 557 patients undergoing CABG without prophylactic CEA/CAS, 95% of 476 postoperative strokes could not be attributed to carotid disease.[63–65] Accordingly, most of the evidence suggests no causal relationship between a significant (asymptomatic) unilateral stenosis and postoperative stroke in the majority of cardiac surgical patients. This would suggest that other aetiologies play a more important role, particularly aortic arch atheroembolism.

✅✅ In a meta-analysis of 190 449 patients undergoing CABG,[66] the risk of stroke was 1.7% (95% CI 1.5–1.9).

✅✅ A meta-analysis observed that three 'carotid' factors were predictive of post-CABG stroke: (i) carotid bruit, (ii) a prior history of stroke or TIA and (iii) the presence of a severe carotid stenosis or occlusion.[66]

✅ In an updated meta-analysis (which excluded symptomatic patients, those with bilateral stenoses and patients with unilateral carotid occlusion), patients undergoing isolated CABG in the presence of a unilateral, asymptomatic stenosis incurred a 2% risk of procedural stroke. It is unlikely that prophylactic CEA/CAS could confer significant benefit, although it would still be appropriate to consider prophylactic intervention in CABG patients with bilateral severe asymptomatic disease.[67]

Table 10.10 details 30-day outcomes from a series of meta-analyses[62,68–70] regarding the roles of synchronous/staged CEA or CAS in CABG patients. In practice, the majority will involve patients with asymptomatic unilateral carotid stenoses.

✅ Morbidity and mortality rates after staged/synchronous CEA + CABG were considerably higher than when CEA or CAS were performed on their own. In a cohort of predominantly asymptomatic patients with unilateral stenoses, the procedural risks probably exceed the risk of performing isolated CABG, suggesting that cardiac surgery patients with unilateral, asymptomatic carotid stenoses will gain little additional benefit by performing staged or synchronous CEA/CAS.

Table 10.10 • Perioperative morbidity and mortality following staged/synchronous carotid interventions in patients undergoing cardiac surgery*

Parameter	n	Death % (95% CI)	Stroke % (95% CI)	MI % (95% CI)	Death/stroke % (95% CI)	Death/stroke/MI % (95% CI)
Synchronous CEA + CABG with CEA done pre-bypass	5386	4.5% (3.9–5.2)	4.5% (3.7–5.3)	3.6% (2.8–4.4)	8.2% (7.1–9.23)	11.5% (10.1–13.1)
Synchronous CEA + CABG with CEA done on bypass	844	4.7% (3.1–6.4)	3.8% (2.0–5.5)	2.9% (1.3–4.6)	8.1% (5.8–10.3)	9.5% (5.9–13.1)
Synchronous CEA + OPCAB	324	1.5% (0.3–2.8)	n/a	n/a	2.2% (0.7–3.7)	3.6% (1.6–5.5)
Staged CEA – then CABG	917	3.9% 1.1–6.7)	2.7% (1.6–3.9)	6.5% (3.2–9.7)	6.1% 2.9–9.3)	10.2% (7.4–13.1)
Reverse staged CABG then CEA	302	2.0% (0.0–6.1)	6.3% (1.0–11.7)	0.9% (0.5–1.4)	7.3% (1.7–12.9)	5.0% (0.0–10.6)
Staged CAS then CABG	2196	4.8% (3.3–6.8)	5.4% (4.5–6.5)	4.2% (3.2–5.6)	8.5% (7.3–9.7)	11.0% (9.4–12.9)
Same-day CAS + CABG	531	4.5% (2.9–7.0)	3.4% (2.0–5.9)	1.8% (0.9–3.7)	5.9% (4.0–8.5)	6.5% (4.6–9.3)

*Based on a series of themed meta-analyses.[62,68–70]
CABG, coronary artery bypass graft; CAS, carotid artery stenting; CEA, carotid endarterectomy; n/a, not available; OPCAB, off-pump coronary artery bypass.

Emergency CEA

In the 1960s, emergency CEA for acute stroke was associated with significant mortality and morbidity, due to haemorrhagic transformation of ischaemic infarction. This led to the abandonment of this strategy and a recommendation that patients should wait 6 weeks before undergoing CEA in order to stabilise the area of infarction. This is clearly at odds with current recommendations to expedite CEA. A meta-analysis has, however, shown that procedural risks for early CEA in patients with minor stroke and full/partial recovery were similar to those in patients for whom surgery was deferred.[71]

Although several single-centre studies have demonstrated feasibility of CAS in the early period after onset of symptoms,[72] a pooled analysis of data from the Carotid Stenting Trialists' Collaboration showed that the risk of CAS as compared to CEA is greatest in patients treated within 7 days of symptoms.[38] It was also seen that patients suffering from periprocedural complications underwent stenting significantly earlier compared with patients whose treatment was uneventful. CAS therefore does not seem to be the treatment of choice in emergency cases.

✅ Emergency re-exploration (i.e. immediate) should be reserved for those patients who suffer an acute thrombotic occlusion of the carotid artery after either CEA or CAS. Urgent CEA (<24 hours) is recommended in patients with stroke-in-evolution, stuttering hemiplegia or crescendo TIAs. There is no evidence that patients with an extensive neurological deficit should be considered for early intervention.

Vertebral artery revascularisation

The vertebrobasilar (VB) territory is affected in 15–25% of ischaemic strokes. In the past, it was believed that the majority of VB strokes were haemodynamic. However, the New England Posterior Circulation Registry observed that 40% were embolic (cardiac (60%), artery to artery (40%)); 32% were haemodynamic, while 28% had miscellaneous causes (trauma, dissection, aneurysm, arteritis, osteophyte compression[73]). Of those TIAs secondary to vertebral/basilar artery stenoses or occlusions; 62% were located within the extracranial vertebral artery (VA) (origin 39%; near VA origin 30%; V2/V3 segment 31%), 30% affected the intracranial VA, while 8% affected the basilar artery. The Vertebral Artery Stenting Trial (VAST) found no evidence that VA stenting conferred any benefit over medical therapy in recently symptomatic patients, although relatively few were treated within 14 days of symptom onset.[74]

In the past, most VB reconstructions involved open surgery (vein bypass or transposition onto the CCA). However, angioplasty (with/without stenting) is assuming an increasing role, especially in the upper limits of the extracranial VA and intracranial vessels. A meta-analysis of 993 patients (27 studies) undergoing VA angioplasty (99% stented) showed a technical success rate of 99%, a 30-day stroke rate of 1.1% and a 1% risk of recurrent VB stroke at 2 years. Restenosis rates were three times higher in patients receiving bare-metal stents, compared with drug-eluting stents.[75] These exceptional results are, however, unlikely to reflect 'real world' practice, but they do support a strategy wherein endovascular interventions are considered the first-line intervention.

Three VB related syndromes are worthy of mention. An occlusion/severe stenosis at the subclavian artery origin may cause reversed flow down the ipsilateral VA to perfuse the arm (subclavian steal). Arm exercise may precipitate forearm claudication or dizziness. Intervention is usually recommended in patients with symptomatic lesions, especially involving the dominant arm. Both surgery and endovascular interventions carry a small risk of procedural stroke. At present, the latter is generally the first choice intervention.

A similar syndrome (coronary steal) occurs in patients who have undergone CABG using the internal mammary artery (usually the left). Should a proximal subclavian stenosis be missed preoperatively (or develop subsequently) angina can be precipitated by arm exercise. In this situation, the angina can be treated by carotid–subclavian bypass or angioplasty/stenting. There is no evidence that either strategy is preferable.

Third, it is traditionally believed that rotational (positional) dizziness/vertigo follows osteophyte compression of the extracranial VA. Recent evidence suggests that this is almost always never the case[76] and an alternative aetiology should be sought.

Surgical management of carotid disease – carotid endarterectomy

Anaesthesia

CEA under locoregional anaesthesia is the only reliable method for predicting who needs a shunt, but it will not prevent thromboembolism (the main cause of intraoperative stroke).

✅✅ An updated Cochrane review,[77] which combined data from 14 RCTs (4596 patients), showed that CEA under locoregional anaesthesia did not confer significant reductions in 30-day stroke (3.2%), compared to CEA under general anaesthesia (3.5%).

Technique

CEA is usually performed using loupe magnification with the extended head turned away from the side of the operation and placed on a rubber ring. An incision is made over the anterior border of the sternomastoid and dissection continued down to the carotid bifurcation after division of the common facial vein.

> ✔ A meta-analysis of four non-randomised trials and two RCTs (740 CEAs) found no evidence that retrojugular (versus antegrade) exposure was associated with reductions in perioperative death (0.6% vs 0.5%) or stroke (0.9% vs 0.7%).[78]
>
> ✔✔ A meta-analysis of four RCTs found no evidence that carotid sinus nerve blockade reduced hypotension, hypertension or arrhythmias after CEA.[79]

The distal ICA is mobilised 1 cm beyond the upper limit of the plaque, facilitated by ligation and division of the sternomastoid vessels, which tether the hypoglossal nerve (with/without division of digastric). If surgeons are worried about the need to proceed higher in the neck, access can be facilitated (preoperatively) by nasolaryngeal intubation or temporomandibular subluxation. The latter must be planned in advance as it cannot be performed once the operation has started. The main cranial nerves (hypoglossal, vagus) are identified. With high dissections, the glossopharyngeal nerve is at risk. Contrary to classical teaching, however, most postoperative swallowing problems do not follow glossopharyngeal nerve injury, but are secondary to damage to the motor branches of the vagus which cross the ICA anteriorly, just distal to the hypoglossal nerve.

> ✔ Any patient who has undergone a contralateral CEA, neck dissection or thyroidectomy must undergo a preoperative check of recurrent laryngeal and hypoglossal nerve function. Bilateral injuries can be fatal.

Following systemic heparinisation, clamps are applied to the ICA, CCA and ECA. A longitudinal arteriotomy is made across the plaque and into the distal ICA. If a shunt is to be deployed it is inserted now.

> ✔ A Cochrane review of six RCTs (1270 CEAs) concluded that no meaningful recommendations could be made regarding shunting strategies because of poor-quality data. The choice of whether to selectively, routinely or never shunt is, therefore, left to the discretion of the surgeon.[80]

> ✔ If the surgeon is a 'selective shunter', the only way of knowing who needs a shunt is to perform CEA under locoregional anaesthesia.

The endarterectomy plane is developed using a Watson–Cheyne dissector and it is conventional to divide the plaque proximally and then mobilise it towards the distal ICA. The upper end usually feathers, but can be tacked down. Loose intimal fragments are removed in a radial, as opposed to axial, direction. An alternative technique is 'eversion' endarterectomy. Here the ICA origin is transected and reimplanted after eversion of the atheromatous core.

> ✔ Systematic reviews suggest that eversion endarterectomy confers similar benefits to traditional endarterectomy provided the arteriotomy is closed with a patch. Patched CEA and eversion CEA are associated with better early and late outcomes than where the arteriotomy is routinely primarily closed.[81,82]

Perioperative monitoring and completion assessment

The aim of monitoring is to prevent cerebral ischaemia before permanent neurological injury occurs. The simplest is a subjective assessment of ICA backflow or stump pressure, but this may bear little relation to intracranial perfusion in the presence of circle of Willis abnormalities. TCD is probably the most versatile of methods and uses a low-frequency (2 MHz) pulsed-wave ultrasound beam directed through the temporal bone. This permits insonation of the MCA, which receives 80% of ICA inflow. The quality of the signal depends on the thickness of the cranium and an inaccessible window may be present in about 10% of patients.

A single monitoring modality, however, is no guarantee of protection. During CEA, TCD fulfils only four roles: (i) diagnosing embolisation during carotid dissection (unstable plaque), (ii) ensuring mean MCA velocity remains >15 cm/s, (iii) ensuring the shunt is working and (iv) diagnosing the very rare case of on-table thrombosis following flow restoration.[83] Neurological activity can be monitored using locoregional anaesthesia and this is the gold standard for determining who needs a shunt. However, it will not prevent thromboembolic complications. Neurological activity can be evaluated indirectly by EEG or sensory-evoked potential (SEP) measurement. Once perfusion falls below 18 mL/100 g brain per minute there is loss of high-frequency activity on the EEG, whereas below 15 mL/100 g brain per minute the EEG becomes isoelectric.[84]

✅ The surgeon should remember that just because an EEG trace is flat, it does not mean that a neurological injury is inevitable, as this only occurs once perfusion falls below 10 mL/100 g brain per minute.[84] Loss of EEG function is a warning that insertion of a shunt or elevation of systemic blood pressure may be beneficial.

The advantage of SEP measurement is that it reflects the function of the afferent pathway from peripheral nerve (usually the median nerve) to the somatosensory cortex. Ischaemia causes a reduction in the amplitude of the primary cortical wave and prolongation of central conduction time.

The role of completion assessment is to identify technical error (incomplete endarterectomy, intimal flaps, luminal thrombus, residual stenoses, wall irregularities). The most important is exclusion of luminal thrombus, which originates from bleeding from transected vasa vasorum. Quality control techniques include TCD, completion angiography, DUS, CW-Doppler and angioscopy. TCD ensures optimal shunt function and is the only method capable of diagnosing embolisation, on-table thrombosis and postoperative occlusion. Angiography (which must be biplanar) provides anatomical data, but requires ionising radiation and can only be performed after restoration of flow (i.e. any thrombus could be swept distally). The latest colour DUS probes are smaller and more accessible because of the development of L-shaped probes but usually require the presence of a technician in theatre. The principal advantage of angioscopy is that it is performed *prior* to restoration of flow. Its main role is to identify the 3–5% of patients with residual luminal thrombus and the 1% with large intimal flaps.[83]

Operative complications

Cranial nerve injuries

✅✅ Cranial nerve injuries are an important source of morbidity, but very few are permanent or disabling.

In NASCET, the incidence of injury to the mandibular branch of the facial nerve was 2.2%, to the vagus 2.5%, to the spinal accessory nerve 0.2% and to the hypoglossal 3.7%. The overall rate of cranial nerve injury was 8.6%, although 92% were minor and fully recovered within 4 weeks.[85] In CREST, the risk of cranial nerve palsy following CEA was 4.7% (2% unresolved at 30 days), compared to 0.3% after stenting. By 1 year, however, cranial nerve injury did not impact on quality of life in patients randomised to CEA in CREST.[47]

Wound complications

In NASCET, 132 CEA patients (9.3%) developed wound complications, of which 76 (58%) were minor, 52 (39%) moderate, while only 4 (3%) were classed as severe.[85] Early vein patch rupture complicates <1% of CEAs, but is virtually abolished provided saphenous vein is harvested from the groin.

Perioperative stroke

Perioperative stroke is classed as intraoperative if the patient recovers from anaesthesia with a new deficit and postoperative if the event occurs thereafter. In historical series, intraoperative stroke predominated and was more likely to affect patients with a combination of cerebral infarction and partial/total haemodynamic compromise. This suggests that high-risk patients are more vulnerable to otherwise minor changes in perfusion or emboli, so that the margin for technical error is reduced or possibly non-existent.

Intraoperative stroke has been virtually abolished at the Leicester Royal Infirmary (0.3% in 2500 cases), a feature attributed to removing luminal thrombus (identified by angioscopy) prior to flow restoration.[83] The commonest causes of postoperative stroke are: (i) ICA thrombosis (especially in the first 6 postoperative hours), (ii) hyperperfusion syndrome and (iii) intracranial haemorrhage (ICH). ICH and the hyperperfusion syndrome complicate 1–2% of CEAs and are more common in patients with severe bilateral extracranial disease in association with impaired cerebral vascular reserve, defective autoregulation and poor collateral flow patterns.

✅ It is essential that emergency medical units recognise the importance of rapid BP treatment in the CEA patient who presents with seizures, usually 5–7 days after surgery. These patients have a high risk of suffering ICH and the mainstay of management is control of seizures and aggressive blood pressure control.

The strategy for managing perioperative stroke depends on: (i) timing (intraoperative/postoperative), (ii) whether it follows thrombosis, embolism or haemorrhage and (iii) the severity of the deficit. The more extensive the deficit, the more likely that the ICA/MCA has occluded. For those without access to TCD or duplex, the surgeon has to assume that any deficit following recovery from anaesthesia or in the first 24 hours is thromboembolic and the patient should be re-explored. Although re-exploration will not benefit patients with MCA branch embolism or haemodynamic stroke, this cannot be avoided. The management of MCA embolisation will be discussed in the section on CAS. For those with access to TCD, decision-making is easier. The immediate priority is to identify patients with ICA thrombosis, as they require immediate exploration. Provided flow is restored within 1 hour, good neurological recovery can be expected.

✅ TCD features of early carotid thrombosis include flow reversal in the ipsilateral anterior cerebral artery, enhanced flow in the ipsilateral posterior cerebral artery and, most importantly, flow velocities in the ipsilateral MCA that mimic those observed during carotid clamping.

✅ The administration of 75 mg clopidogrel the night before surgery (in addition to regular aspirin) was found to virtually abolish stroke due to postoperative carotid thrombosis.[83]

Long-term follow-up and restenosis

The annual risk of late ipsilateral and contralateral stroke after CEA and CAS is about 1%.[40–43,56–60] A number of centres perform serial DUS surveillance after CEA and CAS although a definite association between recurrent stenosis and late ipsilateral stroke has never previously been demonstrated. A recent meta-analysis of DUS surveillance data after carotid interventions in patients who were randomised within 11 RCTs found no evidence that an asymptomatic 70–99% restenosis after CAS was associated with a higher risk of late ipsilateral stroke (0.8% at mean 50 months follow-up), compared with 2.0% in CAS patients without a significant restenosis (OR 0.87 (95% CI 0.24–3.21).[86] By contrast, CEA patients with an untreated asymptomatic restenosis >70% incurred a 4.5% risk of late ipsilateral stroke at a mean of 37 months, compared with 1.5% in CEA patients with no evidence of a significant restenosis (OR 4.38 [95% CI 2.08–9.25]).[86] However, once the perioperative risk of redo CEA or CAS was factored in, very few CEA patients with asymptomatic restenoses >70% will gain benefit from reintervention.

✅✅ Meta-analyses suggest that the average annual risk of recurrent stenosis (50–100%) is 1.5–4.5%,[87] with the highest risk being the first 12 months.

✅ Patients who present with recurrent TIA/stroke after CEA and who have a 50–99% recurrent stenosis should be considered for treatment by CAS or redo CEA.

Patch infection

Patch infection complicates <1% of CEAs. If infection is suspected, the CCA must be controlled below the original incision. The prosthetic patch should be removed and replaced (where possible) with vein (bypass/patch). Infected prosthetic patches should not be treated by insertion of further prosthetic material, as there is a very high risk of reinfection.[88] Ligation should only be considered as a last resort (uncontrollable haemorrhage) and preferably if some form of monitoring (e.g. TCD, awake neurological testing at the original procedure) suggests that collateral flow is satisfactory.

✅ No abscess overlying a CEA wound should be incised before being seen by a vascular surgeon.

Endovascular treatment of carotid disease

Assessing suitability for CAS

Careful case selection is mandatory for safe practice and most patients being considered for CAS require 'overview' anatomical imaging (arch to the circle of Willis) with either CTA or MRA. Absolute contraindications include an occluded ICA (except in cases of acute stroke with a so-called tandem occlusion of both ICA and ipsilateral MCA) or visible thrombus. Anatomical factors that increase the technical difficulty of CAS include those related to access to the ICA (low carotid bifurcation/short CCA, tortuous CCA, diseased CCA and disease or occlusion of the ECA), the configuration of the aortic arch (severe arch atheroma, severe arch origin disease, type III arch and bovine arch) and characteristics of the target vessel (pinhole stenosis, angulated origin of the ICA, angulated distal ICA and circumferential calcification of the ICA).[89,90] A difficult origin to the brachiocephalic artery/left CCA or severe CCA tortuosity are relative contraindications. Tortuosity of the ICA above the stenosis (**Fig. 10.6**) may prevent use of filter or distal occlusive protection systems. This tortuosity potentially can be turned into a kink or occlusion by a stent. The absence of (occlusive) disease of the ECA is essential to enable placement of a long guidewire in the ECA to perform an exchange of the diagnostic catheter for a long introduction sheath or guiding catheter. ECA patency is also a prerequisite for the use of proximal embolic protection devices that use an occlusive ECA balloon (see below).

✅ A multispeciality Delphi consensus has provided recommendations for case selection based on anatomical criteria, and is aimed specifically at the novice (a practitioner with <50 CAS experience). The expected level of difficulty is presented as a traffic-light table (green for straightforward and red for high level of expected difficulty).[89]

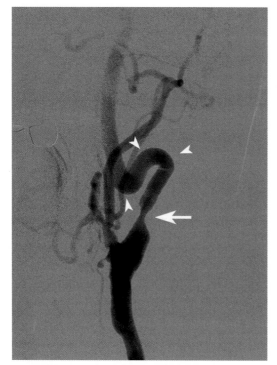

Figure 10.6 • Digital subtraction angiogram of the left carotid bifurcation demonstrating a high-grade stenosis (*arrow*) and severe tortuosity of the distal left internal carotid artery (*arrowheads*) that may preclude the use of distal protection devices (filters and distal balloons).

Dual antiplatelet therapy

It is routine practice to prescribe DAPT prior to CAS; 75 mg of clopidogrel is commenced 1 week prior to intervention in addition to 75 mg aspirin daily. In recently symptomatic patients, 300–600 mg clopidogrel (depending on body weight) is given at least 15 hours pre-intervention. The dual antiplatelet regime should continue for at least 28 days post-procedure, i.e. the presumed time-frame for endothelialisation of the stent.

✓✓ Randomised trials have confirmed the benefit of perioperative dual antiplatelet therapy prior to CAS.[91]

CAS technique

The most commonly used access route is via the common femoral artery. Brachial, radial or direct carotid approaches are alternatives if there is a difficult arch ('type III' or 'bovine'). In a type III arch, the origin of the brachiocephalic is significantly lower than a horizontal line drawn across the highest point of the arch. In a 'bovine' arch, there

is a conjoint origin to the brachiocephalic and left CCA.

During the procedure, anticoagulation should be administered in order to reduce the risk of thrombus formation associated with the presence of intra-arterial sheaths, catheters and guidewires. Usually a bolus of heparin is given. The required dose of heparin ranges from 75 to 100 units/kg. In a standard patient, a single dose of 5000–7500 units will usually be sufficient to provide adequate coverage throughout the entire CAS procedure, provided it does not take more than 45 minutes and (therefore) ACT measurement is not routinely necessary. The effect of heparin is generally allowed to subside in a physiological way, and protamine sulphate reversal is not usually recommended. Lesion access depends on anatomy, experience and choice of protection. Methods include: (i) exchange technique (ipsilateral ECA accessed with a selective catheter and hydrophilic guidewire with subsequent exchange for supportive exchange-length guidewire over which a long sheath is advanced); (ii) co-axial technique with advancement of a dedicated catheter and long 6-Fr sheath over a wire into the CCA, thus avoiding interaction with the bifurcation; and (iii) 'direct probing' with an 8-Fr guiding catheter that is positioned just beyond the ostium of the great vessel of interest (helpful in patients with a type III arch), and which is therefore slightly more vulnerable to catheter prolapse and loss of secure access during the procedure.

The stenosis is then either crossed with a distal cerebral protection device (CPD) or after deployment of a proximal CPD (see 'Cerebral protection devices'). Stent delivery systems are mostly 5-Fr or 6-Fr compatible. Occasionally it is possible to cross the lesion with the delivery system without predilatation, but plaque 'snow-ploughing' must be avoided. Severe stenoses (80–90%) require 3-mm predilatation in order to permit safe passage of the stent-delivery system. Stent length should be chosen such that it will cover the carotid artery over at least 5 mm proximal and 5 mm beyond the stenosis. Extreme elongation or kinks situated close to the stenosis should also be taken into account when choosing stent length, in order to avoid arterial redundancy and increasing the amount of kinking. One must avoid placing the distal end of the stent into kinks and tortuosities of the ICA, because these kinks cannot be eliminated and tend to be displaced distally. The stent diameter should be oversized by at least 1 mm to the reference vessel diameter. In the event that the stent needs to extend from the CCA into the ICA (i.e. covering the origin of the ECA), a tapered stent should be used. The stent is delivered across the stenosis using road mapping (when filter protection is used) or by reference to a 'control' image with bony anatomy once flow arrest/flow reversal has been established. Once deployed, the stent can be dilated to ensure good apposition against the arterial wall. It is important to avoid aggressive postdilatation as emboli are generated during this phase of the procedure. Many practitioners are comfortable with leaving some degree of residual stenosis. This is on the understanding that most Nitinol stent systems will continue to expand after deployment and because the 'potato masher effect' should be avoided. Atropine (0.6–1.2 mg) or 200 µg glycopyrrolate (synthetic derivative with less cardioaccelerator effect) is delivered just before balloon dilatation and stent placement either via the sheath or intravenously to block the carotid sinus baroreceptors.

✅ Atropine/glycopyrrolate will cause short-term unilateral mydriasis if administered via the arterial sheath. Staff looking after the patient upon return to the ward should be notified about this harmless finding.

Angiography is performed in at least two planes after completion of the procedure with attention directed towards excluding plaque prolapse into the lumen through stent interstices (or platelet/thrombus aggregates) (**Fig. 10.7**). This requires gentle re-ballooning or 'double scaffolding' (placement of a second stent inside the first). Plaque prolapse may be less likely to occur with dual-layer or micromesh stent systems. Spasm (usually well tolerated) is managed by careful cephalad movement of the filter, the administration of diluted nitroglycerine (100–200 µg) or (200 µg diluted in a 10 mL solution injected slowly as a 2–3 mL bolus) into the long sheath and timely completion of the procedure. A full filter (causing sluggish flow) requires aspiration with a 0.014-inch compatible rapid-exchange system. Proximal CPD devices avoid these issues, but a proportion of patients are intolerant, leading to yawning, lack of responsiveness, obtundation or seizure. This can be dealt with by either intermittent flow reversal or by stopping flow reversal and using a distal filter.

An evaluation of 627 protected CAS procedures has yielded important information regarding the timing of complications during (after) CAS.[92] At 30 days there were 10 major strokes (two fatal), 18 minor strokes (2.9%) and one cardiac death. Four major strokes occurred in phase 1 (catheterisation of the arch, target vessel and CCA) and six in phase 3 (stent deployment, pre- and postdilatation). It was concluded that a large proportion of major strokes (4/10) during CAS occurred during catheterisation and that these could not have been prevented by the use of a protection device.

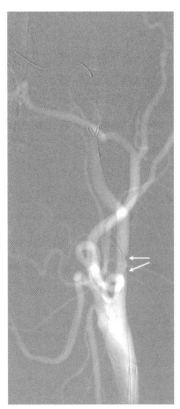

Figure 10.7 • Plaque prolapse through the interstices of a closed-cell stent (Abbott XAct; *arrows*). This was treated by placing a second stent inside the first, i.e. 'double scaffolding'.

Cerebral protection devices

There are three types of CPD. No RCTs have determined whether CPDs reduce the risk of post-CAS stroke. A Cochrane Review on stenting for symptomatic carotid artery stenoses (based on outcomes from EVA-3S, SPACE and ICSS)[93] concluded that for the outcome of death or any stroke within 30 days after treatment, there was no evidence that the use of filter-type CPDs was beneficial. By contrast, a meta-analysis of 22 non-randomised studies ($n = 11655$) reported significantly lower rates of perioperative stroke/death favouring the use of CPDs (OR 0.57 (95% [CI 0.43-0.76], $P < 0.01$).[94] Notwithstanding the conflicting data, most CAS practitioners currently use some form of cerebral protection during the procedure. A recent meta-analysis has shown no difference in outcome between proximal and distal CPDs.[95]

Distal protection devices

Distal balloon occlusion

Although the rationale is simple, there are a number of disadvantages. Angulated lesions may be difficult to cross, the distal balloon can damage the ICA wall, 10% of patients are intolerant of ICA occlusion and the stenosis cannot be imaged whilst the ICA is occluded. These devices are not widely used anymore.

Distal filter devices

These devices can be divided into mesh-like filters, or filters that make use of a porous membrane that can be eccentric or concentric. These devices are either premounted onto a wire that comes with the delivery system (wire-mounted filters) or are inserted over a previously positioned guidewire (bare-wire filters). The filter is placed in a way similar to the placement of a bare guidewire. Predilatation before passage of the filter is typically not performed. Care should be taken to deploy the filter in a segment of the ICA that is straight, in order to allow for proper wall appositioning of the filter. Furthermore, the filter should be placed at a distance from the stenosis that allows the tip of the stent delivery system and distal part of the stent to cross the lesion. In cases of severe tortuosity (where the filter cannot be advanced), the use of an adjunctive wire ('buddy wire') will help to straighten out the ICA, thus facilitating passage of the protection device. The filter is retrieved following final stent dilatation. There is the potential for filter through-flow (controlled by pore size) and filter peri-flow. Self-limiting spasm of the ICA is relatively common (**Fig. 10.8a–c**).

Flow reversal/flow arrest (endovascular clamping)

The working principle of proximal CPDs is by either completely interrupting or reversing blood flow in the ICA. In this way, 'endovascular clamping' can be achieved, with cerebral perfusion relying on collateralisation via the circle of Willis. These devices cannot be used in all cases, because complete occlusion/flow reversal is not tolerated by up to 30% of patients.[96] Embolic particles can be aspirated, and the systems offer the advantage that the ICA stenosis is only crossed once the protection device is in place and thus all manipulation needed to cross the lesion is performed during protection. The currently available proximal CPD systems create occlusion of the ECA and ICA with separate balloons.

MoMa (Medtronic-Invatec) consists of an 8-Fr or 9-Fr sheath that provides an effective working channel of 5-Fr or 6-Fr, respectively, with two balloons that can be inflated independently (**Fig. 10.9a–e**). The distal balloon is located close to the sheath tip and is used to occlude the ECA. The proximal balloon is located on the body of the sheath and is inflated within the CCA. When inflated, both balloons prevent antegrade flow from the CCA and retrograde flow from the ECA, leading to complete flow cessation. The device is advanced into the ECA. The distal ECA balloon should be placed proximal to the origin of the superior thyroid artery in order to provide flow interruption/reversal. Once the

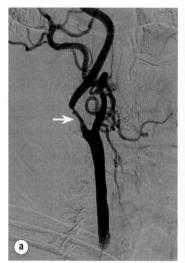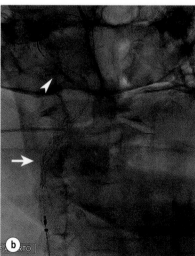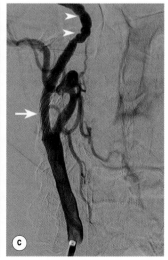

Figure 10.8 • (a) DSA image of high-grade symptomatic stenosis (*arrow*) of the right internal carotid artery (RICA). The straightforward anatomy allows use of a distal filter-type protection device. **(b)** Fluoroscopic image after placement of dual layer stent (*arrow*); filter device is still in place (*arrowhead*). **(c)** Completion DSA showing restoration of flow, with smooth stent surface (*arrow*). Note non-flow limiting spasm in the distal RICA at the level of the previous position of the embolic protection device (*arrowhead*). In this case, no treatment was necessary.

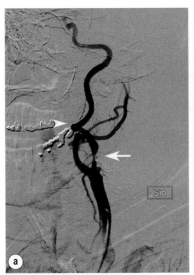
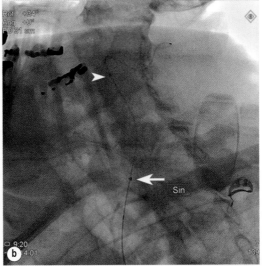
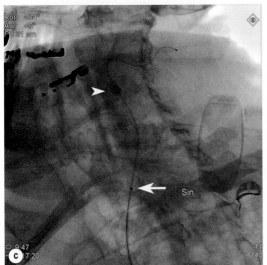
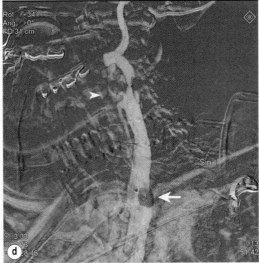
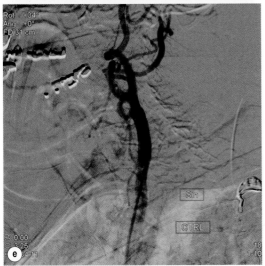

Figure 10.9 • **(a)** DSA of left carotid bifurcation showing high-grade stenosis of the left internal carotid artery (LICA) (*arrow*). Note tortuosity of the distal LICA (*arrowhead*), rendering the use of a distal cerebral protection device (CPD) unfavourable. **(b)** Fluoroscopic image with MoMa device inserted over a guidewire into the left external carotid artery (ECA). Markers for the distal ECA balloon (*arrowhead*) and proximal common carotid artery (*arrow*) are clearly visible. **(c)** Fluoroscopic image with distal ECA balloon inflated (*arrowhead*), proximal balloon marker indicated by arrow. **(d)** Roadmap image with both distal (*arrowhead*) and proximal (*arrow*) protection balloons inflated. The roadmap image is used for stent positioning. **(e)** Completion DSA after stent placement and removal of proximal CPD.

device is in place, the stenting procedure can be performed. Following CAS, three 20-mL syringes of carotid blood are aspirated and checked for debris before deflating the distal and then the proximal balloons, thus re-establishing cerebral blood flow.

The NeuroProtection System (WL Gore) is composed of a 9-Fr sheath with an effective working lumen of 6-Fr and an inflatable balloon at its tip and a separate balloon wire. After positioning the sheath within the CCA, the balloon wire is inserted and placed in the proximal ECA (as with the MoMa device). Both balloons are inflated, leading to flow cessation. After this, the proximal part of the sheath is connected to the contralateral femoral vein. This allows reversal of blood flow from the cerebral circulation, down the ICA and through the sheath into the femoral venous system via a filter with a pore size of 180 μm. In contrast to to the MoMa system (where complete flow cessation is obtained), the procedure is performed in reverse-flow mode. At the end of the procedure, 10–20 mL of carotid blood is aspirated before balloon deflation.

The ENROUTE system (formerly called MICHI) involves flow reversal via a mini CCA incison between the heads of sternomastoid and does not require occlusion of the ipsilateral ECA in order to achieve flow reversal into the femoral vein. This is achieved by means of low-resistance, wide-bore dialysis tubing that completes the extracorporeal circuit. Direct access via the CCA cut-down avoids wire and sheath manipulation within the aortic arch.

Does stent design influence outcome?

A systematic review of 32 studies (1363 procedures) found that closed-cell stents significantly reduced new white lesions on diffusion-weighted MRI, compared with open-cell stents.[97] A small RCT comparing Wallstent and the expanded polytetrafluoroethylene (ePTFE)-covered Symbiot stent (stopped early due to excessive restenosis in the covered stent limb) demonstrated significantly fewer microemboli with the covered stent.[98] The Belgian/Italian registry detailed outcomes following 3179 procedures in a mixed population (largely asymptomatic) and found that stent 'free-cell area' impacted on stroke/death rates. There was a statistically significant benefit for the XAct, the WallStent and the NexStent compared with the open-cell Precise, Protégé, Acculink and Exponent.[99] Another European registry sought to corroborate these findings and demonstrated a similar trend towards a lower rate of procedural events when a closed-cell stent was used in symptomatic patients.[100] In SPACE, the closed-cell WallStent was associated with significantly better outcomes than open cell Acculink or Precise stents,[101]

while ICSS also observed better outcomes where CAS was performed using closed-cell designed stents.[102]

Periprocedural haemodynamic problems

Haemodynamic depression

Haemodynamic instability is common during CAS and is probably baroreceptor-mediated. Early CAS literature suggested that without anticholinergic prophylaxis, the incidence of intraprocedural hypotension was 17–22%, while 28–71% developed bradycardia. Postprocedural hypotension is common (usually lasting about 24 hours) but is usually benign. Treatment is reserved for symptomatic patients or those in whom sustained hypotension may cause cardiovascular compromise (e.g. patients awaiting CABG or aortic valve replacement). Treatment in symptomatic or 'at-risk' patients includes antimuscarinic and/or selective alpha agonists. A recent study evaluated the use of vasopressors in the critical care unit (CCU) for the treatment of persistent post-CAS hypotension in 623 patients.[103] The authors concluded that in patients with a systolic BP ≤90 mmHg, especially those protracted cases where the BP was low for ≥24 hours, there was a significant increase in the risk of stroke/death/MI.[103] Furthermore, compared with the the mixed alpha/beta-agonist dopamine, the more selective alpha-agonists (norepinephrine and phenylephrine) were associated with a shorter infusion time and reduced CCU lengths of stay and fewer major adverse events. Patients that develop clinically significant haemodynamic instability are more likely to experience periprocedural stroke, as compared to patients that are haemodynamically stable (8% vs 1%, respectively). Patients that received prophylactic anticholinergic therapy did not show any increase in procedural stroke, even if they developed clinically significant haemodynamic instability. Haemodynamic disturbances are an important cause of stroke during both CEA and CAS in ICSS. In CAS patients, it was the most frequent cause of stroke, and is probably related to carotid sinus manipulation and baroreceptor dysfunction related to stenting.[104]

Hyperperfusion and intracranial haemorrhage

The incidence of ICH is not significantly different to that following CEA, despite the obligatory use of DAPT. Patients most commonly complain of headache, although stroke-like signs due to oedema may also occur. The most important risk (with the hyperperfusion syndrome) is progression to ICH, with or without seizures. Hypertension associated with carotid baroreceptor or microvascular failure at the level of the blood–brain barrier, reflecting perfusion breakthrough into a recent infarct or spontaneous haemorrhagic conversion, caused by showers of microemboli may occur after stent placement. Prophylactic pharmacotherapy (short-acting beta-blockers) is considered in patients deemed high risk, and may reduce the incidence of hyperperfusion syndrome and ICH.[105] A total of 54 cases of CAS-associated ICH have been reported and a pooled analysis suggests that the incidence of ICH is 0.63% (95% CI 0.38–0.97%).[106]

✔ Intraprocedural haemodynamic instability is an important cause of stroke. Baseline systolic BP >180 mmHg in a patient without prior good control of BP is an independent risk factor for an increased incidence of intra- and periprocedural hypotension/hypertension. If hypotension develops, the magnitude of BP drop correlates linearly with the severity of subsequent neurological insult. Permissive tolerance of an elevated systolic BP in patients with good BP control is supportive during CAS procedures with proximal protection. Withholding angiotensin-converting enzyme inhibitors and calcium antagonists prior to the procedure generally allows a pressure that will withstand 'endovascular clamping'. A procedural systolic BP of ≥160 mmHg generally supports the use of proximal embolic protection.

Management of post-CAS and CEA stroke

The endovascular treatment of acute stroke has been demonstrated to provide significant clinical benefit over intravenous thrombolysis in five RCTs[107] and many of these endovascular techniques can now be applied to treating acute stroke after CEA or CAS (especially embolisation of the MCA mainstem).[108,109]

Distal embolism

In cases of stroke secondary to macro-emboli, these can be removed mechanically or via thrombolysis.[108,109] Mechanical removal has a theoretical advantage over thrombolytic therapy because it carries a lower risk of bleeding (especially in cases where hyperperfusion is more likely to occur) and because the material that may be dislodged can be expected to be more organised and/or non-thrombotic.[108] Mechanical removal of embolic material from the intracranial branches of the ICA is possible using neuro-interventional retrieval systems. Proximal devices include aspiration catheters, while distal devices include spiral-shaped or basket-like devices. These are typically introduced through a guiding catheter or long introduction sheath and are advanced beyond the point of occlusion in an undeployed state. Aspiration of thrombus from the CCA or cervical portion of the ICA can be performed with diagnostic or guiding catheters (diameter 4-Fr to 7-Fr). In order to obtain a vacuum, it is important to use catheters without side-holes. The catheter should be advanced until it contacts the thrombus, and slight negative pressure should then be applied using a syringe. For aspiration thrombectomy (at the intracranial level), microcatheters can be used. Aspiration catheters should have a large inner lumen and should be kink-resistant (provided by micro-braiding). One specific advantage of aspiration catheters is that they can be used in situations where there is limited space beyond the occlusion where distal retrieval devices cannot be used (e.g. distal MCA mainstem branches or bifurcations).

In the absence of dedicated retrieval devices, restoration of antegrade flow can be achieved by fragmenting the embolus using balloon angioplasty or guidewire manipulation.[108,109] Wire fragmentation should be performed using a flexible hydrophilic-tipped guidewire (0.008 in to 0.010 in). The wire tip should be formed into a J-shape in order to avoid vessel perforation. Penetration and fragmentation of the thrombus can be achieved by gently advancing and rotating the wire. Balloon angioplasty tends to be relatively ineffective, due to the spongy nature of the clot/embolus that tends to recoil. In cases of recoil, additional stent placement at the level of the (residual) embolus may be performed. In order to be able to reach the lesion, flexible stents and stent delivery systems should be used. A major disadvantage of the fragmentation technique (and to a lesser extent stenting) is the relatively high risk of distal embolisation.

Intra-arterial thrombolysis is an effective therapy for acute thrombotic occlusion of cerebral vessels.[108,109] The site of occlusion, type of thrombus and presence of leptomeningeal collateralisation influences the chance of recanalisation. Typically, occlusions of the proximal carotid terminus and M1 segment of the MCA respond poorly to intra-arterial thrombolysis, mainly due to the large clot burden, which requires a longer time to achieve complete thrombolysis. Although a thrombus in the MCA mainstem may be successfully treated, clinical success may be negatively influenced by non-recanalisation of smaller lenticulostriate branches. Thrombolytic agents include urokinase and recombinant tissue plasminogen activator (rTPA), and these are delivered through a super-selectively placed microcatheter. An infusion microcatheter (<3.0-Fr) with a single end-hole should be placed into the proximal third of the thrombus using a steerable microguidewire. Using a so-called coaxial catheter technique, the microcatheter is advanced through a Y-connector, attached to a diagnostic catheter with a lumen of at least 0.038 in. The Y-connector also allows for continuous flushing of the microcatheter with heparinised saline. If intrathrombus positioning of the microcatheter is not possible, the tip of the catheter needs to be placed as close to the proximal aspect of the embolic occlusion as possible for thrombolytic infusion. A superselective angiogram needs to be performed through the microcatheter to confirm correct positioning of the catheter. High-dose urokinase regimens are generally administered (500 000 IU urokinase with half being administered as a single bolus). Alternatively, continuous infusion (without a bolus) of up to 1 250 000 units of urokinase over 90 minutes can be performed. rTPA may be given as a 5-mg bolus, followed by slow-infusion (maximum dose 20 mg). It is important to perform serial angiograms (every 15 minutes) and to continue thrombolytic therapy until complete recanalisation has been achieved (to a maximum of 1 hour). If the proximal thrombus dissolves, the tip of the microcatheter needs to be advanced into the next portion of residual clot. Mechanical disruption of the clot can be performed in cases where no advancement of lytic activity is observed. As mentioned previously, intra-arterial thrombolysis increases the risk of haemorrhagic complications. Selective intra-arterial administration of 5 mg abciximab (ReoPro, Lilly Pharmaceuticals, Indianapolis, IN, USA) followed by a bolus of 5 mg abciximab intravenously has also been used for the treatment of neurological sequelae due to distal embolisation after carotid artery angioplasty and stent placement.

Thrombosis

Thrombosis occurring during the CAS procedure seems to be associated with the use of embolic protection devices (e.g. filters), but acute thrombosis of the stented target lesion has also been described. A large embolic load may block the filter completely, leading to proximal flow stasis. In addition, thrombus forming on the wire of the filter system has been described, despite maximum anticoagulation. Treatment consists of local administration of abciximab or aspiration of thrombus, followed by retrieval of the filter device using the guiding catheter or sheath already in place. Care should be taken not to close the filter system completely, as its embolic contents may be squeezed out and embolise distally.[108,109]

Acute stent thrombosis is a potentially fatal complication, with an incidence of 0.5–2%. It seems to be more common in patients not receiving DAPT. Treatment consists of intra-arterial thrombolysis or administration of intra-arterial abciximab.[108,109] Intra-arterial thrombolysis involves administration of urokinase or rTPA as described earlier. A successful dosage regime of 0.25 mg/kg of abciximab intra-arterially, followed by a continuous intravenous infusion (9 µg/min for 12 hours) has been successfully used. Alternatively, intracarotid injection of 5 mg rTPA, followed by systemic administration of 5 mg rTPA and intracarotid administration of a half-dose bolus of abciximab (0.125 mg/kg) is an alternative. In cases where additional endovascular therapy or systemic pharmacological treatment does not resolve the occlusion in a timely fashion, conversion to surgery using either thrombendarterectomy with stent removal and patch closure or thrombectomy using aspiration after transverse arteriotomy of the ipsilateral CCA should be considered.

Dissection

Dissection is a rare complication during CAS. Dissection can be related to stent placement and balloon angioplasty (as in other vascular territories), as well as being caused by distal balloon CPDs. In cases where flow reduction is limited, a wait-and-see policy may be employed. In cases of severe flow impairment, treatment consists of either inserting a second stent, or urgent surgical repair, which will involve removal of the stent and carotid bypass.[108,109]

Key points

- 'Best medical therapy' and risk factor control is mandated in everyone.
- There is compelling evidence that recently symptomatic patients benefit from treatment (medical therapy, intervention) in the early time period after onset of symptoms.
- The beneficial role of CEA is supported by level 1 evidence in selected asymptomatic and symptomatic patients. In symptomatic patients, the benefit conferred by CEA is dependent on being performed early with a low operative risk and requires surgeons to quote their own operative risks rather than trial data.

- Since the last edition, randomised trials have shown that CAS has emerged as an alternative to CEA in selected patients. The decision as to which treatment strategy should be implemented in individual patients will depend on unit experience, recency of symptoms, patient age and overall cardiovascular risk.
- Interventions should not be delayed in order to achieve a lower procedural risk. The highest risk period for stroke is the first few days after onset of symptoms. CAS is not currently indicated in the very early time period after onset of symptoms..

🌐 Full references available at **http://expertconsult. inkling.com**

Key references

3. Menon R, Kerry S, Norris JW, et al. Treatment of cervical artery dissection: a systematic review and meta-analysis. JNNP 2008;79:1122–7. PMID: 18303104.

8. Rothwell PM, Eliasziw M, Gutnikov SA. for the Carotid Endarterectomy Trialists Collaboration. Analysis of pooled data from the randomised controlled trials of endarterectomy for symptomatic carotid stenosis. Lancet 2003;361:107–16. PMID: 12531577.

19. Executive Committee for the Asymptomatic Carotid Atherosclerosis Study. Endarterectomy for asymptomatic carotid artery stenosis. JAMA 1995;273:1421–61. PMID: 7723155.

23. MacMahon S. Antihypertensive drug treatment: the potential, expected and observed effects on vascular disease. J Hypertens 1990;8(Suppl):S239–44. PMID: 2151335.

24. Kalra L, Perez I, Melbourn A. Stroke risk management: changes in mainstream practice. Stroke 1998;29:53–7. PMID: 9445328.

25. Heart Protection Study Collaborative Group. MRC/ BHF Heart Protection Study of cholesterol lowering with simvastatin in 20536 high-risk individuals: a randomised placebo controlled trial. Lancet 2002;360:7–22. PMID: 12114036.

31. Rothwell PM, Eliasziw M, Gutnikov SA. for the Carotid Endarterectomy Trialists Collaboration. Endarterectomy for symptomatic carotid stenosis in relation to clinical subgroups and timing of surgery. Lancet 2004;363:915–24. PMID: 15043958.

32. Rothwell PM, Eliasziw M, Gutnikov SA. Sex difference in the effect of time from symptoms to surgery on benefit from carotid endarterectomy for transient ischaemic attack and minor stroke. Stroke 2004;35:2855–61. PMID: 15514193.

66. Naylor AR, Mehta Z, Rothwell PM. Stroke during coronary artery bypass surgery: a critical review of the role of carotid artery disease. Eur J Vasc Endovasc Surg 2002;23:283–94. PMID: 11991687.

67. Naylor AR, Bown MJ. Stroke after cardiac surgery and its association with asymptomatic carotid disease: an updated systematic review and meta-analysis. Eur J Vasc Endovasc Surg 2011;41:607–24. PMID: 21396854.

68. Naylor AR, Cuffe R, Rothwell PM, et al. A systematic review of outcomes following staged and synchronous carotid endarterectomy and coronary artery bypass. Eur J Vasc Endovasc Surg 2003;25:380–9. PMID: 12713775.

69. Naylor AR, Cuffe R, Rothwell PM, et al. A systematic review of outcomes following synchronous carotid endarterectomy and coronary artery bypass: influence of patient and surgical variables. Eur J Vasc Endovasc Surg 2003;26:230–41. PMID: 14509884.

70. Fareed K, Rothwell PM, Mehta Z, et al. Synchronous carotid endarterectomy and off-pump coronary bypass: an updated systematic review of early outcomes. Eur J Vasc Endovasc Surg 2009;37:375–8. PMID: 19211276.

87. Frericks H, Kievit J, van Baalen JM. Carotid recurrent stenosis and risk of ipsilateral stroke. A systematic review of the literature. Stroke 1998;29:244–50. PMID: 9445358.

91. McKevitt FM, Randall MS, Cleveland TJ. The benefits of combined anti-platelet treatment in carotid artery stenting. Eur J Vasc Endvasc Surg 2005;29:522–7. PMID: 15966092.

11

Vascular disorders of the upper limb

Jean-Baptiste Ricco
Romain Belmonte

Introduction

Arterial diseases of the upper limb are relatively rare in comparison with those involving the lower extremity. The good collateral supply around the shoulder and elbow explains why chronic occlusive disease is commonly asymptomatic, but acute occlusion due to embolism can result in limb-threatening ischaemia. In addition, thoracic outlet syndrome, subclavian–axillary vein thrombosis and occupational vascular problems need to be considered. In this chapter we do not review vasospastic disorders, connective tissue disease, vasculitis and Raynaud's disease, as these are covered in Chapter 12, nor vascular trauma, which is covered in Chapter 9. The main causes of upper limb vascular disease are summarised in Box 11.1.

Clinical examination

Vascular assessment of the upper limb should include the thoracic outlet. Palpation and auscultation of the supraclavicular region may help to detect a cervical rib, a subclavian artery stenosis or aneurysm. The arm pulses should be examined with the arm placed in the neutral position and then in abduction and external rotation (surrender position) to detect arterial thoracic outlet compression. Pulse palpation is important and must include the axillary, brachial, radial and ulnar pulses. The nail folds should be examined for infarcts and splinter haemorrhages. The blood pressure should be measured in both arms, preferably using a hand-held Doppler. A difference of more than 15% is abnormal.

Examination in cases of hand ischaemia is not complete unless Allen's test is performed. The examiner compresses the radial and ulnar arteries at the wrist. The examiner then asks the subject to clench the fist to empty the hand of blood. The radial artery is then released and the hand is observed for return of colour. The test is then repeated for the ulnar artery. The test is normal if refilling of the hand is complete within less than 10 seconds from either side. Any portion of the hand that does not blush is an indication of incomplete continuity of the palmar arch.

Occlusive disease

Occlusive lesions of the brachiocephalic and subclavian arteries occur in relatively young patients with mean ages ranging from 50 to 60 years. These lesions are less frequent than those involving the carotid bifurcation.[1] Atherosclerosis is the predominant cause in Europe, with Buerger's disease and Takayasu's arteritis rarely seen. The symptoms of occlusive disease of the upper extremities include muscle fatigue and ischaemic rest pain. Digital necrosis or atheroembolisation is less common than in the lower extremities, accounting for no more than 5% of patients with limb ischaemia.[2]

Brachiocephalic artery

Stenotic lesions of the brachiocephalic artery are uncommon and may be asymptomatic in 13–22% of patients.[3,4] Symptomatic patients may present

Box 11.1 • Causes of upper limb vascular diseases

Arterial obstruction

Large artery
Atherosclerosis
Radiotherapy
Thoracic outlet syndrome
Arteritis (giant cell, Takayasu's)

Small artery
Atherosclerosis
Connective tissue disease
Myeloproliferative disease
Buerger's disease
Vibrating tools

Arterial vasospasm

Large artery
Ergot-containing medications and other pharmacological causes

Small artery
Raynaud's disease
Vibrating tools

Embolism: proximal sources
Heart
Ulcerated arterial plaques (aortic arch, brachiocephalic and subclavian arteries)
Aneurysm (brachiocephalic, subclavian, axillary, brachial, ulnar arteries)
Thoracic outlet syndrome

Subclavian–axillary vein thrombosis
Primary: Paget–Schroetter syndrome (thoracic outlet syndrome)
Secondary: catheter, hypercoagulable states

Hypercoagulable states
Heparin antibodies
Deficiencies of antithrombin III, proteins C and S
Antiphospholipid syndrome
Malignancy
Cryoglobulinaemia
Aneurysms

with ischaemia of the right upper extremity, carotid territory symptoms or vertebrobasilar symptoms.[5] The diagnosis is suspected by physical examination (i.e. right supraclavicular/cervical bruit, absent right subclavian or axillary pulse) and confirmed by duplex scanning, conventional angiography, or computed tomographic angiography (CTA) or magnetic resonance angiography (MRA). Most patients (61–84%) with brachiocephalic artery occlusion have multiple lesions of the aortic arch vessels.[6] Stenotic lesions of the brachiocephalic artery may be approached by median sternotomy with direct bypass grafting from the aortic arch, or indirectly by extra-anatomical bypass such as subclavian–subclavian, contralateral carotid–carotid or subclavian–carotid bypass.

Aorto-brachiocephalic bypass

✔✔ Extra-anatomical bypasses have a lower morbidity and mortality but direct bypasses from the aortic arch are more durable. In total, the combined postoperative death and stroke rate for direct reconstruction of the supra-aortic trunks ranges from 2.6% to 16% (Table 11.1). The primary patency is about 90% with a 72% survival rate at 10 years.[7]

A median sternotomy is used with extension into the neck. The left brachiocephalic vein is identified (**Fig. 11.1a**). A partial occluding clamp is applied to the ascending aorta proximal to the brachiocephalic artery to avoid the risk of fracturing atheromatous plaque (**Fig. 11.1b**). An 8–10-mm prosthetic graft is anastomosed at this site with deep suture placement in the aortic wall (**Fig. 11.1c**). Once the anastomosis is completed, a clamp is applied across the graft and systemic heparin is given. The brachiocephalic artery is clamped, sectioned and the proximal stump oversewn. The patent distal artery is spatulated and the graft attached in an end-to-end fashion (**Fig. 11.1d**). Air is evacuated from the graft by back-bleeding the subclavian artery, then flow is released into the arm and then into the carotid artery. The mortality of direct bypass ranges from 5.8% to 8% in Kieffer's and Berguer's series,[3,4] with a primary patency rate at 5 years of 94% in both series.

Brachiocephalic endarterectomy

The proximal location of the disease with extension into the aortic arch makes this technique hazardous. Attempts to remove an orifice lesion may initiate an aortic dissection or distal embolisation. For this reason, bypass or endovascular therapy are preferred for all brachiocephalic lesions where treatment is indicated, except perhaps for those located in the distal segment.

Endovascular treatment

Percutaneous transluminal angioplasty (PTA) and stenting of the brachiocephalic artery is being performed with increased frequency. The approach may be percutaneous from either the femoral or brachial artery or through an anterolateral cervical approach with clamping of the right common carotid artery to avoid atheroembolisation during angioplasty. Because of a relatively small number of cases, most papers concerning angioplasty of the brachiocephalic artery include results for the subclavian artery. Only four series report PTA of the brachiocephalic artery alone[9–12] (Table 11.2).

Table 11.1 • Direct reconstruction of the supra-aortic vessels: complications and late patency

Authors, year	No. patients	Mean follow-up (mth) [range]	Complications (%)	Primary patency (%)
Takach et al., 2005[8]	113	61.2±6 [3–264]	Death: 2.7 Stroke: 2.7 MI:* 1.8	10 years:* 94.4±±4
Berguer et al.,[4] 1998[4]	100	51±4.8 [1–184]	Stroke + death: 16 Morbidity: 27	5 years:† 94±3
Uurto et al.,[7] 2002	76	158 [6–136]	Death: 2.6 Morbidity: 19.7	1 year: 95 5 years:‡ 91 15 years:‡ 89

*22 patients were followed at 10 years.
†34 patients followed at 5 years.
‡54 patients followed at 5 years and 25 at 15 years.
MI, myocardial infarction.

The benefit of adjuvant stenting is not well established.[9,10,13] Open surgery gives better midterm results but angioplasty is much less invasive.

Subclavian artery

Symptomatic lesions of the subclavian artery are associated in 72% of cases with concomitant lesions of carotid and vertebral vessels.[1] The indications for intervention are those of vertebrobasilar insufficiency and marked upper extremity ischaemia. Atheroembolisation is quite common in this location.[14] If surgery is contemplated and the ipsilateral common carotid artery is healthy, carotid–subclavian bypass or carotid–subclavian transposition is the method of choice.

Carotid–subclavian bypass

Access is achieved by a horizontal supraclavicular incision with division of both heads of the sternomastoid muscle. Scalenus anterior and the phrenic nerves are exposed, and then scalenus anterior is divided near its insertion into the first rib (**Fig. 11.2a**). On the left side, the thoracic duct is ligated. The carotid sheath is opened, safeguarding the vagus nerve. After heparinisation, the common carotid artery is clamped as low as possible. A vein or polytetrafluoroethylene (PTFE) graft is then anastomosed to the lateral aspect of the common carotid artery in an end-to-side fashion (**Fig. 11.2b**). Use of a prosthetic graft seems to give better results than the vein graft in this location.[15] The graft under arterial tension is then passed behind the jugular vein. Graft length should be cautiously estimated and the graft anastomosed end-to-side to the superior aspect of the distal subclavian artery. If the proximal subclavian lesion is ulcerated, it should be excluded by ligation. If the distal subclavian artery is too diseased for distal implantation, the graft should be passed behind the clavicle and implanted on the axillary artery exposed via a short infraclavicular incision.

> ✓✓ Prosthetic carotid–subclavian bypass has an excellent patency. Postoperative mortality is less than 1%, with a primary patency of 95% at 10 years.[16,17]

Carotid transposition

Reimplantation of the subclavian artery into the common carotid artery is an alternative that avoids graft material but requires a more extensive cervical dissection. Dissection should avoid the recurrent laryngeal nerve, which is closely related to the posterior aspect of the subclavian artery. A curved clamp is applied across the subclavian artery, which is transected and the proximal stump oversewn. The site of anastomosis to the common carotid artery should be chosen to avoid kinking and angulation of the vertebral artery. The clamps on the common carotid artery should be rotated anteriorly to present the posterolateral surface for anastomosis with the subclavian artery (**Fig. 11.3**). An ellipse is excised from the wall of the common carotid artery and the subclavian artery anastomosed in end-to-side fashion.

> ✓✓ Subclavian–carotid reimplantation is an excellent technique that seems to give better results than the subclavian–carotid bypass in the series of Cinà et al.[18] (Table 11.3). Postoperative mortality is less than 1%, with a long-term patency of 100% in the series of Sandmann et al.[19] and Kretschmer et al.[20]

Crossover grafts

Subclavian revascularisation may also be achieved by crossover subclavian–subclavian or axillo-axillary bypass. These grafts are relatively simple

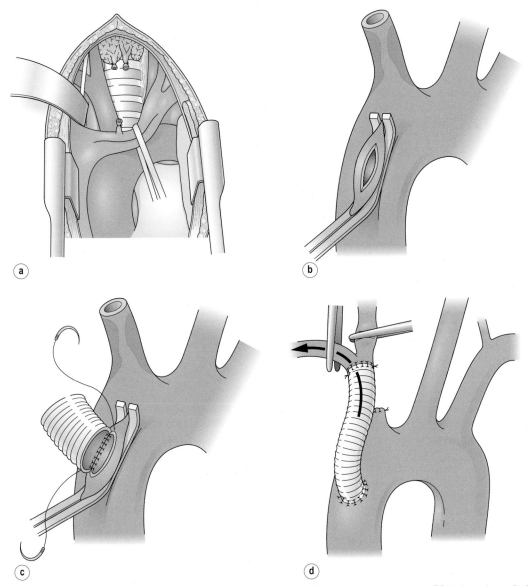

Figure 11.1 • **(a)** The left brachiocephalic vein is retracted to expose the brachiocephalic artery. **(b)** A clamp is applied laterally to the ascending aorta. **(c)** A polyester graft is implanted on the ascending thoracic aorta proximal to the brachiocephalic artery. **(d)** Completed bypass. Flow is released into the arm and then into the common carotid artery.

to construct, although their greater length and reversed angle of take-off may reduce durability. Furthermore, problems may arise if subsequent median sternotomy is needed for coronary bypass. The donor and recipient arteries are exposed by a short supraclavicular incision on either side (**Fig. 11.4**). A tunnel is created from one side of the neck to the other passing behind the sternomastoid muscles and anterior to the carotid vessels. Crossover axillo-axillary bypass is easier to perform but the graft should pass subcutaneously over the sternum, with risks of compression or erosion. The postoperative death rate for crossover axillo-

axillary bypass is 1.6% with a 5-year primary patency of 86.5% in the series of Mingoli et al.[21]

Endovascular treatment

PTA of subclavian artery stenoses is a relatively safe and often simple procedure to perform. Access is usually obtained from the femoral artery or from the brachial artery and the lesion dilated to 5–8 mm (**Fig. 11.5**). Because there is usually retrograde flow in the vertebral artery, stroke is rare. When there is no retrograde flow, an occlusion balloon may be placed in the vertebral artery from the arm while the stenosis is dilated. Simple stenoses are adequately

Table 11.2 • Angioplasty of the brachiocephalic artery: postoperative complications and late patency

Authors, year	No. patients	Mean follow-up (mth) [range]	Complications (%)	Primary patency (%)	Secondary patency (%)
Paukovits et al., 2010[9]	72	42.3 [2–103]	Total: 8.3 Death: none TIA: 2.6 Access site bleeding: 5.2	12 mth: 100 24 mth: 98 ± 1.6 96 mth: 69.9 ± 8.5	12 mth: 100 24 mth: 100 96 mth: 81.5 ± 7.7
Van Hattum et al., 2007[10]	30	n/a Median = 24 [4 weeks – 92]	Total: 10.0 Death: none TIA: 4.0	24 mth: 79	n/a
Hüttl et al., 2002[11]	89	n/a [12–117]	Neurological: 5.6 Local: 3.0	6 mth: 98 ± 2 1 year: 95 ± 3	100 98 ± 2
Mordasini et al., 2011[12]	18	32.4 [4–110]	Neurological: 11.1	n/a	n/a
van de Weijer et al., 2015[13]	51	52 [2–163]	None	Restenosis-free survival 1 year: 94.1% 2 year: 90.2%	n/a

n/a, not available.

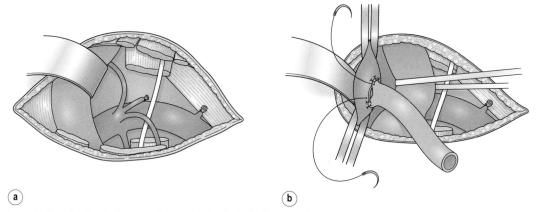

Figure 11.2 • (a) Cervical approach for carotid–subclavian bypass. The sternomastoid muscle is divided and the subclavian artery is exposed by sectioning the scalenus anterior. **(b)** A PTFE graft is anastomosed to the lateral aspect of the left common carotid artery.

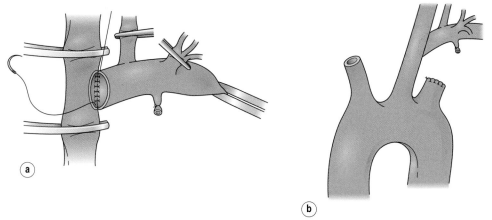

Figure 11.3 • Carotid–subclavian transposition: **(a)** clamps on the common carotid artery are rotated anteriorly to present the posterolateral surface for anastomosis with the subclavian artery; **(b)** end-to-side anastomosis completed.

Table 11.3 • Carotid transposition: postoperative complications and late patency

Authors, year	No. patients	Mean follow-up (mth) [range]	Complications (%)	Primary patency (%) at mean follow-up
Cinà et al., 2002[18]	27	25 ± 21	Morbidity: 11.1	100
Schardey et al., 1996[15]	108	70 [1–144]	Stroke: 1.8 Morbidity: 15	100*

*84 patients followed.

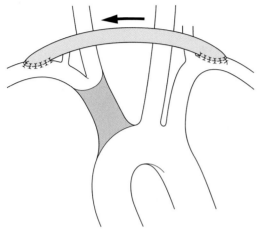

Figure 11.4 • Brachiocephalic artery occlusion. Revascularisation by a cross-subclavian PTFE graft. Tunnelisation is done behind the sternomastoid muscles and anterior to the carotid vessels.

dilated by balloon. Occlusions are more difficult to cross and less frequent in most endovascular series;[22–24] they often require catheterisation from the brachial artery with the use of balloon or self-expandable stents.

☑☑ PTA with or without stenting is an appropriate treatment for symptomatic patients with localised subclavian artery stenosis with a 2-year primary patency of 90% in most series[22–24] (Table 11.4), but a long-term patency inferior to that obtained with carotid–subclavian bypass or transposition.[25]

Upper arm arteries

Patients with chronic atherosclerotic occlusion of the axillary or brachial arteries usually present with fatigue on using the arm. Some of these patients have radiation-induced occlusive disease. Severe ischaemia with rest pain or digital necrosis is uncommon unless there have been repeated episodes of embolism due to proximal ulceration or aneurysmal degeneration. Direct reconstructive surgery is feasible since the occlusive lesions tend to be segmental with preserved distal patency.

Axillobrachial occlusions can be managed by a bypass procedure if symptoms justify it. These sites can usually be approached by limited incisions and the bypass tunnelled subcutaneously between the two incisions (**Fig. 11.6**). In these cases, autogenous saphenous vein is the preferred graft material. When unavailable, basilic or cephalic vein may be considered. Upper limb bypass using saphenous vein has a 5-year patency rate of 60–90%.[26] PTFE has a lower patency rate at this level.

Lower arm and hand arteries

The causes of chronic occlusion in the forearm or hand vessels include atherosclerosis, Buerger's disease, immunological and connective tissue disorders (see Chapter 12) and occupational trauma. Arch-CTA scan to exclude proximal embolic disease, and selective arteriography are essential in evaluating these patients with distal disease. Most of these patients can be managed conservatively. Avoidance of cold and abstinence of tobacco are essential. Vasodilator or sympatholytic agents may also be employed. Patients with digital necrosis may require local debridement or amputation if gangrene is extensive. Some patients with radial, ulnar or palmar arch occlusion and critical ischaemia may be managed, if run-off is present, by vein graft bypass using microsurgical techniques. Cervico-dorsal sympathectomy by thoracoscopy may also be considered in patients with severe distal forearm ischaemia. However, results of sympathectomy have often been disappointing, particularly in patients with diffuse arteritis.

Aneurysmal disease

True aneurysms of the upper limb arteries are uncommon. The subclavian artery is the most frequent site, usually caused by thoracic outlet compression. These patients may present with distal ischaemia, embolisation or acute thrombosis. False aneurysms from trauma or infection often produce motor or sensory impairment because of brachial plexus compression. As described later, subclavian artery aneurysms are best managed by a combined

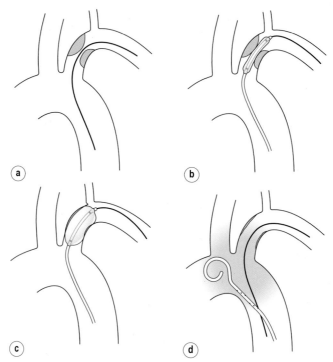

Figure 11.5 • Retrograde approach from the brachial artery by percutaneous puncture, or cut-down if stenting is necessary: **(a)** the guidewire is placed through the subclavian stenosis; **(b)** balloon is advanced over the guidewire and balloon angioplasty performed; **(c)** arteriography completed by withdrawing the balloon with the same catheter; **(d)** more accurate arteriographic control can be achieved by using a second transfemoral pigtail catheter positioned in the aortic arch. From Schneider PA. Endovascular skills; 2003. Reproduced by permission of Informa Healthcare.

Table 11.4 • Angioplasty of the subclavian artery: postoperative complications and late patency

Authors, year	No. patients	Mean follow-up (mth) [range]	Complications (%)	Primary patency (%)
De Vries et al., 2005[22]	110	34 [3–120]	Stroke + death: 4.5 Local: 3.6	2 years:* 89 3 years:† 89
Berger et al., 2011[23]	72	82 [3–299]	Death: 19.6 Local: 4.9 Transient monoplegia: 1.5	10 years: 85.2
Soga et al, 2015[24]	553	39 [1–129]	Death: 0.7 Stroke : 1.8	1 year: 90.6 2 years: 83.4 5 years: 80.5
Özdemir-van Brunschot, 2016[25]	47	n/a	n/a	1 year: 72 5 years: 54

*64 patients followed at 2 years. †36 patients followed at 3 years.
n/a, not available.

supraclavicular and infraclavicular approach. Aneurysms of the brachiocephalic artery are rare. In the series of Kieffer et al.[27] the perioperative death rate was 11%, most deaths occurring in patients operated in an emergency setting.

An aberrant right subclavian artery arising from the descending thoracic aorta is a common anomaly. Rarely, the artery compresses the oesophagus against the trachea, producing a condition described as dysphagia lusoria. Aneurysmal degeneration, known as Kommerell's diverticulum, may also occur. The largest experience has been reported by Kieffer et al.[28] Because of the possibility of rupture, resection of the aneurysmal artery with aortic

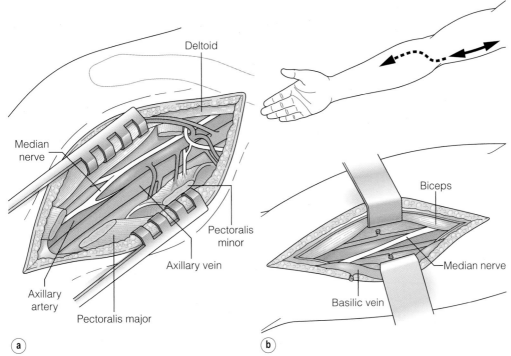

Figure 11.6 • **(a)** Axillary artery approach. The pectoralis minor muscle is divided and the neurovascular bundle is exposed. If access to the axillobrachial junction is needed, the pectoralis major tendon should also be resected. **(b)** Brachial artery approach. Incision along the medial border of the biceps. If necessary, the bicipital aponeurosis is divided to expose the brachial artery division.

prosthetic reconstruction via a thoracic approach is recommended. As this technique carries a relatively high postoperative mortality, hybrid procedures with aortic stent grafts are more commonly used with success.[29,30]

Upper arm artery aneurysms

Axillary artery aneurysms are usually caused by blunt or penetrating trauma. Degenerative or congenital aneurysms are rare in this location. False aneurysms of the axillary artery occur with humeral fractures and anterior dislocation of the shoulder. These aneurysms can lead to neurological complications because of compression of the brachial plexus. Duplex scan and arteriography allow an accurate diagnosis. The axillary artery is exposed by a delto-pectoral incision with division of the pectoralis minor. The aneurysm is resected followed by interposition of a reversed saphenous vein graft. Stent grafts have been used for emergency control of upper limb aneurysms but their long-term integrity is often compromised by compression between the first rib and clavicle or by excessive arterial flexion.[31]

Lower arm and hand artery aneurysms

Radial artery aneurysms are usually due to inadequate compression or infection following removal of an intra-arterial blood pressure cannula. If the Allen test shows good filling of the hand from the ulnar artery, then the radial artery can simply be ligated above and below the aneurysm. If not, reconstruction using a vein graft is required.

Ulnar artery aneurysm or hypothenar hammer syndrome

It is important to recognise an ulnar artery aneurysm because it may lead to digital necrosis. The condition known as hypothenar hammer syndrome develops in workers who suffer repetitive trauma to their hands, including carpenters and pipe fitters. Those who play sports such as volleyball or karate are also at risk. The pathophysiology is related to the vascular anatomy of the hand. The distal ulnar artery is vulnerable to external trauma between the distal margin of Guyon's canal and the palmar aponeurosis. Over this short distance, the artery lies anterior to the hook of the hamate bone and is covered only by the palmaris brevis muscle and the skin. Trauma of the ulnar artery at this level causes thrombosis or aneurysm formation and distal embolisation in the fourth and fifth fingers, with pain, coldness and cyanosis. The thumb is always spared because of its radial blood supply. Angiography with magnification is essential in these patients.

When the ulnar artery is chronically thrombosed, calcium channel blockers may be helpful. In all cases, patients should avoid further hand trauma.

> ✓✓ Surgical therapy includes microsurgical arterial reconstruction with or without adjunctive preoperative thrombolytic therapy to restore patency to digital arteries. Resection of the aneurysm with the placement of an interposition vein graft is the treatment of choice. Satisfactory long-term results have been reported by Vayssairat et al. using this approach.[32]

Upper limb embolism

Embolic arterial occlusion is the major cause of acute upper limb ischaemia; upper limb emboli represent 20–32% of major peripheral emboli.[33] A cardiac origin is found in 90% of cases and is related to arrhythmia, myocardial infarction, valvular disorder or ventricular aneurysm. Non-cardiac sources include ulcerative atherosclerotic plaques or aneurysms in the arch or subclavian–axillary arteries and thoracic outlet compression. The brachial bifurcation is the most frequently involved site for an embolus to lodge. Clinical examination and duplex scan can locate the level of the arterial occlusion. Preoperative conventional angiography or CTA is indicated in order to exclude a proximal arterial embolic lesion if a cardiac source is not evident or if the subclavian pulse is either absent (due to dissection or occlusion) or unduly prominent (due to a subclavian aneurysm or underlying cervical rib). Immediate systemic heparinisation is essential to limit the propagation of thrombus and to prevent recurrent embolism.

Most emboli can be retrieved through a distal brachial transverse arteriotomy. This site has the advantage that both forearm arteries can be directly cannulated. An S-shaped incision is made under local anaesthesia in the antecubital fossa and the brachial artery division exposed by dividing the bicipital aponeurosis. A transverse arteriotomy is made proximal to the bifurcation. It is important to clear both forearm vessels with a 2-Fr Fogarty catheter (**Fig. 11.7**). Heparin saline is then instilled distally, and after confirming proximal patency the arteriotomy is closed with 6/0 Prolene interrupted sutures. Completion on-table angiography should be

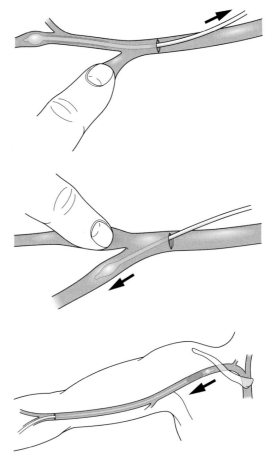

Figure 11.7 • Brachial artery embolectomy. A transverse arteriotomy is performed. A Fogarty catheter is directed into the radial and ulnar arteries in turn, using alternate digital compression and/or Silastic slings. A subclavian–axillary embolectomy is carried out by retrograde catheterisation from the antecubital fossa.

performed. If there is retained distal thrombus, the ulnar and radial artery can be opened at the wrist and a 2-Fr Fogarty catheter passed distally. Alternatively, intraoperative thrombolysis can be used (see Chapter 8). Emboli in the axillary or subclavian arteries may also be removed by the same approach, using transbrachial retrograde catheterisation. However, sometimes a large proximal embolus cannot be removed via the brachial arteriotomy, in which case an axillary or subclavian embolectomy will be required. Percutaneous thromboaspiration with or without local thrombolysis via a femoral approach has also been used in this situation.

Other causes of acute ischaemia

The pharmacological causes of upper extremity ischaemia are summarised in Box 11.2. Inadvertent

Box 11.2 • Upper extremity ischaemia due to pharmacological agents

Ergot poisoning
Beta-blockers
Drug abuse, cocaine use
Dopamine overdose
Cytotoxic drugs

arterial injection by drug abusers often results in intense vasospasm due to particulate microembolism. Intra-arterial infusion of prostacyclin analogues such as iloprost or other vasodilators may help. Forearm compartment syndrome is rare except in this situation and requires fasciotomy. Limb loss is common.

Thoracic outlet syndrome

Thoracic outlet syndrome describes a variety of symptoms caused by compression of the brachial plexus or subclavian vessels at the thoracic outlet. In more than 90% of all cases of thoracic outlet syndrome,[34] symptoms are neurological with pain and weakness resulting from C8 or T1 root compression. Arterial or venous symptoms resulting from compression are uncommon, accounting for 5% of cases in large published series.[35] Standards have been reported by the Society of Vascular Surgery.[36]

Neurogenic thoracic outlet compression syndrome (N-TOCS)

The neurovascular bundle may be compressed between the first rib and the clavicle because of a low-lying shoulder girdle or loss of muscle tone. Other anatomical factors include congenital fibromuscular bands crossing the thoracic outlet that tent up the brachial plexus, and abnormalities/hypertrophy of the scalene muscles. Bony lesions may also be the cause. These include cervical ribs, a broad first rib, and fracture or exostoses of the first rib or clavicle. The scalene triangle is the commonest site of nerve compression. It contains the brachial plexus and the subclavian artery. N-TOCS probably represents a repetitive stress injury as there are well-defined at-risk occupations (e.g. typists) and sports (e.g. swimming). Most patients with N-TOCS are in the 25- to 45-year age group and 70% of them are women. The symptoms are arm pain, paraesthesia and weakness, with involvement of all the nerves of the brachial plexus or with specific patterns related to the upper plexus (median nerve) or lower plexus (ulnar nerve).

Diagnosis

Positive findings on clinical examination include supraclavicular tenderness and paraesthesia in the ipsilateral upper extremity in response to pressure over the scalene muscles. Rotating the head and tilting the head away from the involved side often produces radiating pain in the upper arm. Abducting the arm to 90° in external rotation and repeated slow finger clenching in this position often reproduces the symptoms (Roos' test). Diagnostic tests include a scalene muscle block, and a good response to this test correlates well with successful surgical decompression.[37] Neurophysiology testing is helpful in excluding other sites of nerve compression, e.g. cervical root and carpal tunnel. Duplex scanning is a useful surrogate marker if it shows arterial compression in stress position. Cervical spine films may detect cervical or abnormal first ribs but will not detect non-bony causes of compression. Magnetic resonance imaging is more useful for excluding cervical disc lesions than confirming N-TOCS.

Treatment

Therapy for N-TOCS should always begin with non-operative treatment, including postural exercises and physiotherapy. Patients should avoid heavy lifting and working with the arm above shoulder level. Conservative treatment should be continued for several months. Many patients will improve significantly and will not require surgery. Indications for surgery include failure of conservative therapy after several months and persisting disabling symptoms that interfere with work and activities of daily living. The goal of surgery is to decompress the brachial plexus. A cervical rib can usually be removed via a supraclavicular approach.

Transaxillary resection of first rib

The technique described by Roos[38] is indicated for neurogenic complications of N-TOCS and can be summarised as follows. The patient is placed in the lateral position leaving the arm free. The assistant elevates the shoulder by applying upward traction on the upper arm. This manoeuvre opens the costoclavicular space and pulls the neurovascular bundle away from the first rib. A horizontal skin incision is made at the lower border of the axillary line over the third rib (**Fig. 11.8**). The intercostal nerve emerging from the second intercostal space should be preserved. The fascial roof of the axilla is opened to expose the anterior portion of the first rib. Scalenus anterior is separated from the artery and sectioned at its attachment to the first rib (**Fig. 11.9**). The tendon of the subclavius muscle is divided with care because of its close relation with the subclavian vein. The scalenus medius is then pushed off the rib. The intercostal muscles are similarly detached from the lower part of the rib. The rib is then sectioned at the chondrocostal junction and maintained by bone-holding forceps

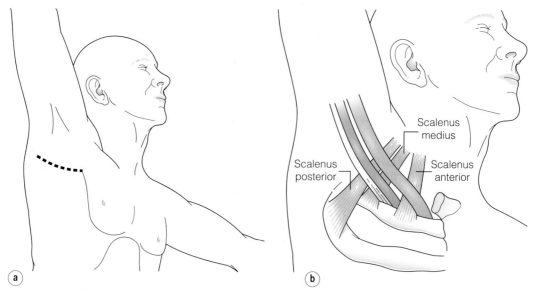

Figure 11.8 • Transaxillary resection of the first rib: **(a)** operative position and skin incision; **(b)** the neurovascular bundle is pulled away from the first rib by traction on the arm.

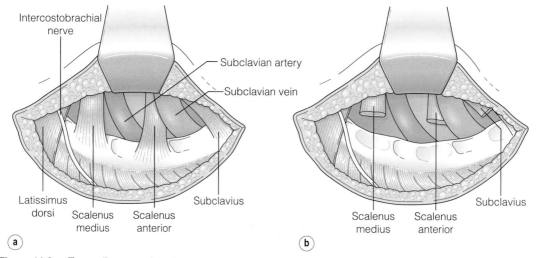

Figure 11.9 • Transaxillary resection of the first rib: **(a)** exposure of the first rib, scalene muscles and subclavian–axillary vessels; **(b)** detachment of the scalenus anterior, medius and subclavius muscles from the first rib.

to distance it from the neurovascular bundle (**Fig. 11.10**). The T1 root is displaced medially. The rib is then divided and excised to within 1–2 cm of the vertebral transverse process using rongeurs. The stump must be smooth since sharp bony spicules may lacerate the plexus. Serum saline is then injected in the wound to ensure that the pleura is intact. The wound is closed in the usual way with suction drainage.

Complications of transaxillary rib resection include subclavian vein or artery injury, extrapleural haematoma or brachial plexus injury caused by traction of the arm or damage to the T1 root

retraction. Good illumination and visualisation are crucial to this approach and can help with both.

Other operative techniques for N-TOCS include a supraclavicular approach. Axelrod et al.[39] reported the results of surgery in 170 patients operated for N-TOCS. No major operative complication occurred in those patients who underwent decompression via a supraclavicular approach. Only 11% of patients experienced minor complications, most commonly the need for chest tube placement because of pneumothorax. At short-term follow-up (10 months), most patients had improved pain levels (80%) and range of motion (82%). However,

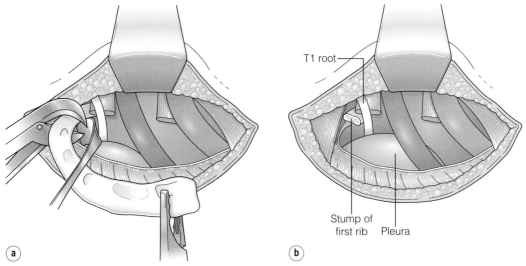

Figure 11.10 • Transaxillary resection of the first rib. **(a)** Exposure of the first rib. The rib has been disarticulated at the chondrocostal junction. T1 root is protected by a retractor. **(b)** Extraperiosteal resection of the first rib is complete.

at long-term follow-up (47 months), residual symptoms were present in 65% of patients, and 35% took medication for pain. Nonetheless, 64% said they were satisfied with the result. Scali et al.[40] performed a long-term follow-up after first rib resection (average 8.7 years). An equivalent or better functional outcome was observed in 72.7% of the patients. Cordobes-Gual et al.[41] showed the importance of a precise questionnaire (DASH) to evaluate the functional recovery after N-TOCS surgery.

> ✔ Controversy still exists concerning the surgical treatment of N-TOCS, and a randomised study of thoracic outlet surgery versus conservative treatment is lacking for this indication.

Arterial thoracic outlet compression syndrome

Arterial complications are often associated with bony abnormalities, including a complete cervical rib or fracture callus of the first rib or clavicle. The initial arterial lesion is fibrotic thickening with intimal damage and post-stenotic dilatation, leading to aneurysmal degeneration with mural thrombus and the risk of embolisation. Most emboli are small and located in the hand vessels, with pallor, paraesthesia and coldness suggestive of Raynaud's syndrome. If unrecognised, severe digital ischaemia with gangrene may occur. Early recognition of this condition is essential and a duplex scan should be performed in all patients with unilateral Raynaud's syndrome and asymptomatic patients with a cervical bruit.

Loss or reduction of the radial pulse during Adson's manoeuvre (abduction and external rotation of the shoulder) is not very reliable as it is found in 9–53% of healthy volunteers.[34] The arteriographic changes may be obvious but sometimes minimal, with moderate dilatation beyond a bony abnormality at the thoracic outlet and radiological evidence of distal embolisation (**Fig. 11.11**). Subclavian stenosis is not always evident on anteroposterior view and oblique stress views are often necessary.

Surgical management

Subclavian lesions associated with cervical ribs can usually be repaired via a supraclavicular approach, after excision of the cervical rib or better by a combined supraclavicular and infraclavicular approach.

Combined supraclavicular and infraclavicular approach

The combined supraclavicular and infraclavicular approach offers a complete exposure. The infraclavicular dissection is commenced first with an S-shaped incision. Pectoralis major is detached from the upper sternum and clavicle (**Fig. 11.12**). The subclavius is resected and the artery and the axillary vein are then freed behind the clavicle. Via a supraclavicular incision, the clavicular head of the sternomastoid and the external jugular vein are divided to expose the scalenus anterior and the phrenic nerve. The scalenus anterior is then sectioned near the first rib. The subclavian artery and vein are freed (**Fig. 11.13**). The intercostal muscles are detached from the first rib and the rib is disarticulated at the costochondral junction. The rib is then sectioned without attempting to reach

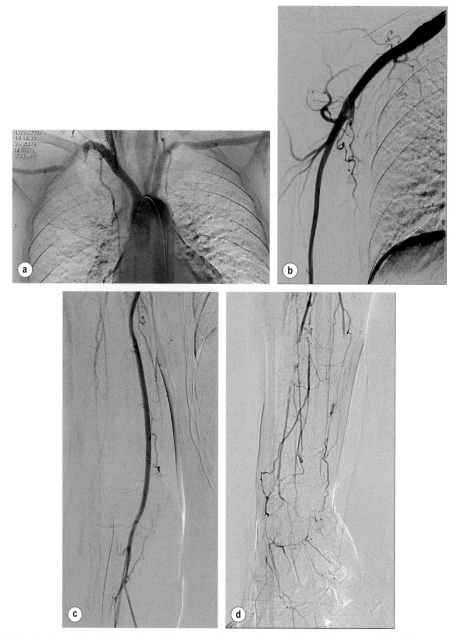

Figure 11.11 • Angiography of a thoracic outlet compression syndrome with arterial compression. **(a)** Right subclavian artery compression when the arm is abducted to 90° in external rotation. **(b)** Poststenotic dilatation of the right subclavian artery. **(c)** Right brachial artery. **(d)** Distal arterial embolisation.

the posterior segment. Access to the rib stump is achieved via the supraclavicular exposure by reflecting the brachial plexus laterally and the artery medially. The scalenus medius is then detached from the first rib and, after protecting the T1 root, the rib is sectioned near the transverse process.

In patients with aneurysm or poststenotic dilatation secondary to first rib or cervical rib, there is often sufficient length of artery to permit resection of the

arterial lesion and direct anastomosis (**Fig. 11.14**). When arterial lesions are more extensive, graft replacement is required using reversed great saphenous vein or PTFE if no vein is available. Intraoperative angiography is recommended in all cases. In patients with a recent distal embolic event, catheter embolectomy should be attempted. If embolectomy is impossible, a distal bypass using the great saphenous vein may be needed to

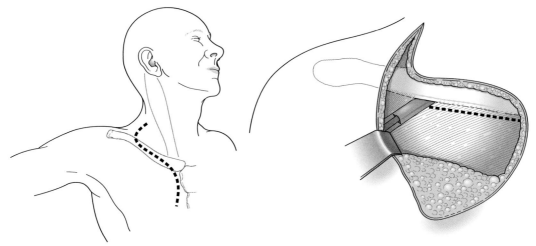

Figure 11.12 • Combined supraclavicular and infraclavicular approach for first rib resection when extensive arterial or venous reconstruction is required. Skin incision and section of the pectoralis major from the clavicle.

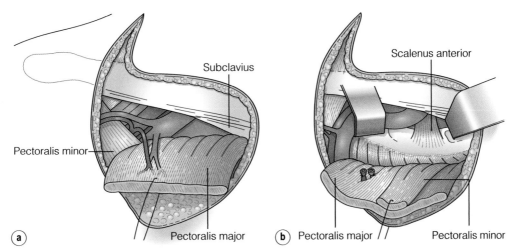

Figure 11.13 • Combined supraclavicular and infraclavicular approach. **(a)** Exposure of the proximal axillary vessels. The axillary vessels are held aside with a retractor to show the first rib and insertion of the scalenus anterior. **(b)** The infraclavicular dissection with detachment of the intercostal muscles from the first rib. The anterior portion of the rib will be removed and the first rib stump will be shortened via the supraclavicular exposure, not shown here.

revascularise one of the forearm arteries. Additional sympathectomy may also be considered where there is an extensive long-standing distal embolic occlusion. Difficulty in clearing the distal arterial bed accounts for the incomplete revascularisation observed in advanced cases with disabling ischaemic sequelae.

✓✓ Arterial reconstruction and first rib or cervical rib resection are indicated in all patients with arterial complications of thoracic outlet syndrome.

Subclavian–axillary vein thrombosis

Spontaneous or effort-related venous thrombosis in a fit young patient is known as Paget–Schroetter syndrome, the first cases being published separately by these two authors over a century ago. Hughes, who in 1949 collected 320 cases and recognised the distinct entity, coined the eponym. As the indications for central venous access have increased, so has the incidence of catheter-related subclavian–axillary vein thrombosis (SVT).[42]

Acute deep venous thrombosis (DVT) of the upper limb has many causes, with treatment and

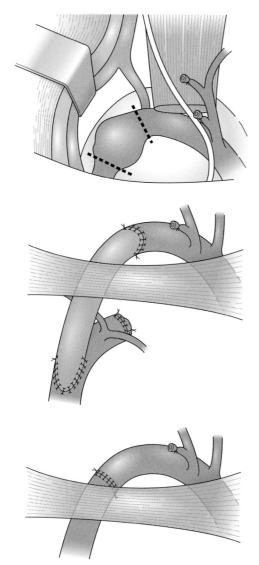

Figure 11.14 • Combined supraclavicular and infraclavicular approach. Exposure of the subclavian and axillary vessels. Depending on the extent of arterial resection, end-to-end anastomosis or graft replacement is done.

prognosis depending on the specific cause. SVT can be divided into two groups, primary and secondary. Primary SVT (Paget–Schroetter syndrome) is due to anatomical venous compression in the thoracic outlet during exercise (V-TOCS) and comprises about 25% of all cases. Secondary SVT is the result of multiple aetiological factors, although in most series trauma due to central venous catheters dominates this category (40% of all cases of SVT). SVT is responsible for 1–4% of all cases of DVT. Monreal et al.[43] reported a 15% incidence of pulmonary emboli in 30 consecutive patients with SVT who were investigated with ventilation–perfusion scanning.

Primary SVT

In a review of the literature, Hurlbert and Rutherford[44] reported a male-to-female ratio of 2:1, with an average age of 30 years for patients with primary SVT that represents only 3.5% of all cases of thoracic outlet compression syndrome (TOCS). Venous thrombosis is seen three times more frequently in the right than the left upper limb, but bilateral venous compression also occurs frequently. Thrombosis is probably caused by repetitive trauma from compression. Virtually every patient with primary SVT has some degree of upper extremity swelling associated with pain that worsens with exertion. Some patients may have cyanosis of the arm. Unlike lower-extremity DVT, symptoms in the upper extremity are more related to venous obstruction than reflux. Venous outflow through the collateral vessels is limited, resulting in venous hypertension, swelling and occasionally venous claudication. Venous gangrene is an extremely rare complication of SVT.

Diagnosis

Clinically, the arm may be swollen and cyanosed, with dilated shoulder girdle collateral veins. Duplex is the first-line investigation and has a sensitivity of 94% and a specificity of 96% compared with venography.[45] MRA has poor sensitivity for non-occlusive thrombi and short-segment occlusion. CTA has been used to diagnose upper-extremity DVT but its specificity and sensitivity are undetermined. Venography is still considered as the reference in evaluating SVT (**Fig. 11.15**). The basilic vein is the preferred site for injection, with the arm abducted at 30°. The catheter used for the venogram should be left in position as it can be used for subsequent thrombolysis and/or heparin infusion. The cephalic vein is not used because it joins directly with the subclavian vein and may miss an axillary vein thrombosis.

Treatment

For many years, treatment of SVT relied on rest and elevation of the upper limb with anticoagulant therapy. However, the morbidity associated with this conservative treatment is high. More recently, investigators have realised that many patients with SVT have compression at the thoracic outlet. Initially, in patients with primary SVT, subclavian vein patency was restored by open thrombectomy associated with first rib resection.[46] Although now supplanted by thrombolysis, open thrombectomy has proved effective and should be considered in patients with contraindications or failure of thrombolysis therapy. Catheter-directed techniques of thrombolysis allow for immediate venous evaluation and assess extrinsic compression with positional

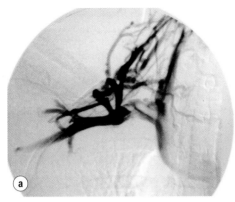
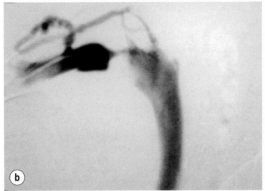

Figure 11.15 • (a) Venogram via basilic vein demonstrating subclavian–axillary vein thrombosis with collaterals. **(b)** Thrombolysis revealed an underlying stenosis of the subclavian vein. This was treated by excision of the first rib and vein patch.

venography after thrombolysis.[47] However, Sheeran et al.[48] have shown that recanalisation of the vein by thrombolysis without decompression of the thoracic outlet has poor outcomes, with 55% of patients remaining symptomatic. Conversely, Machleder[49] reported the success of combined treatment, with 86% of 36 patients becoming asymptomatic. The appropriate time interval between thrombolysis and thoracic outlet decompression is still debated. Machleder waited 3 months, whereas Lee et al.[50] recommended immediate first rib resection within 4 days after thrombolysis. Waiting too long risks repeat thrombosis, whereas operating immediately risks bleeding due to the thrombolytic agent.

> ✓✓ Patients with thoracic outlet syndrome and SVT should have early treatment with thrombolysis followed by first rib resection.[51]

Specific problems may arise in some patients after thrombolysis. In a small group, no residual lesion or compression is seen on positional venography after thrombolysis. In these cases, anticoagulation therapy is recommended without thoracic outlet decompression. In other patients, intrinsic stenosis is seen on venography after thrombolysis (**Fig. 11.15**). In these cases, operative vein bypass or patch angioplasty with first rib resection is needed and should be performed in the days after thrombolysis because the risk of repeat thrombosis appears to be quite high. In this setting, percutaneous balloon angioplasty with or without stenting has been suggested. The results of this technique without thoracic outlet decompression are poor, with a primary patency of 35% at 1 year.[52] Obviously, this technique does not obviate the need for surgery because thoracic outlet decompression is still needed. Even after thoracic outlet decompression, some venous stenoses are resistant to dilatation

or present intrinsic elastic recoil. Various types of stents have been used to treat residual stenoses, but are associated with a worse prognosis than balloon angioplasty alone after vein decompression.[53]

> ✓✓ Stenting in primary SVT is not appropriate. As surgery is usually needed for thoracic outlet decompression, it seems logical to repair the subclavian vein with patch angioplasty or a short autogenous bypass at the same time.

In a significant number of patients, seen more than 10 days after the onset of primary upper-limb DVT, late thrombolysis fails. Most of these patients should be treated conservatively with anticoagulation unless the occlusion is short. In these cases, open thrombectomy with vein reconstruction and first rib resection can be done with acceptable results.[54] The technique involves internal jugular vein transposition or cephalic vein bypass with a temporary arteriovenous fistula. Prosthetic bypass has shown inferior results in this location.

Secondary SVT

The main cause of secondary SVT is central venous catheterisation (CVC). Overall, one-third of patients with central-line catheters develop SVT, although only 15% of them are symptomatic. The aetiology of catheter-associated thrombosis is multifactorial, but may be related to the fibrin sheath that forms around the catheter. The method of insertion, size, composition and duration of use of the catheter are also important. A reduced rate of thrombosis has been found with soft and more flexible catheters. Large catheters used for haemodialysis have a higher incidence of SVT. Another risk factor is the type of fluid infused through the catheter.

Cancer chemotherapeutic agents are aggressive to vascular endothelium and may increase the risk of thrombosis. Furthermore, many patients with central-line catheters also have systemic risk factors for thrombosis, i.e. malignancy, sepsis, congestive heart failure and prolonged bed rest.

Symptomatic patients have oedema and distended veins around the shoulder. Pulmonary embolism is not uncommon, with 16% of patients positive on ventilation–perfusion scan.[55] Therapy guidelines are based on observational reports as no controlled studies are available. In all cases, anticoagulation using intravenous heparin via the affected arm is indicated to prevent clot extension until the catheter is removed. Thrombolytic therapy has a role in reopening thrombosed catheters. Prevention of thrombus formation has been emphasised, and for high-risk patients it may be advantageous to administer low-dose coumadin[56] or low-molecular-weight heparin to reduce the risk of catheter-associated thrombosis. A further discussion about CVC management can be found in Chapter 16.

Key points

- Vascular diseases of the upper limb are rare in comparison to those involving the lower limbs, except for arterial embolism.
- Clinical examination, including the Allen test, is important.
- There are good midterm results of endovascular treatment of supra-aortic trunk stenoses.
- The long-term results of carotid bypass or carotid transposition are excellent.
- It is important to consider arterial disease in the work environment, e.g. hypothenar hammer syndrome.
- There is controversy concerning the diagnosis and treatment of N-TOCS.
- The combined supraclavicular and infraclavicular approach for first rib resection and arterial bypass is of value in the treatment of patients with arterial thoracic outlet compression syndrome.
- Early thrombolytic therapy followed by surgical thoracic outlet decompression is indicated in patients with primary SVT.

🌐 Full references available at **http://expertconsult. inkling.com**

Key references

2. McCarthy WJ, Flinn WR, Yao JST, et al. Result of bypass grafting for upper limb ischemia. J Vasc Surg 1986;3(5):741–6. PMID: 2939264.
   Between 1978 and 1984, the authors performed 33 bypass grafts to relieve hand and forearm ischaemia in 27 patients. A reversed saphenous vein graft was used in 22 cases and PTFE in the remaining 11 procedures. Follow-up of 31 grafts from 6 to 72 months (mean 35.5 months) revealed an overall patency rate of 73% at 2 years and 67% at 3 years. More proximal grafts fared better: the 2-year patency rate was 83% for grafts at or above the brachial artery but only 53% for bypass distal to the brachial bifurcation.

3. Kieffer E, Sabatier J, Koskas F, et al. Atherosclerotic innominate artery occlusive disease: early and long-term results of surgical reconstruction. J Vasc Surg 1995;21(2):326–37. PMID: 7853604.
   During a 20-year period (1974–93), the authors operated on 148 patients with brachiocephalic (innominate) artery atherosclerotic occlusive disease. Approach was through a median sternotomy in 135 (91%) patients. Endarterectomy was performed in 32 (22%) patients, whereas 116 (78%) patients underwent bypass. Eight (5.4%) patients died in the perioperative period. There were five (3.4%) perioperative strokes. Mean follow-up was 77 months. Survival was 51.9% at 10 years. The probability of freedom from ipsilateral stroke was 98.6% at 10 years. The primary patency rate was 98.4% at 10 years. In conclusion, surgical reconstruction of brachiocephalic artery atherosclerotic occlusive disease yields acceptable rates of perioperative complications with excellent long-term patency and freedom from neurological events and reoperation.

16. Vitti MJ, Thompson BW, Read RC, et al. Carotid-subclavian bypass: a twenty-two-year experience. J Vasc Surg 1994;20(3):411–8. PMID: 8084034.
    A retrospective review of 124 patients who underwent carotid–subclavian bypass from 1968 to 1990 was done to assess primary patency and symptom resolution. Graft conduits were PTFE in 44 (35%) and Dacron in 80 (65%) cases; 30-day mortality was 0.8%, 30-day primary patency was 100%. Primary patency rate was 95% at 10 years. Survival rate was 59% at 10 years. Symptom-free survival rate was 87% at 10 years. Carotid–subclavian bypass appears to be a safe and durable procedure for relief of symptomatic occlusive disease of the subclavian artery.

28. Kieffer E, Bahnini A, Koskas F. Aberrant subclavian artery: surgical treatment in thirty-three adult patients. J Vasc Surg 1994;19(1):100–11. PMID: 8301723.

The authors reviewed their experience with surgery for aberrant subclavian arteries (ASA). During a 16-year period they surgically treated 33 adult patients with ASA. Twenty-eight patients had a left-sided aortic arch with a right ASA, whereas five had a right-sided aortic arch with a left ASA. Eleven patients had dysphagia caused by oesophageal compression, five patients had ischaemic symptoms, 10 patients had aneurysms of the ASA and seven patients had an ASA arising from an aneurysmal thoracic aorta. In all cases the distal subclavian artery was revascularised, most often by direct transposition into the ipsilateral common carotid artery. The cervical approach was combined with a median sternotomy or a left thoracotomy in 17 patients. Aortic cross-clamping was required in 12 patients to perform the transaortic closure of the origin of the ASA with patch angioplasty or prosthetic replacement of the descending thoracic aorta. Cardiopulmonary bypass was used in six patients. Four patients died after operation. Satisfactory clinical and anatomical results were obtained in the remaining 29 patients. Provision should be made for cardiopulmonary bypass in patients with aneurysm of ASA or associated aortic aneurysm.

31. Sullivan TM, Bacharach JM, Perl J, et al. Endovascular management of unusual aneurysms of the axillary and subclavian arteries. J Endovasc Surg 1996;3(4):389–95. PMID: 8959496.

Aneurysms of the upper extremity arteries are uncommon and may be difficult to manage in emergency with standard surgical techniques. The authors report the exclusion of three axillary–subclavian aneurysms with covered stents. Palmaz stents were covered with either PTFE (two cases) or brachial vein and deployed to exclude pseudoaneurysms in one axillary and two left subclavian arteries. Endovascular exclusion of axillary and subclavian aneurysms with covered stents may offer a useful alternative to operative repair in patients with ruptured aneurysm or significant comorbidities.

32. Vayssairat M, Debure C, Cormier J-M, et al. Hypothenar hammer syndrome: seventeen cases with long-term follow-up. J Vasc Surg 1987;5(6):838–42. PMID: 3586181.

The authors report 17 patients who had either ulnar thrombosis or ulnar aneurysm; most also had embolic occlusions of the digital arteries. Main pathological findings were thrombosis on the intima and fibrosis in the media. The authors adopted a surgical procedure consisting of resection with end-to-end reconstruction for patent aneurysms to avoid downstream emboli and more conservative treatment when the ulnar artery was thrombosed. No patient required digital amputation and all except one improved and were able to live and work normally.

39. Axelrod DA, Proctor MC, Geisser ME, et al. Outcomes after surgery for thoracic outlet syndrome. J Vasc Surg 2001;33(6):1220–5. PMID: 11389421.

This study determined whether there is an association between psychological and socio-economic characteristics and long-term outcome of operative treatment for patients with sensory N-TOCS. Multivariate logistic regression models were developed as a means of identifying independent risk factors for postoperative disability. Operative decompression of the brachial plexus via a supraclavicular approach was performed for upper-extremity pain and paraesthesia, with no mortality and minimal morbidity in 170 patients. After an average follow-up period of 47 months, 65% of patients reported improved symptoms and 64% of patients were satisfied with their operative outcome. However, 35% of patients remained on medication and 18% of patients were disabled. Preoperative factors associated with persistent disability include major depression, being unmarried and having less than a high-school education. Operative decompression was beneficial for most patients. The impact of the preoperative treatment of depression on the outcome of TOCS decompression should be studied prospectively.

42. Rutherford R. Primary subclavian–axillary vein thrombosis: consensus and commentary. Cardiovasc Surg 1996;4(4):420–3. PMID: 8866074.

Fifteen multiple-choice questions concerning options in the management of primary subclavian–axillary vein thrombosis (SVT) were discussed by a panel of experts and then voted upon by 25 attending vascular surgeons with experience in SVT. The large majority favoured or agreed upon: (i) early clot removal for active healthy patients with a need/desire to use the involved limb in work or sport; (ii) catheter-directed thrombolysis as initial therapy; (iii) further therapy based on follow-up positional venography; (iv) surgical relief of demonstrated thoracic outlet compression after a brief period of anticoagulant therapy; (v) conservative therapy if post-lysis venogram showed either no extrinsic compression or a short residual occlusion; and (vi) intervention for residual intrinsic lesions with over 50% narrowing.

43. Monreal M, Lafoz E, Ruiz J, et al. Upper-extremity deep venous thrombosis and pulmonary embolism. Chest 1991;99(2):280–3. PMID: 1989783.

The authors prospectively evaluated the prevalence of pulmonary embolism in 30 consecutive patients with proved DVT of the upper extremity. Ten patients had primary DVT and 20 patients had catheter-related DVT. Ventilation–perfusion lung scans were routinely performed at the time of hospital admission in all but one patient. Lung scan findings were normal in 9 of 10 patients with primary DVT. In contrast, perfusion defects were considered highly suggestive of pulmonary embolism in four patients with catheter-related DVT. The authors conclude that pulmonary embolism is not a rare complication in upper-extremity DVT and that patients with catheter-related DVT seem to be at higher risk.

49. Machleder HI. Evaluation of a new treatment strategy for Paget–Schroetter syndrome: spontaneous thrombosis of the axillary–subclavian vein. J Vasc Surg 1993;17(2):305–17. PMID: 8433426.

The authors conducted a study to determine an acceptable treatment approach to primary subclavian vein thrombosis. A retrospective review evaluated 11 patients in an 8-year period. All patients with occlusion received urokinase therapy and underwent surgical decompression within 5 days of thrombolytic therapy. Five percutaneous transluminal angioplasties were attempted before operative intervention. Eleven decompressions were performed. All patients received coumadin for 3–6 months after the operation. Urokinase therapy established wide venous patency in 9 of 11 extremities treated, with the remaining two requiring thrombectomy. One patient who underwent transluminal angioplasty before the operation had rethrombosis, and the remaining four showed no improvement in venous stenosis after the intervention. Eight of nine extremities treated by first rib resection and one of two treated by scalenectomy were free of residual symptoms at follow-up. The authors conclude that preoperative use of percutaneous balloon angioplasty is ineffective and should be avoided in this setting. Surgical intervention within days of thrombolysis enables patients to return to normal activity sooner.

51. Urschel Jr. HC, Razzuk MA. Paget–Schroetter syndrome: what is the best management? Ann Thorac Surg 2000;69(6):1663–8. PMID: 10892903.

The authors evaluated the results of 312 extremities in 294 patients with Paget–Schroetter syndrome to provide the basis for optimal management. Group I (35 extremities) was initially treated with anticoagulants only. Twenty-one developed recurrent symptoms after returning to work, requiring transaxillary resection of the first rib. Thrombectomy was necessary in eight. Group

II (36 extremities) was treated with thrombolytic agents initially, with 20 requiring subsequent rib resection after returning to work. Thrombectomy was necessary in only four. Of the most recent 241 extremities (group III), excellent results accrued using thrombolysis plus prompt first rib resection for those evaluated during the first month after occlusion (199). The results were only fair for those seen later than 1 month (42). The authors conclude that early diagnosis (less than 1 month), expeditious thrombolytic therapy and prompt first rib resection are critical for the best results.

56. Bern MM. Very low doses of warfarin can prevent thrombosis in central venous catheters. Ann Intern Med 1990;112(6):423–8. PMID: 2178534.

The goal of this study was to determine whether very low doses of warfarin are useful in thrombosis prophylaxis in patients with central venous catheters. Patients at risk for thrombosis associated with chronic indwelling central venous catheters were prospectively and randomly assigned to receive, or not to receive, 1 mg of warfarin beginning 3 days before catheter insertion and continuing for 90 days. Subclavian, innominate and superior vena cava venograms were done at onset of thrombosis symptoms or after 90 days in the study. A total of 121 patients entered the study and 82 patients completed the study. Of 42 patients completing the study while receiving warfarin, four had venogram-proven thrombosis. All four had symptoms from thrombosis. Of 40 patients completing the study while not receiving warfarin, 15 had venogram-proven thrombosis and 10 had symptoms from thrombosis ($P < 0.001$). In conclusion, very low doses of warfarin can protect against thrombosis without inducing a haemorrhagic state. This approach may be applicable to other groups of patients.

12

Primary and secondary vasospastic disorders (Raynaud's phenomenon) and vasculitis

Andrew R.I. Melville
Jill J.F. Belch

Introduction

There are many inflammatory and vasospastic disorders that can present with ischaemia and thus come to the attention of the vascular clinician. These include Raynaud's phenomenon (RP), the connective tissue diseases and conditions that cause vasculitis (the vasculitides). Due to the systemic nature of these conditions and their overlapping, often non-specific presenting features, diagnosis can be challenging. Management can be complex and is usually multidisciplinary. The aim of this chapter is to provide the vascular clinician with a grounding of knowledge in these conditions so that the initial diagnosis can be made. It describes their most common manifestations, necessary investigations (with particular emphasis on diagnostic autoantibody tests) and briefly delineates their treatment, with emphasis on recent advances.

Raynaud's phenomenon

Vasospasm is the key feature of RP. Maurice Raynaud's original description was of episodic digital ischaemia induced by cold and emotion.[1] The classic manifestation of pallor preceding cyanosis and rubor reflects initial vasospasm, followed by deoxygenation of static venous blood (cyanosis), then reactive hyperaemia (rubor). This full triphasic colour change is not essential for the diagnosis of RP, and a history of cold-induced blanching (with or without subsequent reactive hyperaemia) may be sufficient. Other stimuli can provoke attacks, such as chemicals (including drugs and those in tobacco smoke[2]), trauma and hormones. In addition to the digits, vasospasm may involve the nose, tongue, ear lobes and nipples. There is evidence to suggest that vasospasm may be systemic in distribution: a decrease in lung,[3] oesophageal[4] and myocardial[5] perfusion has been shown after cold challenge, and patients have a higher incidence of other conditions linked with vasospasm, such as migraine, irritable bowel syndrome and angina.

Inconsistent terminology has been a major problem for clinicians managing RP. We advocate the use of the terms primary Raynaud's phenomenon (PRP) where there is no underlying connective tissue disease, and secondary Raynaud's phenomenon (SRP) where there is. The terms Raynaud's disease and Raynaud's syndrome cause confusion and are best avoided.

The prevalence of PRP varies between populations. A recent meta-analysis of observational studies suggests a prevalence of approximately 5% in the UK.[6] PRP usually develops in the second or third decade and is commoner in women than men. Evidence suggests that genetic factors confer susceptibility to PRP: a twin study found a significantly higher concordance rate for monozygotic over dizygotic twins,[7] and a genome wide association study identified some candidate genes.[8] However, the true influence of genetics remains unclear. The prevalence of SRP depends on that of the underlying disorder, which itself varies between populations.

Many patients with mild disease never present to their general practitioners. Of those who do, most will have PRP. Patients with severe disease are likely to be referred to a hospital specialist. Given that an early marker for SRP is the severity of vasospastic attacks, hospital specialists are likely to see a greater proportion of SRP. Recognising SRP allows early monitoring and management of the underlying disorder, but this can be challenging as RP may precede an associated systemic disease by more than 20 years.

Conditions associated with SRP are shown in Box 12.1. Of the connective tissue diseases (CTDs), systemic sclerosis is the most frequent association.

Occupational RP is well recognised. A relatively common form is hand–arm vibration syndrome (HAVS, previously known as vibration white finger). Those typically affected are workers using vibrating tools such as chainsaws, pneumatic road drills and buffing machines. An estimated 4.2 million men and 667 000 women in Great Britain have occupational exposure to hand-transmitted vibration.[9]

> ✓ By using lighter chainsaws and reduced vibration, the frequency of HAVS in Finnish forest workers was reduced from 40% to 5%.[10]

Box 12.1 • Conditions associated with Raynaud's phenomenon

Connective tissue diseases
Systemic sclerosis
Systemic lupus erythematosus
Rheumatoid arthritis
Mixed connective tissue diseases
Sjögren's syndrome
Dermatomyositis/polymyositis

Obstructive
Atherosclerosis
Buerger's disease (thromboangiitis obliterans)
Microemboli
Thoracic outlet syndrome (especially cervical ribs)

Drug therapy
Beta-blockers
Cytotoxics, e.g. bleomycin
Ciclosporin
Ergotamine and other antimigraine therapies
Sulfasalazine

Occupational
Vibration white finger disease
Vinyl chloride disease
Ammunition workers (outside work)
Frozen food packers

Miscellaneous
Hypothyroidism
Phaeochromocytoma
Cryoglobulinaemia
Reflex sympathetic dystrophy
Malignancy
Hyperviscosity syndromes

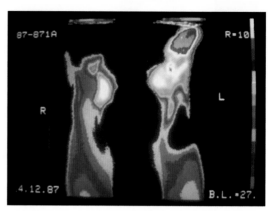

Figure 12.1 • Thermography demonstrating Raynaud's phenomenon of the toes, worse on the right. The image shows a temperature gradient from the midfoot to the toes on the left (L) and an absence of blood flow to the toes on the right (R), as detected by an infrared camera.

Vasospasm in HAVS has been described in the toes as well as the fingers (**Fig. 12.1**) and is likely related to vibration-induced damage of the endothelium.[11,12] The duration of exposure is important, as symptom severity and length of exposure are correlated.[10] The latency period between exposure and disease is usually more than 5 years of full-time work. Resolution of symptoms may occur in up to one-third of cases if there is a change of job early in the disease course.[13]

In the UK, HAVS has been a proscribed industrial disease since 1985. Patients may be eligible for industrial injuries disablement benefits if they fulfil certain criteria.[14] Specific daily time limits for different machines have been proposed and are being implemented opportunistically, often by use of points systems. Recently it has been suggested that prolonged exposure to vibrating computer game controls could also cause HAVS.[15]

Further examples of occupation-related RP include vinyl chloride disease, which is estimated to occur in 3% of exposed workers and can persist long after retirement,[16] and nitrate exposure related to ammunitions work, where habituation to vasodilatory nitrates means that RP can develop away from the work environment.

The remaining conditions associated with RP can be subdivided into those that worsen pre-existing RP (e.g. drugs, hypothyroidism, phaeochromocytoma) and those that mimic RP through microvascular occlusion (e.g. atherosclerosis, hyperviscosity, cryoglobulinaemia). The latter are differential diagnoses that may need to be excluded during work-up. Atherosclerotic obstructive arterial disease is common after the sixth decade, particularly in men. Management centres on identification and treatment of known risk factors, such as hypertension and hyperlipidaemia. Various drugs may precipitate or exacerbate RP (e.g. beta-blockers for angina) and alternative drug therapies may be more appropriate (e.g. calcium channel blockers such as nifedipine). Vasospasm is also a feature of reflex sympathetic dystrophy and thoracic outlet syndrome, particularly occurring in the presence of a cervical rib (see Chapter 11).

Pathophysiology

The pathophysiology underlying RP is not fully understood. Proposed mechanisms can be artificially subdivided into neural, vascular and intravascular, but in reality there is substantial overlap between them.

Neural mechanisms

This largely relates to the influence of the peripheral autonomic nervous system in regulating vascular tone. Thermoregulation usually depends on sympathetic (α-adrenergic) activity at neuroeffector junctions with vascular smooth muscle cells. In patients with RP, changes in the distribution, function and subtype of these receptors have been identified. Studies have found increased α-adrenergic receptor density and sensitivity, and a greater degree of α_2-mediated vasoconstriction over α_1 than healthy controls.[17] The α_{2c} receptor, a further subtype, is upregulated by cold-exposure and has been implicated in RP.[18]

Other neural factors may also be important; for example, altered levels of the synaptic vasoactive substances neuropeptide Y[19] and calcitonin-gene-related peptide[20] have been found. The central nervous system may also contribute to vasospasm but this has proven a difficult area to study.

Vascular mechanisms

The intact endothelium is essential for maintaining normal blood flow. It is a complex organ that produces both vasoconstrictors (e.g. endothelin-1) and vasodilators (e.g. prostacyclin and nitric oxide). Functional abnormalities of the endothelium occur in PRP and SRP, tipping the balance in favour of vasoconstriction. Additional structural abnormalities are seen in SRP.[21]

Factor VIII von Willebrand factor (VWF) antigen is influential in the clotting cascade and in platelet activation, and is usually released following endothelial injury. Levels are increased in RP,[22] which may be pathological. In addition, tissue plasminogen activator levels are reduced in RP, suggesting reduced fibrinolysis.

There is stronger evidence for altered levels of vascular factors in SRP than in PRP, and it is unclear whether this occurs as a consequence or cause of disease. Nonetheless, they are important

drug targets in RP and existing therapies have demonstrated clinical benefit (see below).

Intravascular mechanisms

Healthy blood flow depends on plasma factors and the cellular elements of blood. Abnormalities in various factors have been identified in RP. Abnormally activated platelets produce vasoconstrictors such as thromboxane A_2 and serotonin, and can aggregate to form clumps. Red blood cells (RBCs) appear less deformable in RP and this may impede the microcirculation. Cold temperatures exacerbate this. Activated white blood cells (WBCs) can aggregate within the microcirculation and produce free radicals, which may be prothrombotic.[23] Elevated fibrinogen and globulin levels increase plasma viscosity and further reduce blood flow.

Clinical features

RP is characterised by episodic colour change in the digits due to cold, temperature change or emotion. This is often biphasic or triphasic. The cardinal feature is well-demarcated blanching caused by vasospasm of the digital arteries. Fingers may subsequently turn blue (the cyanotic phase) and/or red (the reactive hyperaemic phase). Reactive hyperaemia may be associated with rewarming paraesthesia and pain. RP can affect selected digits or all the digits, and may be symmetrical or asymmetrical between hands. It is important to screen for clinical features suggestive of SRP (see connective tissue disease section below). As discussed earlier, other extremities such as the ears, tongue and nose can be affected, but a bluish discoloration in isolation is due to acrocyanosis and not RP.

Many people who do not have RP experience cold hands and feet at times, which may be accompanied by mild, poorly demaracated colour change. This likely reflects appropriate cold-induced closure of arteriovenous shunts in the skin, a thermoregulatory mechanism that decreases cutaneous blood flow and limits loss of body heat, and is simply most noticeable in the digits.

Investigations

These should be directed at confirming the diagnosis of RP (if necessary), differentiating between PRP and SRP, and identifying any underlying cause. In the majority of patients, the diagnosis of RP is made clinically from the history and/or examination.

Objective measures of blood flow are not usually required unless the clinical findings are vague. There are a variety of techniques available, many involving cold challenge, but there is no gold standard because of practical difficulties and inter-individual differences. The test we use most involves the measurement of digital systolic blood pressure changes before and after local cooling at 15°C. A pressure drop of >30 mmHg is considered to be significant, but precautions are required to avoid false-negative results. Ideally, patients should not be tested if they have had a Raynaud's attack earlier in the day as they may still be in the reactive hyperaemia stage and relatively protected from further vasospasm. In practice, the test may be carried out 2–3 hours after an attack if there is good clinical recovery. All vasoactive medication should be stopped for 24 hours before testing, and testing should be avoided during mid-cycle in premenopausal women as poor flow can occur during ovulation. Patients should be warm and not vasoconstricted prior to baseline measurements and this is best done by resting in a temperature-controlled laboratory for 30 minutes prior to testing. In warmer weather, additional total body cooling may be required as a warm body may protect a patient from the vasospastic effects of localised digital cooling. Strain gauge plethysmography is the usual method of measuring digital systolic blood pressure. Considerable operator skill is required and flow cannot be measured. Photoplethysmography with more sophisticated Doppler ultrasound equipment allows the measurement of the pressure at which blood flow returns. Computerised thermography uses skin temperature as an indicator of finger blood flow. This technique allows dynamic measurement of all phases of the attack but results must be interpreted with care as skin temperature is also dependent on venous and arterial blood temperature.

Where there is clinical suspicion of SRP, screening tests for an underlying CTD should be performed, including full blood count, urea and electrolytes, urinalysis, ESR and CRP, rheumatoid autoantibodies and antinuclear antibodies (ANA). If the ANA is positive, an anti-ENA screen should be sent to investigate for specific CTDs (anti-topoisomerase, anti-centromere, anti-Ro, anti-La, dsDNA).Investigations for associated conditions may be appropriate, including thyroid function, cryoglobulin screen, myeloma screen, and chest radiograph for cervical rib.

Nail-fold capillaroscopy is important in screening for underlying CTD. Capillary microscopy at diagnostic level can require sophisticated and expensive machines, but a fairly accurate view can be obtained using a dermascope. The dermascope is a high-powered skin magnification device used mainly by dermatologists, and is pocket sized and relatively inexpensive. Normal vessels are not visible but abnormally enlarged vessels, as seen in systemic sclerosis, can be seen (**Fig. 12.2**). The combination of abnormal nail-fold vessels and an abnormal immunological test has been shown to predict progression to CTD; studies suggest that RP

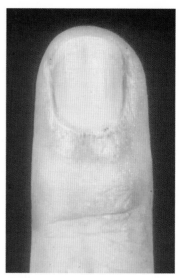

Figure 12.2 • Enlarged nail-fold capillaries in a patient with systemic sclerosis.

patients with both abnormalities are up to 60 times more likely to go on to develop systemic sclerosis (SSc) than those with neither.[24,25] It should be noted that nail-fold changes also occur with trauma and in diabetes mellitus.

> ✔ The diagnostic value of nail-fold capillaroscopy is now fully recognised with a clear diagnostic pattern seen for associated CTD: dilatation and tortuosity of the capillary with patches of so-called 'drop-out' where the vessel has been obliterated by the CTD process.[26]

Other tests, such as laser Doppler flowmetry, are used as research tools but are not helpful in making the diagnosis.[27]

Management

A proportion of patients with mild disease will not require drug treatment. Associated disorders such as hypothyroidism should be treated and causative drugs (e.g. beta-blockers) changed. Good symptomatic relief can be achieved in many patients despite the lack of a cure. A suggested management plan is shown in **Fig. 12.3**.

General measures

Patients should be advised to take precautions in cold conditions to keep their whole body warm. Pocket-sized thermochemical warming agents and electrically heated gloves and socks can provide a portable heat source, but may irritate skin ulcers if

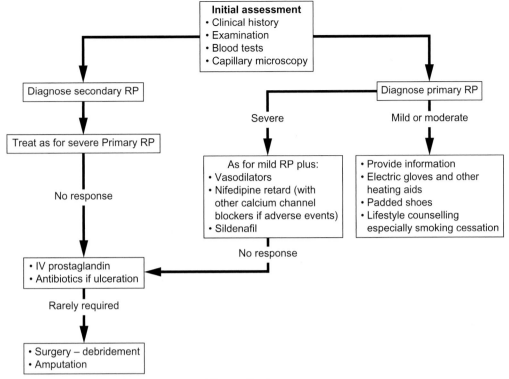

Figure 12.3 • Flow chart for the management of Raynaud's phenomenon.

present. Shoes with cushioned insoles can prevent 'pressure' RP but care must be taken to prevent these making the shoes too tight. These shoes are available from surgical appliance suppliers, are padded and broad fitting and provide warmth whilst also relieving pressure around the toes. Good ulcer care with early and adequate treatment of infection is important. The usual signs of infection may be absent because of poor blood flow, and a high index of suspicion is required. Smokers should be counselled to stop; referral to smoking cessation services may be appropriate. Scleroderma & Raynaud's UK (https://www.sruk.co.uk/) is a trusted source of information for patients, and psychosocial support can be provided by local support groups.

Drug therapy

This should be offered when symptoms are severe enough to interfere with work or lifestyle. Most patients with SRP and some with PRP will fall into this category. A selection of the drugs used in the treatment of RP is shown in Box 12.2.

Calcium channel blockers

These drugs are vasodilatory. Nifedipine is the gold standard and most frequently prescribed, and has additional antiplatelet[28] and anti-WBC activity. Systematic reviews have shown that calcium channel

Box 12.2 • Commonly used drugs in the treatment of Raynaud's phenomenon

Nifedipine

Slow-release or retard preparation preferred, 10 mg b.d. then t.d.s.

Change to 20 mg b.d. then t.d.s. if required

Capsule as 'rescue medication' crushed under tongue if chronic dosing not tolerated

Can be combined at low dose (e.g. 10 mg once daily) with vasodilator if higher dose not tolerated

Naftidrofuryl

Initially 100 mg t.d.s. then 200 mg t.d.s. if required

Inositol nicotinate

Start at 500 mg t.d.s. increasing to forte 750 mg b.d. if required

Maximum dose is 1 g q.i.d.

Administer for a 3-month trial

Pentoxifylline

400 mg b.d. increasing to t.d.s. if required

Moxisylyte (thymoxamine)

40 mg q.d.s. increasing to 80 mg q.d.s.

Discontinue if no response in 2 weeks

blockers (CCBs) can reduce the frequency and severity of attacks in PRP[29] and SRP,[30] and a recent Cochrane review concluded that CCBs reduce the frequency of attacks in PRP.[31] Vasodilatory side-effects (flushing, headache and ankle swelling) are common and may limit their use. Slow-release preparations are better tolerated and should be uptitrated slowly to minimise side-effects. Flushing and headache usually diminish over time. Nifedipine has no licence for use in pregnancy and patients should be advised accordingly. Other CCBs that have been used include amlodipine, diltiazem and isradipine. These tend to have fewer vasodilatory effects but at the expense of efficacy. Verapamil and ketanserin are ineffective.

Other vasodilators

Naftidrofuryl oxalate (Praxilene) is a mild peripheral vasodilator with a serotonin receptor antagonist effect. An oral dose of 200 mg t.d.s. has been evaluated in many studies and mild improvement can be expected in terms of severity of pain and duration of attacks.

A recent meta-analysis comprising six RCTs of PDE_5 inhibitors (sildenafil, tadalafil, vardenafil) showed a significant, modest benefit in RP secondary to SSc.[32] Larger studies are needed. Prazosin and losartan have also been studied in RP secondary to SSc and may have modest benefits.

It is our experience that patients with PRP respond better to vasodilators than those with SRP, the limiting factor often being adverse effects at higher doses. Occasionally, we also find that a combination of a low-dose CCB with a vasodilator such as naftidrofuryl can produce benefit while minimising the adverse effects seen with higher doses of either drug given in isolation.

Prostaglandins

Prostaglandin analogues of PGI_2 (prostacyclin) and PGE_1 have potent vasodilatory and antiplatelet effects but are both very unstable and require intravenous administration. Iloprost is a stable prostacyclin analogue that is effective in RP. It has been shown to reduce the frequency and severity of attacks, reduce ulcer formation and promote ulcer healing.[33] It is given intravenously for 6 hours daily for 3–5 days per treatment. The dose is gradually increased during each 6-hour period to a maximum tolerated dose, which should never be greater than 2 ng/kg per min. It is often less than this, particularly in women, because of flushing, headache or, rarely, hypotension. The same maximum dose is used each day. It is the agent of choice in cases of severe ischaemia or digital ulceration secondary to RP. Alprostadil is a PGE_1 analogue also given parenterally, which small studies suggest may have similar efficacy to iloprost. Studies of oral iloprost in SRP have given encouraging results.[34,35] Oral beraprost seems to be ineffective.

Other treatments

An open-label pilot study comparing fluoxetine (a selective serotonin reuptake inhibitor) with nifedipine in PRP and SRP demonstrated reduced attack frequency and severity.[36] Bosentan is an endothelin-1 antagonist that has been shown to reduce new digital ulcer formation in SSc without improving healing or pain. The usefulness of bosentan and other endothelin-1 antagonists in RP remains under investigation.[37] The cold-induced α_2-receptor (α_{2C}) is another interesting drug target but a recent small study of an antagonist yielded disappointing results.[38] *Ginkgo biloba* extracts may be effective in some cases of PRP.[39] Other treatments under investigation include topical nitrates, botulinum toxin A injections and MLS laser therapy.

Sympathectomy

The evidence for sympathectomy is largely based on case reports and series, some of which are historical. However, it is used in practice where there is critical ischaemia intractable to medical therapy. Chemical sympathectomy (cervical or digital) involves injection of local anaesthetic and may provide temporary relief from ischaemia and pain. Surgical cervical sympathectomy involves incision of the sympathetic chain and has a high complication and relapse rate. Digital sympathectomy involves stripping the adventitia of affected digital arteries. It is preferable to cervical sympathectomy, but long-term data and controlled trials are lacking. Lumbar sympathectomy has an important role in intractable RP of the feet and may be worth considering.

Conclusion

RP is a common condition affecting around 5% of the population. Differentiation between primary and secondary RP is important as identification and treatment of underlying CTD improves long-term outcomes. In severe cases a combination of non-pharmacological aids and drug therapy are used. Achieving satisfactory symptomatic relief can be challenging. New drug targets and treatment strategies are emerging. Surgery may be appropriate when RP is intractable or secondary to a cervical rib. Occupational RP should always be considered and may improve following a change of job or work practices.

Connective tissue diseases

CTDs are the most common group of disorders underlying SRP. Box 12.3 lists these disorders along with their incidence of RP. The severity of

Box 12.3 • Incidence of Raynaud's phenomenon in connective tissue disorders

Systemic sclerosis	95%
Systemic lupus erythematosus	29–40%
Polymyositis/dermatomyositis	40%
Sjögren's syndrome	33%
Mixed connective tissue disease	85%
Rheumatoid arthritis	10%

RP varies widely; some patients experience colour change with minimal discomfort, whereas for others it is their most significant symptom, and can lead to ulcer formation and gangrene. RP is found in the majority of patients with systemic sclerosis (SSc) and mixed CTD. Patients with limited SSc often have very severe RP, requiring hospital referral.

RP may predate the other symptoms of CTDs by years. One study reported that 12.6% of patients referred for assessment of RP progressed to SSc after a median follow-up of 4 years.[25] Another reported a 9% transition in patents presenting with RP alone and 30% from 'possible' secondary RP after a 12.4-year mean follow-up.[40] Clinicians should therefore 'safety net' when reassuring patients with what appears to be PRP.

A comprehensive initial assessment of patients presenting with RP helps identify those most at risk of transition to CTD. Predictive factors include certain clinical features, abnormal nail-fold vessels, and abnormal autoantibody screen.

The presence of RP with an isolated clinical sign associated with CTD, such as sclerodactyly, digital pitting or photosensitivity, should arouse suspicion. Classification criteria for CTDs are not 100% sensitive or specific, and such patients may develop fully established CTD over time.

The age of onset of RP is also important in predicting risk of transition. RP is common amongst young women and most are likely to have PRP. RP associated with definite underlying CTD has a higher median age of onset (36 years in SRP versus 14 years in PRP according to one study[41]). Around 80% of patients over 60 years presenting with new digital ischaemia will have an associated condition,[40] but the incidence of CTD is the same as in the general population, as a higher proportion of these patients have atherosclerosis (29% vs 5% in the total Raynaud's population), and to a lesser extent hyperviscosity syndromes and malignancy. Conversely, RP occurring in very young children, whilst rare, is frequently due to an underlying CTD.

Suspicious symptoms that should alert the clinician to the likelihood of SRP include severe attacks persisting throughout the summer, the recurrence of chilblains in adults, and the presence of digital

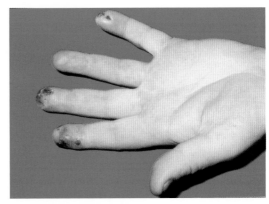

Figure 12.4 • Digital ulceration.

ulceration (**Fig. 12.4**). Digital ulceration does not occur in PRP. Asymmetrical colour change with fewer digits affected and involvement of the thumb suggest SRP rather than PRP.[42]

As above, there have been a number of recent advances in the use of nail-fold capillaroscopy and autoantibodies to detect or predict progression SRP in patients presenting with RP. Attempts have been made to develop algorithms to predict the risk of transition to SSc using a combination of NCM findings and autoantibody results.[43]

Vasculitis

Vasculitis means inflammation of the blood vessel wall. This can be primary or secondary. Secondary vasculitis is caused by a wide range of conditions, including infections, immune reactions, drug reactions and systemic diseases (e.g. rheumatoid, sarcoid and lupus vasculitis). Primary vasculitis is caused by a group of overlapping systemic syndromes of unknown cause: the vasculitides. The term vasculitis is often used in reference to these conditions specifically. They are distinguished from one another by their distribution, clinical features and histology, and are classified according to the size of the vessels affected, as shown in Table 12.1. Multiple blood vessels and organ systems can be involved, and widespread inflammation results in constitutional symptoms, such as fever, weight loss and anorexia. Damage to vessel integrity and tissue ischaemia results in more specific clinical features. Diagnosis is made according to the pattern of clinical features, supported by histology and/or imaging. Biopsy allows histological confirmation and has traditionally been used. Non-invasive imaging techniques allow assessment of the distribution of vasculitis and are increasingly used. These have superseded conventional angiography. Techniques include whole-body contrast-enhanced magnetic

Table 12.1 • Relationship between vasculitis classification and vessel size

Type of vasculitis	Aorta and branches	Large and medium-sized arteries	Medium-sized muscular arteries	Small muscular arteries	Arterioles, capillaries and venules
Takayasu's arteritis	✓				
Buerger's disease (thromboangiitis obliterans)	✓	✓			
Giant cell arteritis (temporal arteritis)	✓	✓			
Polyarteritis nodosa		✓	✓		
Wegener's granulomatosis			✓	✓	
Connective tissue disorders				✓	✓
Rheumatoid vasculitis				✓	✓
Cutaneous vasculitis (leucocytoclastic/allergic)					✓

resonance angiography (CE-MRA) and multislice computed tomography. [18F]fluorodeoxyglucose positron emission tomography/computed tomography (PET-CT) can be used to demonstrate the presence, distribution and activity of vasculitis as well as to monitor its response to treatment.

Classification criteria exist for certain vasculitides. These are meant for distinguishing between vasculitides in the research setting. They are often used in lieu of diagnostic criteria, but are imperfect for this purpose.

Takayasu's arteritis

Tayakasu's arteritis (TAK) is an idiopathic, chronic inflammatory, granulomatous arteritis. It primarily affects the large elastic arteries: the aorta, its major branches and the pulmonary arteries. The most common branches affected are the subclavian, common carotid and renal arteries. Chronic inflammation leads to arterial stenosis as well as occlusion and aneurysm formation, with associated clinical sequelae.

TAK is a rare disease, most commonly described in Japan. The annual incidence in the UK is estimated at 0.8 per million. It has a striking female predominance, affecting women five to nine times more frequently than men. It usually occurs before the age of 50 and most commonly in the second or third decades.[44]

Disease symptomatology can be divided into two phases: the acute systemic phase (pre-pulseless or pre-stenotic) and the chronic obliterative phase. The acute symptoms reflect generalised inflammation and include fatigue, malaise, weight loss and fever. Arthralgia and myalgia are common. The nature of the chronic phase disease depends on which vessels are affected. Hypertension, limb claudication,

cerebrovascular events, renal artery stenosis and mesenteric ischaemia are all recognised. Heart disease, as a consequence of hypertension, coronary disease or aortic valve insufficiency, is also seen, as is pulmonary hypertension secondary to pulmonary artery involvement. Clinical signs include diminished or absent arterial pulses, vascular bruits (e.g. over the aorta or subclavian artery), unexplained hypertension, inequality of blood pressure between arms or between arm and leg, abnormalities on auscultation of the heart and carotid artery tenderness.

There are no specific disease markers or autoantibodies for TAK. An elevated ESR and CRP are usually (but not always) seen during active disease.

Given TAK's rarity and non-specific initial presentation, diagnosis can be delayed by years. By this time irreversible structural changes may have occurred. The American College of Rheumatology classification criteria for TAK (1990) are commonly used for diagnostic purposes; three of six clinical and imaging criteria are required, with 90% sensitivity and 98% specificity.[44] Non-invasive imaging techniques include contrast-enhanced magnetic resonance angiography (CE-MRA) and computed tomography angiography (CTA). These can identify structural changes such as stenoses (**Fig. 12.5**), occlusions, collaterals and aneurysms. PET-CT has an emerging role in detection of vessel wall inflammation characteristic of pre-stenotic disease. Updated diagnostic criteria that reflect these new technologies and facilitate early diagnosis are required.

Biopsy findings reveal inflammation in all arterial layers (panarteritis). There is thickening of the adventitia with nodule formation, leukocyte infiltration of the media with granulomas, and intimal

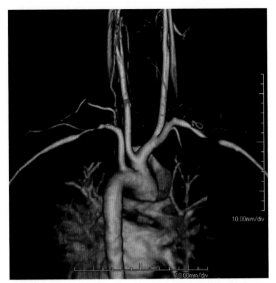

Figure 12.5 • Posterior view of a three-dimensional volume-rendered thoracic aorta magnetic resonance angiogram showing severe bilateral subclavian artery stenoses in a 35-year-old woman who presented with chest pain. In addition there were severe stenoses and occlusions of visceral and lower limb arteries.
Image courtesy of Dr John Bottomley, Sheffield Vascular Institute, UK.

hyperplasia, leading to progressive luminal narrowing. Over time, fibrosis of the intima and media ensues, resulting in stenosis or occlusion.

> ✅ During the acute inflammatory phase immunosuppression with corticosteroids has been found to be effective in halting the angiographic progression.

There are no RCTs of treatments for TAK. Current practice is based on expert opinion, open-label studies and case reports. High-dose steroids are the mainstay of treatment in the acute setting, with subsequent tapering and addition of steroid-sparing agents such as methotrexate or azathioprine. Mycophenalate mofetil, tacrolimus and cyclophosphamide have also been used, and there is growing interest in biologic therapies such TNFα and IL-6 inhibitors.[45] Related comorbidities such as hypertension should be treated aggressively. Assessment of response and monitoring for recurrence is difficult as there is no reliable assessment tool.[46] A combination of clinical assessment, monitoring of inflammatory markers and serial imaging is used. Surgical intervention is reserved for selected complications and should be delayed until after remission. Indications include severe aortic coarctation, arterial stenoses causing critical limb ischaemia or cerebrovascular disease, renal artery stenosis causing accelerated hypertension, and unstable aneurysms. Upper limb claudication usually improves without intervention due to collateralisation. Outcome data are better for bypass grafting than percutaneous angioplasty.[47]

Buerger's disease (thromboangiitis obliterans)

Buerger's disease is a vasculitic syndrome characterised by segmental, non-atherosclerotic, inflammatory thrombotic occlusions of the small and medium-sized arteries and veins of the extremities. The lower limbs are most commonly affected. There is associated migratory superficial thrombophlebitis.

Buerger's disease usually occurs in men less than 45 years of age, although disease in women and older people is recognised. The cause is unknown, but smoking is by the far the most important risk factor and appears to be key in pathogenesis, to the extent that a smoking history is generally regarded as a prerequisite for diagnosis.[48] Periodontitis may also be a risk factor. Altered blood flow parameters, including haematocrit and red cell rigidity, have been detected,[49] and prothrombin gene mutation and anticardiolipin antibodies may confer increased risk of disease.

Thrombus histology differs in acute and chronic disease. Acutely, thrombi are inflammatory and hypercellular, comprising neutrophils, giant cells and microabscesses. Later they become fibrosed ('organised thrombus') and inflammatory cells are absent. Throughout the disease process there is sparing of the internal elastic lamina, and this is key in differentiating Buerger's disease from atherosclerosis and other vasculitides.

The symptoms of Buerger's disease include intermittent claudication, usually of the foot or leg, and rest pain indicative of critical limb ischaemia. Ulceration or gangrene can follow. More than one limb may be involved. Ischaemia of the fingers may mimic Raynaud's phenomenon. Migratory superficial thrombophlebitis occurs in around 40% and may predate symptoms of ischaemia. This manifests as tender nodules overlying veins and is rare in the other vasculitides apart from Behçet's disease. Clinical examination may reveal palpable femoral and popliteal pulses but absent pedal pulses. Allen's test is non-specific but may suggest compromised blood flow to the hand, which in a young smoker raises the suspicion of Buerger's disease. Peripheral nerve involvement is seen in up to 70% of cases.

The diagnosis of Buerger's disease is clinical, supported by non-invasive arteriography. There are no specific disease markers, and ESR, CRP and autoantibody screens are typically normal.

Differential diagnoses, such as atherosclerosis, proximal embolism and immune disorders must be excluded. Imaging reveals angiographically normal vessels, free of atherosclerosis, proximal to the popliteal arteries in the legs and brachial arteries in the arms. Subsequently there are segmental occlusive lesions of the small and medium-sized arteries with more severe disease distally. Corkscrew collaterals may be seen around occlusions. It is wise to image all four limbs, even when symptoms are confined to one, as early disease may be detected in the others. Biopsy is only required in cases of diagnostic uncertainty.

✔ Tobacco abstinence is the cornerstone of management for Buerger's disease. In patients who stop smoking the appearance of new lesions and gangrene requiring amputation are unusual.[50]

The mainstay of management is smoking cessation. Some medical therapies are used but there is a lack of high-quality clinical trials assessing their efficacy. Aspirin and parenteral iloprost have been used to relieve rest pain and promote ulcer healing.[51] Other treatments that have been used include corticosteroids and lumbar sympathectomy. There are small studies of emerging treatments, including intramuscular gene transfer of vascular endothelial growth factor and stem cell therapy. Surgical revascularisation is limited due to the distal and diffuse nature of the disease, but may be beneficial if there is a distinct target lesion. Major and minor limb amputation is fairly common (around 40% in one retrospective study[51]) but rare after successful smoking cessation.

Giant cell arteritis

Giant cell arteritis (GCA) is an idiopathic, systemic, granulomatous large- and medium-vessel vasculitis. It occurs in people over 50 years of age, is commonest in Caucasians of northern European origin, and affects women two to three times more often than men. The overall incidence in people over 50 is 17 per 100 000 per year, making it one of the most commonly occurring vasculitides. GCA is histologically indistinguishable from Takayasu's arteritis, but has different epidemiological and clinical features (e.g. age of onset, ethnic predominance, distribution of disease and acuity of presentation).[52]

GCA is associated with a spectrum of disease, comprising cranial GCA, large vessel GCA and polymyalgia rheumatic (PMR). Constitutional symptoms, such as fever, weight loss and fatigue, are common to all forms. Cranial GCA (GCA affecting the cranial branches of the aortic arch) is the most well recognised. New onset headache occurs in two-thirds of affected patients. This is refractory to standard analgesia and is commonly localised to the area overlying the superficial temporal artery. The artery itself may be tender, hardened and pulseless. Scalp tenderness may be prominent feature of cranial GCA and this is due to involvement of the superficial temporal and occipital arteries. Patients may complain of pain on combing their hair or resting their head on a pillow. Necrosis of the skin of the scalp is an extreme manifestation of the same disease process. Jaw claudication occurs in around half of patients and results from facial and maxillary artery involvement. Tongue claudication is recognised and rarely glossitis and tongue necrosis are seen. Sudden visual loss is the most feared consequence of cranial GCA and is due to disease of the ophthalmic or posterior ciliary arteries. Visual symptoms, such as amaurosis fugax, blurred or double vision, may be warning signs of impending blindness. Associated clinical signs include a new deficit in visual fields or acuity, fundoscopic evidence of optic neuritis or central retinal artery occlusion and a relative afferent pupillary defect. Cerebrovascular events, secondary to carotid or vertebrobasilar artery inflammation, are rarer complications of cranial GCA.[53]

Large vessel involvement by GCA is increasingly recognised and may result in limb claudication. Symptoms of PMR occur in around half of patients with GCA. The conditions are clearly linked and may be caused by the same disease process.[54] PMR is characterised by proximal pain and stiffness due to bursitis and tenosynovitis of the shoulders and pelvic girdle. Peripheral non-erosive arthritis may occur, sometimes accompanied by significant pitting oedema of the hands and lower limbs due to tenosynovitis (RS3PE).

Diagnosis of GCA relies of clinical features, supportive laboratory tests, and biopsy and/or imaging findings. There are no serological tests for GCA, but inflammatory markers (CRP, ESR) are almost invariable raised (2 to 10 times the upper limit of normal). Raised alkaline phosphatase and anticardiolipin antibodies may also be seen in the acute setting. Temporal artery biopsy has traditionally been used to confirm a diagnosis of cranial GCA, with the hallmark finding being transmural granulomatous inflammation (**Fig. 12.6**). However, inflammation occurs intermittently along the length of affected arteries (so called 'skip lesions'), meaning biopsy may be false negative, even when ultrasound guided, in up to 20% of cases. Modern imaging techniques, including Doppler ultrasonography, MRA and CTA, can detect vessel wall inflammation associated with early GCA and are emerging as important diagnostic tools. PET-CT may also have a role in assessing extent of disease.[55] Of note, biopsy or imaging performed

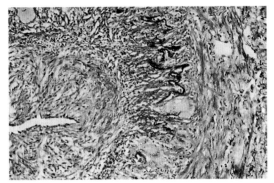

Figure 12.6 • Temporal artery biopsy demonstrating granulomatous inflammation with giant cells (A), transmural mononuclear cell inflammation, disruption of the internal elastic lamina (B), and intimal hyperplasia with narrowing of the lumen (C).

after initiation of treatment may result in false negative findings, but due to the severity of potential sequelae, treatment should not be delayed where clinical suspicion is high.

✅ Corticosteroids are the mainstay of treatment. A rapid response to corticosteroid therapy is strongly supportive of the diagnosis. Ischaemic complications, including blindness, are rare after initiation of steroids.[56]

Patients with suspected GCA should be started on high-dose corticosteroids (usually 40–60 mg prednisolone per day). Intravenous methylprednisolone is often used for patients with visual disturbance, although the evidence that this is more effective than standard treatment at preventing blindness is limited. Patients often require prolonged courses of corticosteroids of up to 2 years. Steroids should be tapered to the minimum effective dose to minimise complications. Calcium and vitamin D should be started contemporaneously as prophylaxis against osteoporosis, along with bisphosphonate therapy for those with pre-existing low bone mineral density. Low dose aspirin is recommended by EULAR, as there is some evidence from retrospective analyses that this can reduce ischaemic complications.[56] Some patients run a relapsing–remitting course and require long-term corticosteroid treatment. Patients with PMR generally require lower doses of corticosteroids. Steroid-sparing agents, including methotrexate, azathioprine, TNFα and IL-6 inhibitors, are sometimes used in GCA but there is no strong evidence that they provide benefit compared with steroids alone.

Polyarteritis nodosa

Polyarteritis nodosa (PAN) is a rare necrotising vasculitis affecting the small and medium-sized muscular arteries. Variants include idiopathic generalised PAN, hepatitis B-associated PAN and single-organ PAN, the commonest of which is cutaneous PAN. Hepatitis B formerly accounted for one-third of cases, but now accounts for only 5%. The overall annual incidence in Europe has fallen to around 1 per million, owing to widespread vaccination against hepatitis B. PAN affects both genders but is commoner in men. The peak incidence is in the fifth and sixth decades, although children and older people are also affected. There is no ethnic predominance. The precise pathogenesis remains incompletely understood.

The presenting symptoms are often indolent and constitutional, including malaise, weight loss, fever and myalgia. Further symptoms and signs depend on the organs affected. Ischaemia (secondary to arterial narrowing), infarction (secondary to thrombosis) and haemorrhage can all occur; the latter two can result in abrupt clinical deterioration. Any organ can be affected other than the lungs, the commonest being the skin and peripheral nervous system. Skin manifestations include nail-fold infarcts, digital infarcts (**Fig. 12.7**), palpable purpura and livedo reticularis (**Fig. 12.8**). Peripheral nervous system manifestations include mononeuritis multiplex, which can present as wrist or foot drop, and polyneuropathy. The kidneys are often involved. Hypertension occurs secondary to renal artery disease, and renal infarcts can cause frank or microscopic haematuria with proteinuria.

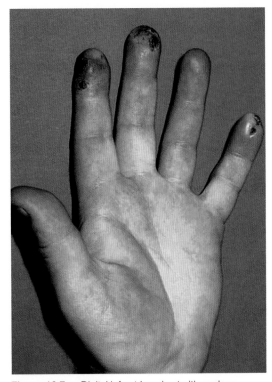

Figure 12.7 • Digital infarct in polyarteritis nodosa.

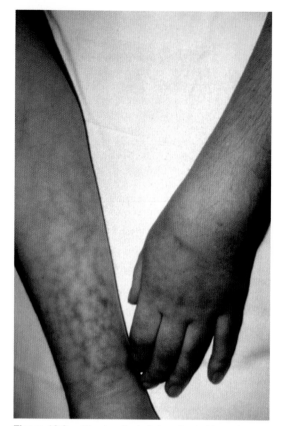

Figure 12.8 • Livedo reticularis in polyarteritis nodosa.

arteries can support the diagnosis. Microaneurysms (classically described as saccular or fusiform) are seen alongside stenotic lesions.

> ✓ Life-threatening or severe disease is treated with high-dose corticosteroids and cyclophosphamide. Less severe disease is treated with corticosteroids alone. A steroid-sparing agent such as azathioprine or methotrexate may be used to maintain remission. However, PAN is usually thought of as a monophasic disease, with only 10% relapse rate. The mainstay of treatment for hepatitis B-associated PAN is antiviral therapy.[59]

Small-vessel vasculitis

Small-vessel vasculitis largely affects the capillaries, intra-parenchymal arterioles and intra-parenchymal venules. The main subcategories are ANCA-associated vasculitis (AAVs) and immune complex-mediated vasculitis.

ANCA-associated vasculitis (AAVs)

This is a group of systemic diseases associated with ANCA (anti-neutrophil cytoplasmic antibodies). The three subtypes are microscopic polyangiitis (MPA), granulomatosis with polyangiitis (GPA, formerly known as Wegener's granulomatosis), and eosinophilic granulomatosis with polyangiitis (EGPA, formerly known as Churg–Strauss syndrome). They are all characterised by necrotising vasculitis with an absence of immune complex deposition ('pauci-immune vasculitis'). ANCA are believed to mediate vasculitis and vessel necrosis by activating circulating neutrophils and complement.[60] GPA and EGPA, but not MPA, are also associated with extravascular inflammation that may be granulomatous (hence the term 'granulomatosis').

The AAVs cause diverse patterns of disease. They can affect single organs, but usually cause multi-organ disease with a range of symptoms and signs. Disease severity can be indolent or rapidly progressive and life-threatening. Disease course tends to be relapsing–remitting.

MPA has an annual UK incidence of 6 per million with a usual age of onset around 50 years. Initial symptoms may be constitutional and non-specific, reflecting widespread underlying inflammation. These include fever, malaise, weight loss, arthralgia and myalgia. Additional clinical manifestations depend on which organs are involved. Necrotising vasculitis results in bleeding and ischaemia of affected vessels. Skin involvement (dermal venulitis) results in palpable purpura, and peripheral nerve involvement (epineural arteritis) results in mononeuritis multiplex. Involvement of the renal glomeruli results in glomerulonephritis, which can be rapidly progressive and lead to renal failure. Alveolar capillaritis can

Glomerulonephritis does not occur. Gastrointestinal symptoms are common due to mesenteric ischaemia and range from non-specific abdominal pain, nausea and vomiting to life-threatening bowel infarction, perforation and haemorrhage.[57] Further manifestations include cardiac disease, orchitis secondary to testicular artery involvement, sensori-neural hearing loss and eye involvement.[58]

Laboratory findings are non-specific. An elevated CRP and ESR is common. There is no serological test for idiopathic PAN, and antineutrophil cytoplasmic antibody (ANCA) is negative.[59] Screening for hepatitis B is imperative.

Diagnosis depends on supportive biopsy or imaging findings and the exclusion of related conditions such as small vessel vasculitis. The organ biopsied should be involved by disease. Where possible, muscle or nerve biopsy is preferred due to better diagnostic yield and safety profile. Histology reveals a mixed inflammatory infiltrate with fibrinoid necrosis largely affecting arterial branch points. Vessel wall injury leads to microaneurysms. Later, intimal hyperplasia and fibrosis of the vessel wall occur. Where biopsy is not feasible, visceral angiography of the renal, hepatic or mesenteric result in pulmonary haemorrhage, which can be severe and diffuse. Gastrointestinal, cardiac, central nervous system and ocular disease are all recognised.

GPA and MPA overlap clinically. GPA affects a similar age group but is more common, with a UK incidence of 11 per million. GPA has additional clinical manifestations due to associated granulomatosis. Upper and lower respiratory tract involvement are common; nasal crusting and sinusitis are classic presenting symptoms of GPA, whilst subglottic stenosis is recognised and pulmonary granulomatosis results in nodules that can cavitate.[61] Damage caused by GPA can result in collapse of the nasal bridge and saddle-shaped deformity. Ear involvement is common and patients may present with otitis media. Eye involvement is more common than in MPA and includes conjunctivitis, uveitis and episcleritis.

EGPA is the rarest of the three (annual UK incidence 1–2 per million). It presents with severe, late-onset asthma, or allergic rhinitis with nasal polyps, and is associated with raised circulating eosinophils. The vasculitic phase occurs after a latency of up to 10 years, and any of the manifestations described for MPA can be seen. Granulomatosis in EGPA occurs as a result of infiltration of organs by eosinophils. The lungs are particularly susceptible ('eosinophilic pneumonitis').

The diagnosis of AAV is clinical, supported by biopsy where feasible. The differential diagnosis is wide: other causes of small vessel vasculitis, malignancy, infections, polyarteritis nodosa, atrial myxoma and cholesterol emboli can all present similarly. The aim of investigations is threefold: to confirm the diagnosis of AAV, to screen for damage caused, and to exclude other conditions. Initial laboratory tests include a full blood count, renal profile, CRP and ESR. Urinalysis (for blood and protein) may provide evidence of glomerulonephritis, and chest radiograph may show a discoid lesion or cavity. If AAV is suspected, ANCA screen should be sent and the major organ systems screened for damage by clinical examination and further tests, including protein:creatinine ratio (to quantify proteinuria), echocardiogram, lung function tests, etc. Tests for other conditions include infection screen (for HIV, Hep B, Hep C), ANA, RF, complement and cryoglobulins.[62]

ANCA target a variety of auto-antigens that originate within neutrophil granules but are expressed on the surface of activated neutrophils. PR3-ANCA (ANCA targeting proteinase 3) and MPO-ANCA (ANCA targeting myeloperoxidase) are associated with AAVs. PR3-ANCA positivity is strongly suggestive of GPA. MPO-ANCA positivity is associated with MPA and EGPA but is less specific, as conditions such as inflammatory bowel disease and primary sclerosing cholangitis can also give a positive MPO-ANCA. ANCA-negative disease is well recognised, particularly in EGPA and single-organ GPA.

ANCA is detected by indirect immunofluorescence using fixed neutrophils, which produces cytoplasmic (cANCA) or perinuclear (pANCA) staining patterns. PR3-ANCA is a cANCA and MPO-ANCA is a pANCA. Other targets for ANCA are known but their clinical significance is unclear.[63]

Biopsy of an affected organ is important in confirming a new diagnosis or relapse but should not delay urgent treatment where the clinical picture is convincing.[64] Common sites for biopsy include the skin, upper and lower respiratory tract and the kidneys. Findings of necrotising vasculitis, or pauci-immune glomerulonephritis for renal biopsies, are confirmatory.

The European League Against Rheumatism (EULAR) has recently issued recommendations for the treatment of AAVs. Potent immunosuppressant drugs are the mainstay. There is superior evidence for GPA and MPA than EGPA, but guidance is the same for all three. New diagnoses and major relapses are treated in the same way. Where disease is organ-threatening or life-threatening, high-dose steroids and either cyclophosphamide (given in pulses to limit accumulation) or rituximab is used. Plasma exchange should be considered in cases of rapidly progressive glomerulonephritis or diffuse alveolar haemorrhage. Where disease is less severe (e.g. simple skin, nasal or skeletal muscle involvement, pulmonary nodules without cavitation or haemorrhage) corticosteroids with methotrexate or mycophenolate mofetil (MMF) are recommended, due to their favourable adverse effect profiles.

Treatment to maintain remission is usually continued for at least 2 years following induction. Agents used include low-dose glucocorticoids, azathioprine, rituximab, methotrexate and MMF. Disease activity is monitored by way of clinical assessment, aided by scoring tools such as the Birmingham Vasculitis Activity Score (BVAS). Increasing activity may necessitate a change in treatment. The role of ANCA titres in monitoring disease activity is unclear.

The effects of active disease should be distinguished from damage caused by disease, which is permanent and can be wide-ranging. Patients may be left with chronic kidney disease, lung disease, destruction of the nasal bridge, neuropathies, visual or hearing loss and skin scarring. Drug treatments themselves, whilst improving survival, are associated with adverse effects, including infections (all), diabetes, hypertension and osteoporosis (corticosteroids) and malignancies (e.g. azathioprine, MMF). Patients tend to be at high risk of cardiovascular events as a result of disease and treatment and cardiovascular disease (CVD) risk factors should be optimised.

Immune complex-mediated vasculitis

Deposition of immune complexes in the small vessels results in inflammation through activation of complement. Examples include IgA vasculitis and cryoglobulinaemia.

IgA vasculitis was formerly known as Henoch–Schonlein purpura. The aetiology is unknown, but deposition of IgA is central to pathogenesis. Production of IgA is increased and clearance is decreased. It is the commonest vasculitis in children. Disease in adults, whilst rare, with an annual incidence of around 1 per 100 000, is more severe, more likely to relapse, and more likely to progress to renal failure. The classic triad of presenting features is palpable purpura, arthralgia (without arthritis) and abdominal pain. IgA nephropathy is a well-recognised cause of end-stage renal failure (ESRF). Microscopic haematuria is an early indicator of glomerulonephritis. The disease course of IgA vasculitis is variable; it is not possible to predict which patients will remit spontaneously and which will progress to ESRF. Treatment is non-evidence-based and controversial[65].

Cryoglobulins are circulating immunoglobulins that precipitate in cool conditions. Type I cryoglobulinaemia is associated with B-cell lympho-proliferative conditions (e.g. multiple myeloma and Waldenstrom's macroglobulinaemia), whilst types II and III (mixed cryoglobulinaemia) are associated with hepatitis C virus (HCV) in around 80% of cases. Clinical features include fatigue, palpable purpura, peripheral nerve involvement (mononeuritis multiplex or polyneuropathy) and glomerulonephritis. Precipitation of cryoglobulins in the peripheries causes acrocyanosis and can mimic Raynaud's phenomenon. The management of cryoglobulinaemia depends on identification and treatment of the underlying condition. Antiviral therapy is the mainstay of treatment in HCV-related disease and is associated with a good prognosis.[66]

Primary cutaneous small-vessel vasculitis

Primary (or idiopathic) cutaneous small-vessel vasculitis is the term applied to small-vessel vasculitis affecting only the skin for which no secondary cause (e.g. drug reaction, infectious cause, systemic disease) is found. It usually manifests as palpable purpura occurring in the lower limbs. The lesions occur in crops, initially appearing as erythematous macules before progressing to purpura, and are usually symmetrical. It is typically self-limiting, with immunosuppressant treatment reserved for the most severe cases.[67]

Key points

- Raynaud's phenomenon can be primary (PRP) or secondary (SRP). Screening for associated conditions is important. PRP is usually a benign condition requiring conservative management only. Management of SRP can be challenging and may involve medical or surgical treatment.
- The systemic vasculitides are a diverse group of conditions that often require multidisciplinary care in specialist centres.

Key references

47. Mason JC. Takayasu arteritis – advances in diagnosis and management. Nat Rev Rheumatol 2010;6(7):406–15. PMID: 20596053.
    Recent review of advances in the clinical management of Takayasu arteritis.

48. Olin JW. Thromboangiitis obliterans (Buerger's disease). N Engl J Med 2000;343:864–9. PMID: 10995867.
    Review of thromboangiitis obliterans covering pathogenesis, clinical features and treatment.

53. Dasgupta B, Borg F, Hassan N. BSR and BHPR guidelines for the management of giant cell arteritis. Rheumatology (Oxford) 2010;49(8):1594–7. PMID: 20371504.
    British Society of Rheumatology guidelines for the management of giant cell arteritis.

54. Dejaco C, Duftner C, Buttgereit F, et al. The spectrum of giant cell arteritis and polymyalgia rheumatica: revisiting the concept of the disease. Rheumatology (Oxford) 2017;56(4):506–15. PMID: 27481272.
    Recent review exploring the overlap between giant cell arteritis and polymyalgia rheumatica.

56. Mukhtyar C, Guillevin L, Cid MC, et al. EULAR recommendations for the management of large vessel vasculitis. Ann Rheum Dis 2009;68(3):318–23. PMID: 18413441.
    EULAR (European League Against Rheumatism) recommendations for the management of large vessel vasculitis.

60. Jennette J.C., Falk R.J., Gasim A.H. Pathogenesis of antineutrophil cytoplasmic autoantibody. Curr Opin Nephrol Hypertens 2011;20(3):63–70. PMID: 21422922.
    Recent review outlining the detailed pathogenesis of ANCA-associated vasculitis.

62. Ntatsaki E, Carruthers D, Chakravarty K, et al. BSR and BHPR guideline for the management of adults with ANCA-associated vasculitis. Rheumatology (Oxford) 2014;53(12):2306–9. PMID: 24729399.
    British Society of Rheumatology guidelines for the management of ANCA-associated vasculitis.

64. Yates M, Watts RA, Bajema IM, et al. EULAR/ERA-EDTA recommendations for the management of ANCA-associated vasculitis. Ann Rheum Dis 2016;75(9):1583–94. PMID: 27338776.
    EULAR recommendations for the management of ANCA-associated vasculitis.

13

Peripheral and abdominal aortic aneurysms

Andrew L. Tambyraja

Introduction

The normal diameter of the aorta varies with age, sex and bodyweight.[1] It decreases in size as it leaves the thorax and enters the abdomen, tapering to its iliac bifurcation. However, the infrarenal aorta enlarges progressively with age. An aortic aneurysm is a permanent localised dilatation of all three layers of the vessel wall of at least a 50% increase in diameter compared to the expected normal diameter of the aorta.[2] If the maximum normal diameter of the aorta is considered to be 2.1 cm, aneurysmal dilatation is said to occur when the diameter exceeds 3.0 cm.

The abdominal aorta is the most commonly affected artery and accounts for 90% of all aneurysms. Of these, 95% will originate below the level of the renal arteries. The aortic arch, thoracic aorta and thoracoabdominal aorta are involved in approximately 10% of aneurysms.

The morphology or shape of aneurysms may be classified as saccular or fusiform, although this description represents a continuous spectrum. Saccular aneurysms affect only a small portion of the aortic circumference while fusiform lesions involve the entire circumference of the vessel.

Epidemiology

The prevalence of abdominal aortic aneurysm (AAA) in men over 65 years is around 7–8%.[3,4] The condition is thought to be six times greater in men than in women.[5] In determining the prevalence of AAA, the frequently asymptomatic nature of the disease is a major confounding factor. Data on prevalence stem from four sources: autopsy surveys, routine mortality and hospital inpatient statistics and population-screening surveys. It should be noted that all of these sources have their limitations and potential for bias; screening surveys offer, potentially, the most accurate estimate of prevalence.

The prevalence of screen-detected AAA in men in England is reported to be between 1.3 and 12.7%.[6] This variation is accounted for by differing criteria for the definition of AAA and the age group screened. If the criterion of aortic diameter >29 mm is used as the definition for AAA, the prevalence in men aged 65 years within the UK screening programme in the year 2014–2015 was 1.2%.[7] These figures are in keeping with data from other European and North American series.[8,9] Interestingly, data from autopsy-based surveys yield similar results. The prevalence of AAA at autopsy in the UK has been reported at 2.3% in men and 1.6% in women.[10]

Ruptured abdominal aortic aneurysm (AAA) accounts for around 10 000 deaths each year in the United Kingdom.[11] This represents a similar number to deaths caused by gastric, oesophageal and prostatic malignancies.[12]

Cause-specific mortality data for England and Wales and Hospital Episodes Statistics for England have shown that AAA mortality and ruptured AAA admission have fallen in England and Wales by around one-third, while non-ruptured AAA admission has remained steady between 2001 and 2009.[13] However, globally, AAA mortality has not declined over a similar time period. National differences can be explained by variations in cardiovascular risk factors. Of these, the reduction in smoking prevalence correlates most closely with declines in AAA mortality.[14]

Epidemiological data on peripheral aneurysm are less readily available. However, the association with AAA is well recognised and approximately 25% of patients with AAA have synchronous femoral or popliteal aneurysms.[15] It is likely that peripheral aneurysm will have similar epidemiological trends to AAA.

Pathophysiology

The cause of aneurysms remains unclear. Historically, aneurysmal change was thought to be underpinned by atherosclerosis. However, because of histological and epidemiological differences it is now recognised that atherosclerosis is a coexistent phenomenon and the majority of AAA (90%) are thought to represent a degenerative or non-specific process.[16]

Abdominal aortic aneurysms exhibit familial clustering. This raises the possibility of both genetic and environmental aetiological factors. Genes encoding for type III collagen, matrix metalloproteinases and protease inhibitors and plasminogen activator inhibitor have all been reported to play some role in AAA development or expansion.[17,18] However, no specific genes have been convincingly implicated to date and it is inferred that susceptibility to the development of AAA is an irreversible process with multiple genetic and environmental risk factors. Genetic influences are attributed to a few gene polymorphisms with large effects.[17]

North American and European data suggest that there is a fourfold increase in risk of having an AAA for the brother of a patient having an AAA.[19,20] Familial abdominal aortic aneurysms are more common when the index case is female and rupture is said to occur at a younger age and more often than with sporadic aneurysms.[21,22]

Established independent risk factors for AAA include male gender, age, hypertension, hyperlipidaemia and smoking.[5,23,24] In particular, the relationship between tobacco use and AAA development is striking. Aneurysms are four times more prevalent amongst smokers than non-smokers and the comparative relative risks of chronic cigarette smokers developing an AAA are threefold greater than their risk of developing coronary artery disease.[5,25] For these reasons, it is thought that smoking is the foremost environmental risk factor for aneurysm development and growth. Interestingly, diabetes is associated with a reduced risk.[26]

Abdominal aortic aneurysms are characterised histologically by destruction of elastin and collagen in the tunica media and tunica adventitia, smooth muscle cell apoptosis with thinning of the medial wall, infiltration of lymphocytes and macrophages, and neovascularisation.[27] Four pathological mechanisms are thought to play central roles in AAA development: proteolyis of connective tissue, inflammation, biomechanical stress and genetic influences.[28]

Proteolysis

Macrophage and aortic smooth muscle cell derived matrix metalloproteinases (MMPs) and other proteases are secreted into the extracellular matrix and are integral to aneurysm formation.[29] Though MMPs are expressed and active during normal physiological aortic remodelling, they mediate degradation of elastin and collagen within the aortic media and internal lamina in AAA pathogenesis.[30] A shift in the balance between MMPs and their inhibitors moves away from normal remodelling activity towards pathological elastin and collagen degradation. Factors initiating and propagating proteolyis in the aorta remain unclear.[31]

Inflammation

Transmural lymphocyte and macrophage infiltration is a histological characteristic of AAA.[27] An inflammatory cytokine cascade released by these cells is thought to stimulate protease activation. The chemotactic trigger responsible for this cellular migration remains uncertain, although it has been proposed that aortic elastin degradation products, interstitial collagen or oxidised low-density lipoprotein, may be antigenic and chemotactic stimuli for macrophages.[31]

Biomechanics

The aortic wall contains smooth muscle, elastin and collagen arranged in concentric layers in order to withstand arterial pressure. Elastin is the principal load-bearing element in the aorta while collagen provides tensile strength and helps maintain the structural integrity of the vascular wall.[32] The normal aorta displays a reduction in the elastin-to-collagen ratio as it passes from the thorax into the abdomen.[31] Thus, the abdominal aorta has less elastin and as a consequence, less load-bearing potential than the aortic arch.

Matrix metalloproteinase-9 expression and activity is increased in the abdominal aorta compared with aortic arch and thoracic aorta. Activation of these proteases is also thought to be brought about by the disruption of normal laminar flow seen in the infrarenal aorta.[33] Furthermore, the attenuation of the vasa vasorum in the infrarenal aorta is proposed to contribute to relative hypoxia of the vessel stimulating MMP activity. These factors are all thought to contribute to the predisposition of the infrarenal aorta to develop aneurysmal change.[25]

Genetics

As already discussed, though multifactorial genetic influences are involved in AAA development, the polymorphisms responsible for aneurysm pathogenesis remain elusive. Similarly, the phenotypic expression of these traits is uncertain. It is proposed that an abnormality of the primary structures of elastin and collagen or a mutation, directly or indirectly, affecting protease and protease-inhibitor activity are implicated.[18]

Clinical features

About 75% of aortic aneurysms are asymptomatic and are discovered incidentally. A small proportion will present with symptoms related to pressure on adjacent structures (dysphagia, ureteric obstruction, caval obstruction).

A small subset of abdominal aortic aneurysm cases may present with the triad of lower back pain, weight loss and raised erythrocyte sedimentation rate. This triad is characteristic of inflammatory abdominal aortic aneurysm, which represents the most extreme end of the spectrum of chronic inflammatory change seen in degenerative aneurysms, and accounts for 10% of all abdominal aortic aneurysms. These cases are further characterised by a thickened aneurysm wall, retroperitoneal fibrosis that may cause obstructive uropathy and dense adhesions to adjacent viscera.

Most of the clinical symptoms due to aortic aneurysm are related to aneurysm rupture or embolism of mural thrombus.

Aneurysm rupture is associated with an estimated overall mortality of 90% and a significant proportion of patients will not reach hospital. Of those that present, most will have a contained retroperitoneal haematoma causing tamponade and resulting in temporary haemodynamic stability. The characteristic triad of abdominal or back pain, hypovolaemic shock and a pulsatile abdominal mass is present in only a few patients and the symptoms may be vague, and an abdominal mass missed. Other symptoms and signs may include groin pain, syncope, paralysis, or flank mass. A ruptured aneurysm should be considered in any elderly patient with unexplained hypotension and abdominal symptoms. The diagnosis may be confused with renal colic, diverticulitis, pancreatitis, or disease affecting the lumbar spine. A small proportion of abdominal aortic aneurysms rupture into an adjacent structure causing a primary aortic fistula; rupture into the vena cava produces a large arteriovenous fistula. In this case, symptoms include tachycardia, congestive heart failure, leg swelling, abdominal thrill, abdominal bruit, renal failure and peripheral ischaemia. Abdominal aortic aneurysms may rupture into the fourth part of the duodenum and presentation may be with a herald upper gastrointestinal bleed followed by massive haemorrhage.

Embolism: patients with embolisation of thrombus from an aortic aneurysm may also present with acute ischaemia of the lower limb due to occlusion of the femoral or popliteal artery. Small aortic aneurysms may also undergo acute occlusion due to thrombosis as the aortic lumen becomes progressively narrowed by the accumulation of mural thrombus; these patients may present with acute bilateral lower limb ischaemia.

Screening

As most AAA are asymptomatic, the majority of patients who suffer rupture will die, B-mode ultrasound is a highly sensitive and specific diagnostic tool, and elective aneurysm repair is an effective prophylaxis against rupture, population screening is appealing. A meta-analysis of four randomised controlled trials of screening elderly men for AAA with 15-year follow-up, has shown a significant and substantial reduction in the risk of death from AAA and the need for emergency surgery with an associated increase in elective repair.[34–36]

☑☑ The Multicentre Aneurysm Screening Study (MASS) trial has provided good statistical evidence to show that the prevalence of aneurysm-related death is reduced significantly in a screened male population aged 65–74 years, with a 53% reduction in those who attended for screening.[34] Because other causes of death overshadow those due to ruptured AAAs, it has not been possible to demonstrate a statistically significant overall survival advantage for the screened population. Nevertheless, the case for extending population-based screening for AAAs is convincing.

In England, the National Health Service AAA screening programme began in 2009. It offers all men aged 65 years an invitation for ultrasound screening. The same screening strategy is employed in Sweden and the rest of the United Kingdom. Interestingly, both programmes have demonstrated an incremental cost-efficiency ratio of £7000 per quality-adjusted life-year (QALY).[37,38] Compared with existing screening programmes for breast and cervical cancer, AAA screening for men remains cost effective.

✓✓ The MASS trial data show that over 4 years the mean incremental cost-effectiveness ratio for screening was £28 400 per life-year gained, equivalent to approximately £36 000 per QALY. It was estimated that this would fall to approximately £8000 per life-year gained at 10 years.[35]

✓✓ Analysis of the 10-year Multicentre Aneurysm Screening Study (MASS) data shows that the NHS AAA Screening Programme (NAAASP) will prevent significant numbers of AAA ruptures and AAA deaths. It also proves that the number of lives saved will greatly outweigh the number of post-elective surgery deaths. The following figures use the 10-year MASS data and assume an 80% attendance for screening and a 5% post-elective surgery mortality: 240 men need to be invited (192 scanned) to save one AAA death over 10 years and each 2080 men invited for screening (1660 scanned) result in one extra post-elective surgery death. This means that over 10 years, for every 10 000 men scanned under the NAAASP, 65 AAA ruptures will be prevented, saving 52 lives. However, there will also be six post-elective surgery deaths involving men whose aneurysm is detected under the screening programme.[35]

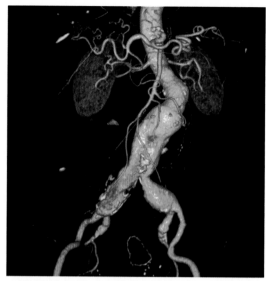

Figure 13.1 • Reconstructed CT aortogram of infrarenal aorto-iliac aneurysm.

Diagnosis

Aortic aneurysms may not be detected by clinical examination. Calcification of the aneurysm wall may be apparent on plain abdominal or chest radiograph, but this method lacks sensitivity and is unsatisfactory for routine use.

B-mode ultrasound is the diagnostic investigation of choice for the detection of AAA, providing accurate assessment of the aneurysm diameter and some indication regarding site.

Computed tomography (CT) is the investigation of choice to delineate abdominal aortic aneurysm morphology and relationship to the visceral and renal arteries (**Fig. 13.1**). CT or magnetic resonance imaging will detect thoracic aortic aneurysms.

Principles of management

The principles of management in asymptomatic abdominal aortic aneurysm are based on an assessment of the risk of aneurysm rupture weighed against the morbidity and mortality associated with surgical repair.

The size and growth of AAA are strongly associated with the amount and duration of smoking; smoking cessation can moderate this risk.[26] The association between hypertension and hypercholesterolaemia and AAA suggests that medical management of these conditions may have a benefit on aneurysm growth.

However, several drugs have been investigated in randomised controlled and non-randomised trials – beta-blockers, ACE inhibitors, angiotensin-receptor blockers and statins. None of these drugs has been shown to confer a benefit.[39] Nevertheless, given the strong association between atherosclerosis and AAA, it is recommended that aneurysm patients receive best medical therapy to reduce the incidence of cardiovascular events.

The natural history of untreated asymptomatic AAA is considered to be one of expansion and potential rupture. Measurement of the maximum anteroposterior diameter of the aneurysm predicts the risk of rupture. Randomised controlled data on abdominal aortic aneurysm of <55 mm diameter has demonstrated a mean risk of rupture of 1% per year.[40] However, there is little randomised evidence to inform the rate of rupture in large aneurysms. A multicentre study of 198 patients with AAA >5.5 cm for whom elective repair was not planned due to medical comorbidity or patient refusal, demonstrated a 1-year rupture risk for AAA of 5.5–5.9 cm of 9.4%, 10.2% for AAA of 6.0–6.9 cm and 32.5% for AAA of >7 cm.[41] Interestingly, the risk of rupture in the smallest AAA diameter cohorts was significantly greater than that reported in randomised controlled trials. This finding has been reported across other studies and it is likely that patients with significant coexistent morbidity are at a higher risk of rupture than their healthier counterparts. The projected annual rates of rupture for AAA from a meta-analysis of 13 studies are shown in Table 13.1.[42] However, some small aneurysms will rupture and some large aneurysms will not.

Table 13.1 • Annual abdominal aortic aneurysm rupture risk in relation to size

AAA size (cm)	Risk of rupture per year (%)
<3.0	0
3–3.9	0.4
4–4.9	1.1
5–5.9	3.3
6–6.9	9.4
7–7.9	24

Adapted from Law MR, Morris J, Wald NJ. Screening for abdominal aortic aneurysms. J Med Screening 1994;1:110–15.

Patients with asymptomatic abdominal aortic aneurysm of 30–54 mm should be kept under regular ultrasound surveillance to monitor growth. Current recommendations for surveillance intervals are 3-yearly for 30–34 mm, annually for 35–44 mm, and every 6 months for 45–54 mm.[43] Elective repair is only recommended in asymptomatic abdominal aortic aneurysm of >55 mm diameter – this applies to both open and endovascular aneurysm repair. The operative mortality associated with elective infrarenal abdominal aortic aneurysm repair is between 1% and 6%.[40,44]

✔✔ The Medical Research Council-sponsored UK Small Aneurysm Trial (SAT) randomised 1090 patients with asymptomatic AAAs of 4.0–5.5 cm diameter to either initial ultrasound surveillance (527 patients) or surgery (563 patients).[40] In the surveillance group, 321 patients eventually underwent surgery due to rapid expansion or growth to above the 5.5 cm threshold. In the early surgery group, the 30-day mortality rate was 5.8%. There was no difference in survival between the groups and the UK SAT concluded that early operative intervention for patients with AAAs of less than 5.5 cm diameter was not indicated. The rupture rate for untreated small aneurysms in this trial was less than 2% per annum. However, the rate was relatively higher in females and this suggests that elective surgery may be indicated for smaller aneurysms in this group of patients. However, at present the data are insufficiently robust to support this conclusion convincingly.

Symptomatic, intact AAA or rapid expansion (>1 cm/year) represents a relative indication for operative repair. It is thought that symptoms of pain attributable to an aneurysm are due to acute expansion or imminent rupture and urgent repair is recommended.

Aneurysm rupture is usually an absolute indication for surgery because without repair, mortality is almost certain. Surgery in some patients may be futile due to comorbidity or poor preoperative clinical condition (unconsciousness, cardiac arrest).

✔✔ The Canadian Aneurysm Study demonstrated an in-hospital mortality rate of 4.7% with a 5-year survival rate of 68%. The UK Small Aneurysm Trial reported a 30-day mortality rate of 5.8% and the recent EVAR-1 trial a 30-day mortality rate of 4.7% in patients fit for surgery.[40,44,45]

Preoperative assessment

Patients with asymptomatic AAAs >55 mm who are candidates for surgical repair require careful risk assessment of their general health and fitness to determine their suitability for surgery. The goals of assessment are: to identify patients in whom the balance of risk favours surgical intervention, to reduce perioperative morbidity and mortality by identifying modifiable comorbidity; to determine suitability for either open or endovascular repair by assessing aneurysm anatomy; to determine patient preferences for management.

Thorough clinical assessment is necessary as it is recognised that perioperative death is related to pre-existing physiological status companion. Most early deaths after AAA repair relate to cardiac events and if pre-existing cardiac disease is identified and treated prior to surgery, survival rates can be improved.

Preoperative assessment often includes:

- Full blood count
- Serum urea and electrolytes
- Liver function tests
- Pulmonary function tests
- Cardiac assessment with resting ECG and echocardiography
- Cardiopulmonary exercise testing
- Multidetector CT aortography.

Further cardiovascular assessment (exercise ECG, dobutamine-stress ECHO, or coronary angiography) may be indicated in patients with a history (or symptoms) of ischaemic heart disease.

In patients with significant and irreversible comorbidity, it is appropriate to continue ultrasound surveillance until aneurysm diameter reaches a size where the risk of rupture outweighs the increased risk of surgical mortality. It may be impossible to justify elective operative repair (regardless of size) in patients with overwhelming comorbidity.

Repair of intact abdominal aortic aneurysm

There are two methods by which abdominal aortic aneurysms may be excluded – traditional open repair and endovascular aneurysm repair (EVAR). Open surgical repair of AAA is a durable and cost-effective procedure. Endovascular aneurysm repair is effective and safe in selected patients, with lower short- and medium-term morbidity and mortality rates than open surgery. Patients with AAAs have a markedly reduced life expectancy in comparison with age- and sex-matched controls. The 5-year survival of patients post open surgery varies from 62% to 72% (compared with 83–90% in age- and sex-matched populations), with the majority of deaths due to coronary artery disease.[45,46]

Open repair

Under general anaesthesia and with perioperative broad-spectrum antibiotic and thromboembolic (heparin [s/c]) prophylaxis, a transverse supraumbilical or midline incision is utilised to allow a transperitoneal approach to the aorta. Alternatively, an oblique left-sided abdominal incision may be used to achieve an extraperitoneal approach to the aorta. Epidural analgesia may also be used to improve postoperative respiratory function. The routine use of cell salvage for intraoperative autologous transfusion is a useful adjunct companion.

At laparotomy, the transverse colon is reflected upwards and the small bowel reflected to the right. Division of the posterior peritoneum exposes the aneurysm. The left renal vein is identified and the neck of an infrarenal aneurysm will be identified. The common iliac vessels are also identified and exposed. Care should be taken to avoid damage to the hypogastric plexus of nerves to avoid postoperative sexual dysfunction.

A bolus of heparin is given intravenously (to reduce the risk of thrombosis in situ and perioperative cardiac injury) after which aortic and iliac clamps are applied. If the aneurysm extends into the common iliac arteries, the vessels may be mobilised to the common iliac bifurcation and control obtained of the internal and external iliac arteries. The aneurysm sac is opened longitudinally and mural thrombus removed. Back-bleeding from the lumbar, median sacral and inferior mesenteric arteries (IMA) may ensue and over-sewing these vessels controls this. The aneurysm may be repaired using a tube (60–70%) or bifurcated prosthetic aortic graft made from sealed or coated, knitted Dacron™. The graft is secured proximally and distally using an inlay technique and end-to-end anastomoses with a monofilament suture.

The lower limbs are reperfused sequentially upon completion of the anastomoses. The anaesthetist should be warned prior to releasing the clamps of each limb because of the hypotension caused by limb reperfusion and the sudden release of anoxic metabolites from the lower limbs into the systemic circulation. The aneurysm sac is closed over the aortic graft to reduce the risk of late postoperative aortoenteric fistulation. The lower limbs and left colon should be inspected to ensure adequate perfusion. Postoperatively patients are extubated and managed in a high-dependency unit. Early procedure-specific complications are mainly cardiac and respiratory in aetiology although renal dysfunction, colonic ischaemia and lower limb problems due to microembolism may also occur. The patient should be encouraged to mobilise early and oral intake can be re-established within 24 hours. In-hospital stay is usually 7–14 days. The 30-day mortality rate has remained around 3–5% for the past 10 years.

Aortic aneurysmal disease extends above the renal arteries to involve a variable length of the thoracic aorta in 5–10% of patients. Transperitoneal suprarenal clamping may be possible for juxtarenal AAA, but more proximal aneurysms require supracoeliac clamping performed by laparotomy with medial visceral rotation or thoracolaparotomy and replacement with a Dacron™ aortic prosthesis as well as reimplantation of the visceral and intercostal arteries. The results of surgery in specialist centres are good but complications such as paraplegia, organ dysfunction and significant mortality may occur.

A few centres have advocated the technique of laparoscopic aortic surgery. There is an absence of any randomised data to support its use outside of a clinical trial.

Operative repair of ruptured abdominal aortic aneurysm

The surgical mortality associated with ruptured AAA is in excess of 40%.[47] Once a ruptured AAA is diagnosed, patients suitable for attempted repair should be transferred to the operating theatre immediately. In general, patients should receive cautious fluid resuscitation with permissive hypotension. Sudden overloading of the intravascular compartment (together with its associated increase in systemic blood pressure) may cause expansion and rupture of a contained retroperitoneal haematoma resulting in potential exsanguination.

In theatre the patient is prepared and draped prior to the induction of anaesthesia; central venous access can be performed after induction. Rapid sequence induction is performed together with rapid entry into the abdomen (limiting the potential hypotensive effects of anaesthesia caused by the loss of tamponade from relaxation of the anterior abdominal wall). The neck of the aneurysm must be identified for clamping despite the significant distortion of anatomy that may be caused by a large retroperitoneal haematoma; iatrogenic injury in this period may prove fatal for the patient. If access to the infrarenal aortic neck is not possible, the aorta may be clamped at the diaphragmatic hiatus or control achieved by passing a balloon occlusion catheter up the lumen of the aorta. These techniques are associated with significant morbidity owing to the resultant visceral and renal ischaemia. When haemorrhage has stopped, aortic repair may be performed as for intact abdominal aortic aneurysms. Aggressive correction of haemostatic variables is recommended to limit the problems of coagulopathy caused by massive haemorrhage and transfusion. Despite improvements in perioperative care, the operative mortality rate from ruptured AAA remains high at around 40%.

EVAR

Endovascular aneurysm repair was first described by Voldos and colleagues in 1986 and Parodi and colleagues in 1991.[48] The premise of EVAR is to exclude the aneurysm from the systemic circulation using a preoperatively sized stent graft; this prevents further expansion and risk of rupture. This minimally invasive technique has resulted in a paradigm shift in the treatment of infrarenal AAA. Between 2000 and 2010, the use of EVAR increased from 5% to 74% of all AAA repairs in the USA.[49]

Indications and eligibility for EVAR

In contrast to open aneurysm repair, suitability for EVAR depends on both aneurysm morphology and patient fitness. It is reported that up to 45% of patients will have an AAA that is morphologically unsuitable for conventional infrarenal endografting.[50] Morphological variables that impact on suitability include length of infrarenal aortic (>10 mm), neck angulation (<60°), neck diameter (<30 mm), smooth parallel neck without significant mural thrombus. In addition, the iliac arteries should be of a calibre wide and straight enough to deliver a stent graft. As endografts evolve, the capability to treat more challenging anatomy may expand (**Fig. 13.2**).

In general, there are four graft constructs for EVAR of infrarenal AAAs: straight aorto-aortic tube endografts, bifurcated systems, aorto-uniiliac systems and combined bifurcated grafts with iliac branch grafts to permit perfusion and sealing in the external and iliac arteries. All devices form their proximal seal in the infrarenal aortic neck with variation in the distal seal zone – aorta, common iliac, external iliac or both external and internal iliac arteries. Aorto-aortic stent grafts were the first described and have a very limited application in contemporary practice in short localised saccular

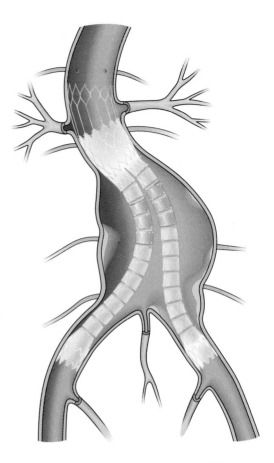

Figure 13.2 • Schematic representation of abdominal aortic aneurysm repair using an aortic stent graft.

aneurysms, postoperative pseudoaneurysm and penetrating aortic ulcers. In conventional AAA, aorto-aortic endografts have an unacceptably high incidence of failure due to aneurysmal change in the seal zone.

Bifurcated grafts offer the most desirable solution by securing seal in vascular segments unlikely to be affected by aneurysmal change and preserving normal anatomical flow. These devices are suitable for around 50% of patients.[51] The remainder of EVAR-eligible aneurysms with more challenging anatomy require either an aorto-uniiliac or iliac branched stent graft. The former may be indicated where there are problems of unilateral iliac access due to tortuosity or stenoses and require occlusion of the contralateral common iliac artery with a plug and revascularisation of the limb with a femorofemoral cross-over graft. Iliac-branched grafts may be indicated in aneurysms that extend into the common iliac arteries and permit preservation of blood flow into the internal iliac arteries using a bifurcated iliac component.

Patient assessment and EVAR technique

The patient should be formally assessed, discussed within a multidisciplinary team and counselled for EVAR as for conventional open surgery. Multidetector CT aortography should be obtained to enable multiplanar reconstruction and sizing of the entire abdominal aorta and iliofemoral segments and provide information regarding arterial access. Informed consent should include the routine morbidity and also the known EVAR-specific complications, including death, reintervention, nephropathy, arterial injury, endoleak (see later) and open surgical conversion. Ideally, the theatre should be capable of endovascular and open procedures and equipped with fixed imaging capability. Mobile C-arm equipment may be utilised if necessary but affords poorer imaging capability and greater radiation dose exposure.

After anaesthetic induction the patient is positioned, prepped and draped. A surgical cut-down to the femoral arteries permits catheterisation of the arterial circulation. A total percutaneous approach facilitated by the use of femoral closure devices may be performed instead. Evidence to justify this approach is emerging with claims of non-inferiority compared to surgical cut-down.[52] After femoral access is achieved, a soft wire and catheter are placed into the ascending aorta and a stiff guidewire is introduced through the catheter. Stiff guidewires are not intended to be 'working' wires and it is not sensible to try to negotiate tortuous iliac vessels with them. After systemic heparinisation, the stent graft body is introduced over the stiff guidewire and the renal arteries are imaged through a diagnostic catheter from the contralateral side. The image intensifier should be angled to optimise the view of the renal arteries and this typically requires a small amount of cranio-caudal and oblique tilt.

The diagnostic catheter is left alongside the graft body as the top stents are released in stages. Further angiographic runs may be performed to ensure accurate positioning relative to the renal arteries. Modular devices require cannulation of the short leg of the main body of the device prior to introduction of the contralateral limb. This is generally performed by a retrograde approach from the contralateral femoral artery using angled catheters. Confirmation of successful cannulation is needed to avoid the error of inadvertently deploying the contralateral limb alongside rather than within the main graft. The iliac limbs are deployed close to the internal iliac origins, which are defined using oblique projections. Substantial overlap at the modular connections is essential to avoid late disconnections. Balloon moulding with a compliant aortic balloon can then be performed to optimise proximal and distal seal zones and junctions of the modular graft components.

Completion angiography is performed to confirm the aneurysm has been excluded and to ensure that

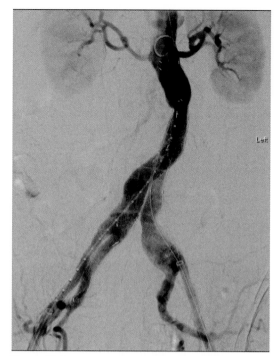

Figure 13.3 • Completion angiogram of right iliac branched endovascular aneurysm repair showing satisfactory exclusion of aorto-iliac aneurysm and freedom from endoleaks.

there has been no encroachment by the fabric of the graft on the orifices of the visceral or internal iliac arteries (**Fig. 13.3**). Every effort must be made to resolve any significant primary type I endoleak before completion of the procedure.

EVAR-related complications and device failure

The physiological advantages of EVAR are reflected by the reduced requirement of postoperative critical care support and incidence of significant cardiac, pulmonary and renal complications. However, in addition to the general causes of postoperative morbidity following AAA repair, EVAR carries some procedure-specific complications.

Endoleak

Endoleak is defined as the persistence of blood flow outside the lumen of an endovascular stent graft but within an aneurysm sac or the adjacent vascular segment being treated by the stent. The leak may be described as primary, originating at the time of EVAR, or secondary, referring to a leak not seen at completion angiography but demonstrated on subsequent surveillance imaging. Endoleaks have been classified according to the source of aberrant blood flow, since this characterises the endoleak and the potential for aneurysm enlargement and eventual rupture (Table 13.2).[53] This is most often seen in type I (**Fig. 13.4a**) and type III (**Fig. 13.4c**) leaks that communicate directly with the aortic lumen, and reintervention is almost always necessary in these patients.

Type II endoleaks (**Fig. 13.4b**) denote continued blood flow into the aneurysmal sac from refilling collateral vessels, typically the lumbar and inferior mesenteric arteries. The clinical significance of type II endoleaks is contentious and there is no standard treatment protocol. Increasingly, they are considered self-limiting and an expectant course of management is recommended. There is some evidence that they are associated with an increased risk of reintervention, but not aneurysm rupture or survival. At the very least, they should be kept under surveillance for signs of aneurysm sac enlargement.[54]

Blood flow across intact graft fabric within 30 days of EVAR defines the type IV endoleak (**Fig. 13.4d**). These leaks typically seal spontaneously and may be seen more frequently with thinner and more porous stent grafts. Type V endoleaks are not true leaks but are defined as aneurysm sac expansion of >5 mm in the absence of a radiologically identifiable endoleak. They are considered to be due to a phenomenon of endotension caused by the accumulation of a transudate due to ultrafiltration of blood across the stent graft material.

Graft migration and dislocation

Successful EVAR depends on the generation of a blood-tight seal between stent graft and healthy native vessel for AAA exclusion. Failure at any attachment site renders the endograft insecure and prone to abnormal movement (migration) that is facilitated by systemic arterial blood pressure. Significant device migration at the seal zones predisposes the patient to endoleak (type I), whereas unwanted mobility of modular systems may lead to component dislocation and potential type III endoleak.

Device migration most likely results from the combined effect of patient and device related factors with a proximal attachment site failure most often described. In view of the significant risk of type I endoleak associated with distal migration of the proximal stent, remedial intervention is almost always indicated. This can usually be achieved with aortic cuff deployment to repair the proximal seal, but occasionally stent revision is required.

Kinking and occlusion

Any distortion (kinking) of the endograft used in EVAR may result in stent stenosis, thrombosis and ultimately device (or limb) occlusion (**Fig. 13.5**). In a review of 4613 EVAR cases submitted to the EUROSTAR registry over an 8-year period, postoperative graft kinking was described in 3.7% cases.[55] Patent, symptomatic kinked stents can usually by treated by balloon angioplasty and adjunctive stenting, whereas occluded limbs typically require surgery.

Other EVAR-related complications

Wire and stent manipulation within the aorta and aneurysmal sac during positioning and device deployment carries the risk of atheroembolisation with potential for organ infarcts and limb ischaemia. Introduction of guidewires, large-bore catheters and the endograft itself risks vessel injury such as rupture or dissection. Delayed presentations or iatrogenic arterial injury may occur, with pseudoaneurysm formation requiring prompt repair.

Surveillance after EVAR

The modes of failure after aortic stent grafting are well documented. It is mandatory that all patients be recruited onto a programme of systematic postoperative surveillance with the aim of detecting causes of late rupture. The principal concerns are endoleak, aneurysm enlargement and migration of stents at the aortic or iliac landing zones or at the modular connections. Options for the method of surveillance include duplex ultrasound, CT, magnetic resonance imaging (MRI) and plain radiography.

It has been shown that ultrasound can be used to detect graft-related (type I) endoleaks reliably.[56] Ultrasound is less effective for the detection of type II endoleaks, but since it is known that type II endoleaks without increased sac diameter are not associated with a significant risk of adverse clinical events, this may be regarded as an acceptable limitation. Plain radiography using a standardised protocol is an effective method for the detection of device migration. Stent fractures and separation of modular components are also relatively easy to identify. It is comparatively

Table 13.2 • Endoleak classification

Endoleak type		Source
I	A: Proximal	Graft attachment site
	B: Distal	
	C: Iliac occluder	
II	A: Simple (single vessel)	Collateral vessel
	B: Complex (>2 vessels)	
III	A: Junctional leak	Graft failure
	B: Mid-graft hole	
	C: Other (e.g. suture hole)	
IV		Graft wall porosity
V	A: Without endoleak	Endotension
	B: With sealed endoleak	
	C: With type I or III leak	
	D: With type II leak	

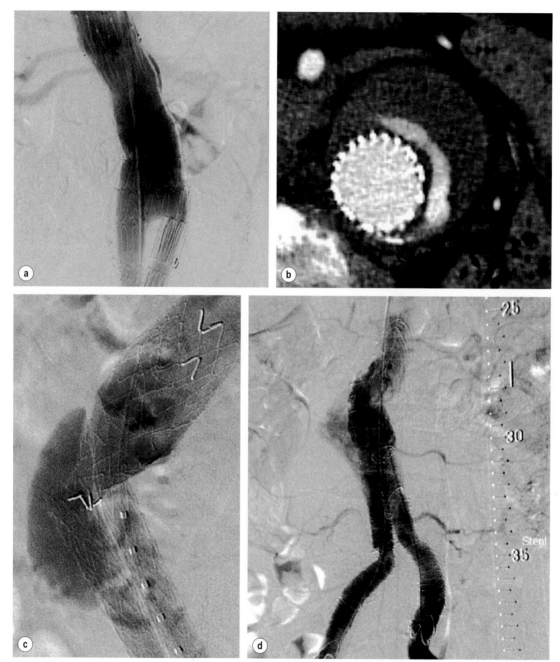

Figure 13.4 • Images showing type I–IV endoleaks post-EVAR. **(a)** Completion angiogram showing a type I endoleak (proximal seal failure). **(b)** Post-EVAR contrast-enhanced CT scan showing a type II endoleak. **(c)** Delayed angiogram showing a type III endoleak (junctional graft failure). **(d)** Completion angiogram showing a type IV endoleak (graft porosity).

inexpensive and usefully complements ultrasound scanning. Used in combination these two methods represent an acceptable alternative to CT for surveillance.

It is generally accepted that surveillance after EVAR should be lifelong. The surveillance intervals vary but typically include baseline imaging with CT and plain radiography at 1 month after EVAR. Most protocols include more frequent surveillance intervals during the first 2 years, with annual surveillance thereafter.[57]

Outcomes after EVAR

There is now a good evidence base from randomised controlled trials in the UK, USA, Netherlands and France to support the use of EVAR in the normal infrarenal AAA population.[58–60]

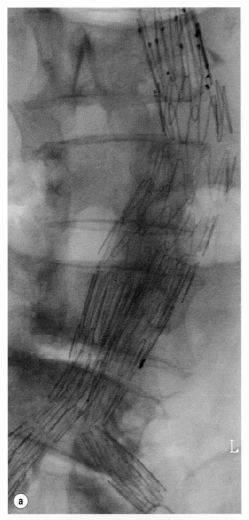

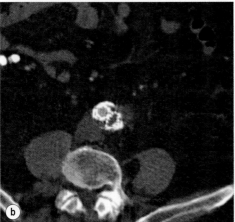

Figure 13.5 • Post-EVAR imaging showing graft kinking and occlusion in the same patient. **(a)** Plain film showing left iliac limb kinking. **(b)** Contrast-enhanced CT scan showing consequent intraluminal occlusion.

✔✔ The UK EVAR-1 trial enrolled 1082 patients with suitable aneurysms (mean diameter 65 mm) that were considered fit enough for elective open AAA surgery and randomised them to either EVAR or conventional open repair (OR). Early outcome analysis revealed significantly lower 30-day mortality for the EVAR group (1.7%) compared to open surgical controls (4.7%). Medium-term study follow-up reported EVAR to be as effective as surgery in protecting from late aneurysm-related death, although there was a significantly higher rate of graft-related complications following EVAR (35% vs 8%). In a smaller but similarly designed study, the Dutch DREAM trial compared outcome following EVAR and OR in 345 fit patients. A significantly lower operative mortality rate post EVAR was confirmed (1.2% vs 4.6%) with reduced incidence of early severe postoperative complications. At 2-year follow-up, however, there was no observed survival advantage after EVAR or OR.[58–60]

The UK EVAR-1 trial demonstrated a clear short-term benefit for EVAR compared with open surgery. Furthermore, EVAR was found to be associated with a shorter hospital stay. However, this survival advantage is eroded over follow-up. By 4-year follow-up, there are no differences in all-cause mortality between patients who had EVAR or open aneurysm repair. The latest 15-year results of the EVAR-1 trial have generated further debate; beyond 8 years follow-up, open-repair has a significantly lower all-cause mortality with an increased aneurysm and cancer mortality amongst EVAR patients. Potential explanations for this finding include poor compliance with EVAR surveillance protocols during the trial follow-up and whether endoleaks in the trial were managed to the level of contemporary standards.[61]

✔✔ The latest 15-year results of the EVAR-1 trial have shown that open repair is associated with a long-term survival benefit when compared with EVAR. After 8 years of follow-up both total and aneurysm-related mortality were significantly higher in the EVAR group than in the OR group (adjusted HR 1.25, 95% CI 1.00–1.56, $P = 0.048$ for total mortality; and 5.82, 1.64–20.65, $P = 0.0064$ for aneurysm-related mortality). After the first 6 months, the increased aneurysm-related deaths in the EVAR group were predominantly from secondary sac rupture (13 deaths [7%] in EVAR vs 2 [1%] in OR). Reinterventions occurred in both groups during follow-up, including in patients who were free from reintervention after 2 years or even 5 years. The rate of reintervention was higher in the EVAR group at all follow-up timepoints. An increased cancer mortality was also observed in the EVAR group.[61]

Renal failure after EVAR is associated with an increased rate of mortality and its aetiology is probably multifactorial. Implicated factors include radiological contrast-associated nephropathy, renal artery trauma, stent-induced stenosis and aortic neck thromboembolism following vessel instrumentation and manipulation. It is rare for the renal ostia to be inadvertently covered by graft fabric, and careful planning and deployment decrease the risk of this occurring. There was concern that the introduction of suprarenal bare-stent fixation would lead to increased rates of renal failure, especially in patients with pre-existing renal impairment; however, studies have failed to demonstrate this.[62]

A large American observational study has also shown that EVAR patients are more likely to undergo AAA-related reinterventions during 4-year follow-up.[63] However, these were less likely to require inpatient hospitalisation compared to reintervention following open aneurysm repair. Among patients who underwent EVAR in the randomised trials, 20–30% required a secondary reintervention over the following 6 years. Cost-analyses from the EVAR-1 trial have shown EVAR to be associated with a higher cost than open repair.[64]

These long-term results raise questions over the durability of EVAR. For the majority of patients EVAR still provides short-term but no long-term benefits but it is clear that lifelong surveillance is necessary to prevent aneurysm-related death. For the very frail patient with multiple comorbidities, if life expectancy is adequate then EVAR after appropriate medical optimisation may bring some benefits; if life expectancy is short, EVAR is unlikely to bring any benefits.[65] Future work modelling the extent of any benefit in subgroups may help clarify this issue. Patient preference is also important in terms of surgical approach. Clinical decision-making skills clearly remain of crucial importance in the management of patients with large aneurysms.

✓✓ The UK EVAR-2 trial randomised 338 medically unfit patients who were anatomical candidates for endovascular AAA repair (>55 mm) to either EVAR or 'best medical therapy' (BMT). The early mortality in the EVAR limb was 9% and at a mean follow-up of 3.3 years there was no difference in the all-cause aneurysm-related mortality between the groups. Many clinicians have adopted these findings as justification not to offer EVAR in the higher-risk population. Caution is advised against this approach to management as closer scrutiny of the

EVAR-2 results reveals some complicating issues. Firstly, there appeared to be an unacceptable delay from randomisation to treatment in the EVAR limb, so that nearly half (9 of 20) of the aneurysm-related mortality was explained by rupture prior to planned AAA repair. Operative (EVAR) mortality was surprisingly high (9%) and the rupture rate in the medically treated group (9 per 100 person-years) was significantly lower than expected, raising concern about disparate medical management between the two groups. Clearly, though, EVAR-2 demonstrates the poor long-term prognosis of the unfit AAA patient irrespective of treatment, with only 62–66% alive at 4 years.

The long-term follow-up of the EVAR-2 trial shows that after 8 years EVAR is associated with much improved aneurysm-related survival (86% at 6 years vs 64% for no intervention), although no clear difference in all-cause survival was observed (30% at 6 years vs 26%). The ability of EVAR to reduce aneurysm rupture (and aneurysm-related mortality) but not to improve survival is the sting in the tail for EVAR. However, after 8 years less than 20% of the patients remained alive, so that the long-term outcome for these patients might carry less weight than for those enrolled in the EVAR trial 1.[65]

The future of EVAR

There is still doubt whether the advantages of EVAR are reproducible in the case of AAA rupture, with several groups advocating its role. Avoidance of laparotomy confers a marked physiological advantage over open repair in an already dire situation. However, the urgency associated with ruptured AAA repair results in little or no time being available to gather the required morphological information prior to EVAR. This is of particular importance since these aneurysms tend to have shorter and wider necks and are therefore more challenging for EVAR with current devices. Furthermore, the requirement of a permanently available on-call endovascular team with access to the appropriate facilities for EVAR is a significant obstacle in most centres.

The IMPROVE trial is the largest randomised controlled trial to determine whether endovascular repair improves the survival of all patients with ruptured AAA. This pragmatic trial randomised patients with an in-hospital clinical diagnosis of ruptured AAA. The trial showed no difference in mortality between EVAR and open repair patients.[66] Similar findings were seen in two other contemporary European randomised controlled trials. Interestingly, the study did demonstrate shorter hospital stays, better quality of life and superior cost effectiveness for patients treated with EVAR.[67]

The UK IMPROVE trial enrolled 613 patients with a clinical diagnosis of ruptured AAA of whom two-thirds were randomised to either open or endovascular repair. Thirty-day mortality was 35% in the endovascular strategy group and 37% in the open repair group. At 1 year, all-cause mortality was 41.1% for the endovascular strategy group and 45.1% for the open repair group The endovascular strategy group and open repair groups had average total hospital stays of 17 and 26 days, respectively, *P* <0.001. Patients surviving rupture had health-related quality-of-life scores in the endovascular strategy compared to the open repair groups at 3 and 12 months. There were indications that QALY were higher and costs lower for the endovascular first strategy.[66]

More than 50% of patients have aneurysm morphology that is unsuitable for conventional endovascular repair.[42] Of these, a significant proportion will have an inadequate length of normal infrarenal aorta above the aneurysm within which to achieve a proximal seal, and account for up to 15% of AAA.[68] Fenestrated endovascular aneurysm repair (FEVAR) was first described in 1999 as an endoluminal solution for patients with an inadequate infrarenal aortic neck.[69] Fabric fenestrations of the endograft, with or without bridging stents, permit perfusion of visceral branch vessels while achieving a secure proximal seal. Fenestrations may be one of three types: scallops, small or large circular fenestrations. Scalloped grafts have a U-shaped defect in the leading edge of the endografts for preserved patency of the most proximal visceral arteries. Both of the other types of fenestration reside in the body of the device fabric. The bare-metal scaffold traverses large fenestrations, whereas small fenestrations lie between stent struts and require secondary stenting to achieve a seal and prevent occlusion (**Fig. 13.6**). Observational data on the use of these devices has shown promise and these devices are now widely used in major vascular centres globally. An Achilles heel of these devices is their bespoke nature, which continues to necessitate a 6–12 week manufacture time for each graft.

Data from the United Kingdom have demonstrated that FEVAR can be performed with a high degree of technical success with good clinical outcomes[70] (**Fig. 13.7a**). Although mortality rates of less than 5% were reported, the selected nature of these data and the lack of long-term follow-up make widespread application of this technique difficult to justify at present. Concerns about these devices include uncertainty regarding the long-term patency of stents in normal branch vessels, the increased

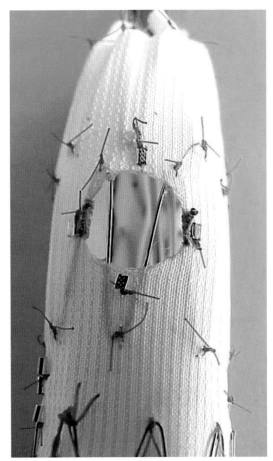

Figure 13.6 • Fenestrated stent graft used for the treatment of perirenal aortic aneurysms.
Courtesy of Cook Medical.

number of modular connections and the possibility that the branches may kink if the aneurysm shrinks (**Fig. 13.7b**). The technology is evolving rapidly and 'off-the-shelf' fenestrated grafts will soon become readily available.

An alternative strategy for short-necked AAA is the use of parallel chimney grafts alongside conventional aortic endografts (**Fig. 13.8**). This technique has gained application as an off-the-shelf, less expensive alternative to custom-made fenestrated graft. Again, promising results have been reported in observational studies and a systematic review reported a 5% 30-day mortality.[71] Nevertheless, concerns persist about the lack of randomised data and longer-term follow-up. Further concerns exist around the potential for endoleaks in the gutters between chimney and aortic grafts.

More recently, polymer technology has been utilised to develop novel solutions for managing

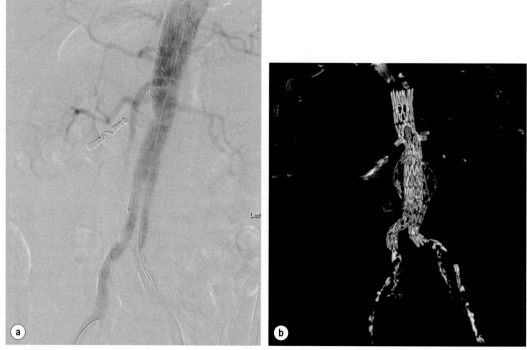

Figure 13.7 • Three-fenestration stent graft with coil embolisation of accessory right renal artery and satisfactory exclusion of juxtarenal abdominal aortic aneurysm. **(a)** Completion angiogram. **(b)** Reconstruction of surveillance CT aortogram.

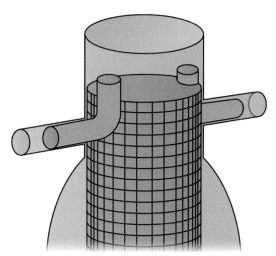

Figure 13.8 • Schematic representation of chimney grafts/snorkels.

AAA. The first method modifies conventional aortic stent grafts to use inflatable polymer rings to create a seal at the neck of the aneurysm. It is argued that this method avoids the constant outward force, and potential for future dilatation, on the aortic neck that a conventional stent graft would exert.[72] A more innovative use of polymers is seen in the technique of endovascular aneurysm sealing (EVAS). The procedure is similar to traditional EVAR; two balloon expandable stents grafts with attached endobags are delivered up each iliac artery and deployed below the renal arteries. A biostable polyethylene glycol polymer is injected through the catheters into the endobags to fill the aneurysm sac, sealing it off from the circulation and holding the stent graft in place. This technique may negate the problem of short aortic necks and type II endoleaks.[73] For both methods, proof of durability is eagerly awaited.

Infected aneurysms

Although much less common than degenerative pathology, infected aneurysms remain an important subgroup of the disease. Since the introduction of antibiotic therapy and concomitant decline of endocarditis, true mycotic aneurysms are now uncommonly seen. Conversely, with increasing intravenous drug abuse (IVDA), post-traumatic infected false femoral aneurysms are now a major clinical problem confronting the vascular specialist. These are discussed in more detail in the section on femoral aneurysms.

Mycotic aneurysms

True mycotic aneurysm results when septic emboli lodge in the vasa vasorum of an artery. This is typically in the setting of infective endocarditis. Patients tend to be middle-aged and may have multiple aneurysms at differing sites. Both normal and abnormal vessels in any territory may be affected although there is a predilection of the aorta, intracranial, visceral and femoral vessels. The causative organisms are usually Gram-positive cocci, in particular *Streptococcus* spp. and *Staphylococcus aureus*.

Microbial aneurysmal arteritis

With an ageing population with attendant increasing prevalence of atherosclerosis, microbial arteritis with aneurysm formation is now more common than true mycotic aneurysm. The pathological process involves blood-borne bacteria seeding into a diseased intima with subsequent suppuration, localised perforation and pseudoaneurysm formation. Unlike mycotic aneurysm, healthy native vessels are not affected. Aortic involvement is typical and pathology in this location is three times more common than in the peripheral circulation (**Fig. 13.9**). The classical infecting microorganisms are the *Salmonella* spp., but others have been reported, including *Escherichia coli*, *Staphylococcus* spp. and *Klebsiella pneumoniae*.

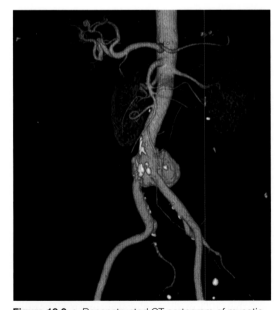

Figure 13.9 • Reconstructed CT aortogram of mycotic saccular aortic aneurysm.

Clinical features and management principles of infected aneurysms

The clinical presentation of an infected aneurysm depends both on the site of involvement and the underlying infective process. Usually, the patient presents with a pyrexia of unknown origin and little else; therefore a high index of suspicion is necessary. Supportive features include positive blood cultures, raised white cell counts, uncalcified aneurysms, vertebral erosion and a first presentation of aneurysm following an episode of bacterial sepsis. Classical radiological or appearances on angiography may or may not be present; and include saccular aneurysms, multilobulated and/or eccentric pathology with a narrow neck.

Following diagnosis, all patients should be commenced on appropriate antibiotics. Traditional management strategy for infected aneurysm has been one of open surgical repair. The principles of such surgery are generic, irrespective of the site and include: haemorrhage control, sepsis control (aneurysm resection, wide debridement, irrigation and drainage); confirmation of diagnosis (specimen culture and sensitivity); and arterial reconstruction, usually with an autologous conduit, e.g. superficial femoral vein for creation of a neo-aorta. In some instances, cadaveric or prosthetic grafts may be used in situ or routed away from the infected field. Postoperatively, the patient should be treated with long-term antibiotics that may be lifelong in some cases. Recently, increasing interest has centred on the use of endovascular stent grafts to treat infected aneurysms. The minimally invasive nature of this approach is appealing, with improved short-term outcomes, but balanced against uncertain long-term outcomes in terms of infection control.[74]

Despite improvements in diagnosis, surgical techniques and pharmacology, the early outcome for patients with infected aortic aneurysm remains poor, with a mortality rate of 23%. Infected post-traumatic false aneurysms are associated with better outcomes (5% mortality), but the lower limb amputation rate may be up to 25–33% if the femoral artery is involved.

Peripheral aneurysms

Iliac aneurysms

Up to 40% of iliac aneurysms occur in association with aortic aneurysms. Isolated iliac aneurysms are comparatively unusual, the prevalence having been estimated to be less than 2% of aorto-iliac aneurysms. They tend to be large (4–8 cm) and typically involve either the common or internal iliac arteries. Aneurysmal disease of the external iliac artery is extremely rare.

Generally accepted guidance is that elective open or endovascular intervention is indicated for asymptomatic iliac aneurysms greater than 3–4 cm in diameter.[75] Symptomatic and ruptured aneurysms require immediate surgical intervention. Once again, treatment may be performed with an open surgical repair with a Dacron™ graft or if anatomy permits, an endovascular stent graft for isolated common iliac aneurysm. Isolated internal iliac aneurysms are usually managed by open surgical ligation or endovascular embolisation.

Common femoral aneurysms

Femoral arterial aneurysms can be divided simply into true or false (pseudo) aneurysms. True aneurysms relate to a distinct pathological process involving all three layers of the femoral arterial wall. False aneurysms are due to a traumatic breach of a vessel wall with an associated contained blood collection with flow.

Both disease processes may be symptomatic or asymptomatic. Symptomatic femoral aneurysms can present as a pulsatile groin mass that may or may not be painful, leg swelling (due to femoral vein compression and deep vein thrombosis) or features associated with chronic ischaemia attributable to aneurysm thrombosis/embolisation. Rupture can occur but is rare. Asymptomatic pathology is usually discovered incidentally on clinical examination or imaging studies of a patient with an aneurysm elsewhere or with chronic ischaemia.

True femoral aneurysms

True femoral aneurysms are the second commonest peripheral artery aneurysm after the popliteal artery. They occur in 2–3% of patients with aortic aneurysms and tend to be a disease of elderly men (male-to-female ratio 30:1). The condition is frequently bilateral and a coexistent generalised aneurysmal process may be manifest in other anatomical sites such as the aorto-iliac or popliteal arteries.

Small, asymptomatic true femoral artery aneurysms can be managed expectantly with clinical assessment at intervals. Surgical treatment is indicated for symptoms and probably for most aneurysms of 3.5 cm or more in size.[76] Usually, a short interposition or inlay tube graft anastomosed proximally at the level of the inguinal ligament and distal to the common femoral bifurcation is required. This is a relatively small operation with durable results.

False femoral aneurysms

The common femoral artery is regularly used for catheterisation of the arterial circulation (e.g. angiography, cardiac catheterisation, EVAR, intra-aortic balloon pumps, etc.). As a consequence, iatrogenic injury leading to false aneurysm is a relatively common occurrence that complicates approximately 1% of transfemoral interventions. The diagnosis should be suspected in any patient with a pulsatile mass at the site of a recent arterial cannulation. Initially a duplex scan should be obtained to both confirm the diagnosis and characterise the false aneurysm. If the pathology is small (<2 cm) and associated with minimal symptoms, simple observation with re-scanning may be justified, as most of these pseudoaneurysms will thrombose spontaneously within 2–4 weeks. Other options include compression therapy (direct pressure and/or ultrasound guided) in an effort to seal the feeding arterial jet. Thrombin injection is an effective treatment with a reported success rate of over 95%. If these measures fail or in cases of tense swelling, threatened skin viability or neurology, open surgical repair is indicated. Unlike non-invasive methods, surgery has the advantage of combining both the arterial repair and field decompression. The former is usually a primary repair of the vessel with a Prolene suture, although formal graft reconstruction is sometimes required.

Infected femoral pseudoaneurysms are now the most common type of infected aneurysm observed in clinical practice, largely explained by increased intravenous drug abuse in recent years. Although the usual microorganism cultured is a *Staphylococcus* species, the infection may be polymicrobial and close liaison with the microbiology team is required for appropriate antibiotic therapy. The surgical strategy for infected femoral false aneurysms depends largely on its cause. For non-IVDA patients, arterial excision and reconstruction with autologous conduit (e.g. long saphenous vein and obturator bypass) following the operative principles for infected aneurysms outlined earlier is preferred. In IVDA patients, arterial excision with ligation alone (i.e. no reconstruction) is advised due to the unacceptable risk of subsequent graft infection with continued drug abuse and likelihood of exhausted superficial veins (**Fig. 13.10a,b**). Ligation of the femoral artery does not necessarily mandate amputation if only one femoral segment is involved. If the femoral bifurcation is excised, however, the risk of limb loss is significant and reconstructive surgery may need to be considered, although this is contentious.

Popliteal artery aneurysms

Popliteal aneurysms are the most commonly encountered peripheral aneurysm, accounting for more than 80% of all peripheral aneurysms. The ratio of popliteal aneurysms to AAAs is approximately

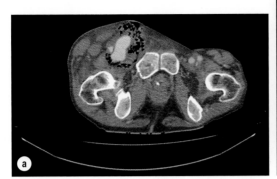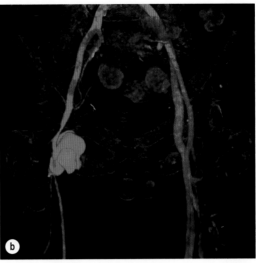

Figure 13.10 • CT angiogram of mycotic false aneurysm of right common femoral artery. **(a)** Cross-sectional image of false aneurysm with gas in soft tissues. **(b)** Reconstructed CT of mycotic aneurysm at common femoral bifurcation.

1:15. Half are bilateral, a third asymptomatic and 40% are associated with AAAs.

Although rupture is rare, 50% of cases present with peripheral limb-threatening ischaemia. In common with aneurysms at all other sites, laminated thrombus develops within popliteal aneurysms. The popliteal artery is continually subjected to flexion and extension, greatly increasing the risk of disintegration and embolisation of this thrombus. In many patients microembolisation of the peripheral circulation occurs silently prior to main vessel occlusion or thrombosis of the popliteal aneurysm itself. For this reason, the viability of the limb may be seriously threatened. Furthermore, compromise of the run-off circulation can impact adversely on the outcome from emergency bypass surgery. The bigger the aneurysm, the more likely there is to be thrombus. The presence of intraluminal thrombus is therefore a more important indication for elective surgical intervention than the size of the aneurysm. Any thrombus detected by ultrasound, CT or MRI constitutes an indication for elective treatment. In the absence of laminated thrombus, it is generally accepted that aneurysms with a diameter of 2 cm or greater warrant consideration for elective surgical repair.

Traditionally, popliteal aneurysms are treated by proximal and distal ligation and bypass using autologous vein undertaken via a medial approach. However, recent studies have identified persistent flow within the popliteal aneurysm in 30% of patients treated in this way. Furthermore, there is a significant risk of continued expansion and even rupture due to pressurisation of the sac resulting

from backflow through geniculate branches. Therefore, a posterior approach and insertion of an inlay graft is to be preferred.[77]

An acutely thrombosed popliteal aneurysm is a clinical emergency. Preoperative or on-table thrombolysis has been used to open up the run-off vessels and thereby facilitate bypass surgery. There is some low-level evidence to suggest that this approach may improve the chances of successful limb salvage.

With the evolution of flexible endografts, endovascular repair is now a viable alternative to open surgery for the treatment of some popliteal aneurysms. Long-term follow-up suggests that in selected patients this is a durable technique, capable of achieving excellent patency rates and limb preservation[78] (**Fig. 13.11a–c**). Further large-scale clinical trials are warranted to help define optimal candidates for this technique.

✓✓ Another important determinant of patient outcome following AAA repair is the ability and experience of the operating surgeon. A recent meta-analysis demonstrated a significantly lower mortality following AAA repair with higher volume surgeons and suggested a minimum caseload of 13 open AAAs per annum for continued practice. With further analysis, this number is likely to rise and, naturally, this has significant implications for the provision of vascular services and would support the argument for fewer, larger, regional vascular centres linked directly to a nationwide targeted AAA screening programme.[79]

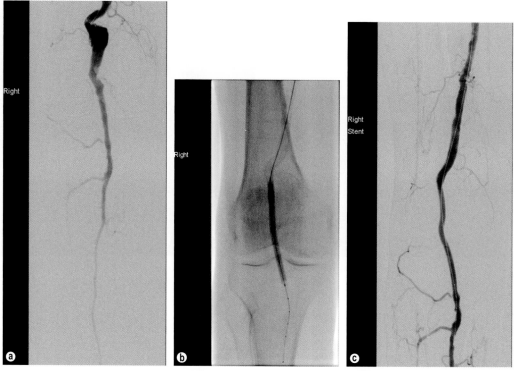

Figure 13.11 • Angiogram of popliteal aneurysm. **(a)** Diagnostic angiogram. **(b)** Balloon moulding of popliteal stent graft. **(c)** Completion angiogram of popliteal stent graft.

Key points

- The prevalence of AAA appears to be declining, as does aneurysm rupture and mortality.
- There are good clinical and cost-effectiveness data to support targeted population-based screening programmes for AAA.
- The UK Small Aneurysm Trial supported a policy of surveillance rather than operation for patients with AAAs of less than 5.5 cm diameter.
- Three principal, randomised controlled trials for abdominal aortic aneurysm have shown marked benefits of EVAR over open repair with respect to 30-day mortality.
- However, the total mortality benefit of EVAR was lost in these randomised controlled trials after 1–5 years.
- Beyond 8 years, open aneurysm repair was associated with better survival and durability than EVAR in the UK EVAR-1 trial
- EVAR requires annual surveillance and has a crude annual reintervention rate of 4%.
- EVAR does not confer a survival advantage in patients who are unfit for open aneurysm repair as 50% will die within 5 years, mostly from comorbidity rather than rupture.
- EVAR has not been shown to be superior, in terms of survival, to open repair in ruptured AAAs. However, it is associated with shorter hospital stay, better quality of life and cost-effectiveness.
- Technological advances have widened the endovascular treatment options for juxtarenal AAAs.
- Infected true aneurysms are associated with a poor prognosis, but their incidence is falling.

Recommended videos
EVAS – https://tinyurl.com/yaolz8ug
EVAR – https://tinyurl.com/y7fyyvjl

Full references available at http://expertconsult.inkling.com

Key references

34. Ashton HA, Buxton MJ, Day NE, et al. The Multicentre Aneurysm Screening Study (MASS) into the effect of abdominal aortic aneurysm screening on mortality in men: a randomised controlled trial. Lancet 2002;360:1531–9. PMID: 12443589.
A UK multicentre population-based screening study of 67 800 men, aged 65–74 years, who were randomly allocated to be invited to attend for ultrasound assessment or not. The primary outcome measure was aneurysm-related death and there was a 42% risk reduction in the invited group.

35. Multicentre Aneurysm Screening Study Group. Screening men for abdominal aortic aneurysm: 10-year mortality and cost effectiveness results from the Multicentre Aneurysm Screening Study. Br Med J 2009;338:b2307. PMID: 19553269.
Cost-effectiveness analysis at 4 years showed that the cost per quality-adjusted life-year (QALY) was £36 000. It is projected that this value will fall to £8000 per QALY within 10 years.

37. Wanhainen A, Hultgren R, Linné A, et al. Outcome of the Swedish Nationwide Abdominal Aortic Aneurysm Screening Program. Circulation 2016;134:1141–8. PMID: 27630132.
Outcome data on 302 957 men aged 65 years invited for AAA screening. There was a 1.5% prevalence and 29% had AAA repair. Screening was associated with a significant reduction in AAA-specific mortality. The number needed to screen and the number needed to operate on to prevent 1 premature death were 667 and 1.5, respectively. Screening 65-year-old men for AAA is an effective preventive health measure and is highly cost-effective in a contemporary setting.

40. The UK Small Aneurysm Trial Participants. Mortality results for randomised controlled trial of early elective surgery or ultrasonographic surveillance for small abdominal aortic aneurysms. Lancet 1998;352:1649–55. PMID: 9853436.
A multicentre randomised controlled trial of 1090 patients with asymptomatic aneurysms of diameter 4.0–5.5 cm who were randomly allocated to early elective surgery or ultrasound surveillance. There was no significant survival advantage at 6 years for those undergoing surgical repair.

44. Greenhalgh RM, Brown LC, Kwong GP. Comparison of endovascular aneurysm repair with open repair in patients with abdominal aortic aneurysm (EVAR trial 1), 30-day operative mortality results: randomised controlled trial. Lancet 2004;364:843–8. PMID: 15351191.
A multicentre randomised controlled trial comparing open and endovascular repair in patients anatomically suitable for either. The 30-day mortality results show an initial survival advantage for patients treated with EVAR.

45. Johnston KW. Non-ruptured abdominal aortic aneurysm: six-year follow up results from the multicentre prospective Canadian aneurysm study. Canadian Society for Vascular Surgery Aneurysm Study Group. J Vasc Surg 1994;20:163–70. PMID: 8040938.
A prospective analysis of 680 patients undergoing elective aneurysm surgery showed that cardiac-related death is the major perioperative risk and cardiac and cerebrovascular events are the major causes of death at 6 years.

58. The UK EVAR trial investigators. Endovascular versus open repair of abdominal aortic aneurysm. N Engl J Med 2010;362:1863–71. PMID: 20382983.
In this large randomised trial, endovascular repair of AAAs was associated with a significantly lower operative mortality than open repair, However, no differences were seen in total mortality or aneurysm-related mortality in the long term. Endovascular repair was associated with increased rates of graft-related complications and reinterventions and was more costly.

61. The UK EVAR trial investigators. Endovascular versus open repair of abdominal aortic aneurysm in 15-years' follow-up of the UK endovascular aneurysm repair trial 1 (EVAR trial 1): a randomised controlled trial. Lancet 2016;388:2366–74. PMID: 27743617.
The 15-year follow-up data from this trial showed that after 8 years, open repair was superior to endovascular aneurysm repair in terms of all-cause mortality and aneurysm-related mortality.

65. EVAR Trial participants. Endovascular aneurysm repair and outcome in patients unfit for open repair of abdominal aortic aneurysm (EVAR-2 trial): randomized controlled trial. Lancet 2005;365:2187–92. PMID: 15978926.
A multicentre randomised trial comparing EVAR and best medical therapy in 338 unfit patients with morphologically suitable AAAs; 30-day mortality was 9% in the EVAR group and at a mean follow-up of 3.3 years there was no difference in either the all-cause or aneurysm-related mortality between groups.

66. Improve Trial investigators. Endovascular or open repair strategy for ruptured abdominal aortic aneurysm: 30-day outcomes from IMPROVE randomised trial. BMJ 2014;348:f7661. PMID: 24418950.

A multicentre randomised trial of 613 patients with ruptured AAA randomised to either an attempted endovascular strategy or open repair. Thirty day mortality was 35% in the endovascular strategy group and 37% in the open repair group. A strategy of endovascular repair was not associated with significant reduction in either 30-day mortality or cost.

70. British Society for Endovascular Therapy and the Global Collaborators on Advanced Stent-Graft Techniques for Aneurysm Repair (GLOBALSTAR) Registry. Early results of fenestrated endovascular repair of juxtarenal aortic aneurysm in the United Kingdom. Circulation 2012;125:2707–15. PMID: 22665884.

A registry study of 318 patients from 14 British centres undergoing fenestrated EVAR. Primary procedural success was achieved in 99%; perioperative mortality was 4.1%. The early reintervention (<30 days) rate was 7% (22/318).

79. Young EL, Holt PJ, Poloniecki JD, et al. Meta-analysis and systematic review of the relationship between surgeon annual caseload and mortality for elective open abdominal aortic aneurysm repairs. J Vasc Surg 2007;46:1287–94. PMID: 17950569.

A meta-analysis involving 115 273 elective open AAA repairs demonstrating significantly lower mortality with higher caseload surgeons. The study suggested a critical case volume threshold of 13 open AAA repairs per annum.

14

Thoracic and thoraco-abdominal aortic disease

Benjamin Patterson
Peter Holt
Ian Loftus

Introduction

Diseases of the thoracic and thoraco-abdominal aorta are less common than infrarenal abdominal aortic aneurysms but their management should be familiar to all vascular surgeons, as they often present acutely and unexpectedly in a variety of settings. This is partly due to the greater utilisation of cross-sectional imaging, which has in turn led to an apparent increase in the incidence of thoracic aortic conditions.[1] Over the last two decades, endovascular repair has become the first-line treatment of choice for most distal arch, descending and thoraco-abdominal aortic pathologies. Despite the move toward minimally invasive strategies, the increasing employment of endovascular repair of the thoracic aorta (TEVAR) has lacked the large randomised trials that underpinned the widespread adoption of standard infrarenal repair (EVAR). Registry data, institutional cases series and national routine data have suggested that endovascular procedures can be offered with low mortality and morbidity rates in comparison with open repair of thoracic pathology, and appear to be equally as effective in preventing aortic-related death.[2,3] Critics of the increase in the repair of thoracic pathology draw attention to the lack of accurate contemporary natural history data for untreated pathology, and also that newer and costly technologies lack data on their long-term durability. In the case of aortic dissection there is continuing controversy over the role of TEVAR in uncomplicated acute and chronic dissection and the ability of this procedure to prevent aortic-related death. The advance of fenestrated and branched stent-graft technology has allowed many patients that were previously not fit enough to undergo treatment by highly invasive open surgery of the thoraco-abdominal aorta to be offered complex TEVAR, although open repair is still recommended for those with connective tissue disorders. This chapter reviews the contemporary treatment of thoracic and thoraco-abdominal aortic disease, excluding the ascending aorta.

Imaging of the thoracic aorta

Computed tomographic angiography (CTA) is the investigation of choice to diagnose aortic pathology and plan subsequent repair. Modern workstations allow reformatting of images in multiple planes with the derivation of luminal centrelines. These techniques can be used to estimate lengths and diameters to a greater degree of accuracy than axial images alone, and are essential if endovascular repair is planned[4] (Fig. 14.1). CTA is also the modality of choice when performing surveillance for patients that have had previous repair. The disadvantages of CTA are the relatively high dose of radiation required and the need for nephrotoxic intravenous contrast.[5,6] In younger patients, such as those with connective tissue disorder who are likely to require some years of surveillance, magnetic resonance angiography (MRA) may be more appropriate, but offers less spatial resolution than CTA. MRA has been used in experimental applications for patients with aortic dissection to characterise flow in the false lumen and this may come to represent an important way to predict disease progression and success of treatment in the future.[7]

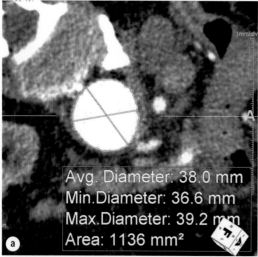

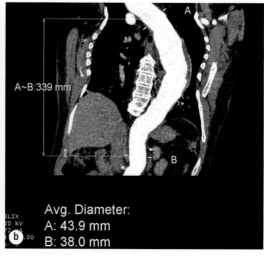

Figure 14.1 • Planning thoracic endovascular intervention using images produced by reconstruction of CT angiographic images of the thoracic aorta. This allows more accurate measurements of lengths and diameters, vital when selecting suitable devices (software shown produced by Terarecon, CA, USA).

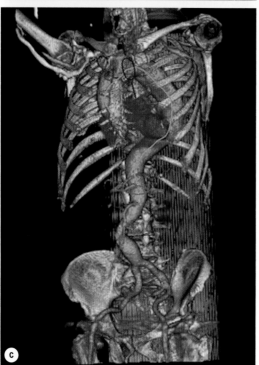

Thoracic aortic aneurysms (TAAs)

Classification and aetiology

The majority of thoracic aortic aneurysms (TAAs) are degenerative or atherosclerotic in nature, although approximately one-quarter are caused by a chronically dilating aortic dissection. Less frequently, aneurysms are related to connective tissue disorders such as Marfan syndrome or Ehler–Danlos syndrome. Mycotic or other inflammatory aneurysms of the thoracic aorta are relatively rare. False aneurysms can be caused by trauma and may present many years after the original precipitating event, or may originate at the site of a previous surgical repair of the aorta. Aneurysms involving the descending aorta and the visceral segment are referred to as thoraco-abdominal aortic aneurysms (TAAAs). The majority of aneurysms are fusiform in morphology. Saccular aneurysms are less common and are usually the result of infection or previous trauma.

Incidence, clinical presentation and indications for treatment

The incidence of aneurysms of the descending thoracic aorta appears to have increased, and in the UK has doubled from 4.4 to 9 per 100 000 patients per year over the last decade.[1] The reason for this apparent increase is probably that thoracic aneurysms are most frequently discovered incidentally on routine chest radiography or cross-sectional imaging to investigate other conditions. Thoracic aneurysms have a strong association with abdominal aortic aneurysms (AAA), and the conditions are concurrent in 23% of men and 48% of women with this condition.[8] Clinical presentations include substernal, back or shoulder pain, superior vena cava syndrome, dysphagia, dyspnoea, stridor and hoarseness and rupture. The risk of rupture increases with the size of the aneurysm, but data regarding estimated annual rupture rates and aortic diameter are sparse and less robust than for the abdominal aorta. The main indications for intervention are symptoms and size. There is controversy regarding the size criteria for treatment of TAAs, and the natural history remains poorly understood.[9] Juvonen et al. reported that the 2-year rupture rate for TAAs was 23% in aneurysms less than 7 cm,[10] whereas Elefteriades observed a 30% 5-year rupture rate when the aorta exceeded 6 cm.[11] A more recent study of 257 patients with TAAs showed that event rates at 1, 3 and 5 years were $4.3\pm1.3\%$, $6.9\pm1.9\%$ and $9.7\pm2.6\%$ for definite aortic events and $6.6\pm1.6\%$, $12.1\pm2.4\%$ and $16.5\pm3.1\%$ for possible events. Those with a starting aortic diameter of <50 mm experienced an event rate of less than 1%, but the rate of definite or possible event rates rose to 2.7 or 8.1% at aortic diameter between 50 mm and 60 mm, and increased exponentially to 37.5 or 62.5% at >70 mm.[12] Most clinicians regard a maximum aortic diameter of 5.5–6 cm as an indication for possible repair in an asymptomatic patient, with the threshold being balanced by the surgical risk. This is reflected in various consensus documents that have been published in recent years.[13] Diameter thresholds should be reduced in patients with defined connective tissue disorders as rupture may occur at smaller aortic diameters.

Technique of surgical repair

The standard method of traditional open surgical repair of TAAs is a left thoracotomy for access, aortic clamping and inlay grafting. In cases involving the aortic arch a two-stage approach may be employed, which is known as an 'elephant trunk' procedure. This comprises open repair of the arch via a median sternotomy and suturing of a surgical graft to the origin of the descending aorta, which is then inverted distally into the aneurysm beyond this point. A second procedure can be performed through a left thoracotomy to continue the repair distally into the chest or an endovascular stent-graft can be deployed into it subsequently. These procedures are technically challenging and physiologically demanding for patients due to the need for aortic cross-clamping of the aorta and organ ischaemia. Several adjuncts are available to achieve these aims, including the use of a Gott shunt, left heart bypass and distal aortic perfusion, selective intercostal shunting and cerebrospinal fluid (CSF) drainage.

Endovascular repair of thoracic aneurysms

Successful endovascular repair is dependent on the presence of suitable access vessels with adequate sealing (or 'landing') zones proximal and distal to the aneurysm. Preoperative CT angiography is assessed to determine which endografts should be used and the mode of access. It is recommended that centreline image reconstruction is employed using vascular-specific software to minimise error during planning.

The optimal proximal landing zones should be between 15 mm and 20 mm along the inner curvature of the aorta, depending on the specific stent-graft manufacturer instructions for use. If the landing zone is considered to be of inadequate length, surgical bypass may be performed to lengthen the effective sealing zone. The supra-aortic trunks that would need to be covered by the endograft determine the Ishimaru zone of the repair (**Fig. 14.2**).[14] If left subclavian artery coverage for an aneurysm extending to Ishimaru zone 2 is required then a carotid subclavian bypass can be employed (**Fig. 14.3**). If Ishimaru zone 1 extent coverage is required, a right-to-left carotid-to-carotid bypass must be employed with or without left subclavian revascularisation. In zone 0 coverage, ascending aorta to innominate and left common carotid bypass via a median sternotomy is performed (**Fig. 14.4**). Different commercially available stent-graft devices are available in different diameters, and these vary from 22 mm to 46 mm. A degree of oversizing is required with respect to the aortic diameter during device selection to ensure sufficient sealing, and it is recommended that this be 15–20%. As a result, the upper and lower limits of landing zone diameter are 40–42 mm and 18 mm, respectively. In many cases more than one device is required, and when calculating the length of coverage then the overlap between adjacent devices recommended by manufacturers should be noted. A recent analysis has suggested that using endografts in unsuitable anatomy may significantly compromise durability.[15]

The TEVAR procedure is usually performed under general or regional anaesthesia, although stents

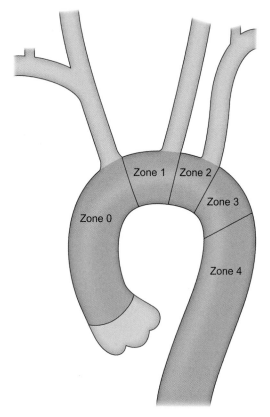

Figure 14.2 • Ishimaru zones describing the proximal extent of the stent-graft landing zone required to achieve an adequate proximal seal.

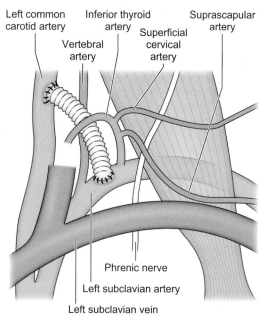

Figure 14.3 • Carotid subclavian bypass performed selectively prior to TEVAR where coverage of the origin of the vessel is required.

can also be inserted using local anaesthesia alone. Transfemoral access is obtained via an arteriotomy or using a percutaneous technique and a 300 mm length of extra-stiff guidewire (e.g. Lunderquist guidewire, Cook, UK) is advanced so that the tip is placed in the ascending aorta. A pigtail angiographic catheter is placed alongside this, and the first device is advanced into position along the stiff wire. Angiographic images are obtained in the correct plane to allow visualisation of the supra-aortic branches. This usually requires a left anterior oblique angulation of the imaging system. The systolic blood pressure should then be reduced to below 100 mmHg peak systolic pressure to allow accurate deployment of the endograft (**Fig. 14.5**). This can be achieved by pharmacological means or overdrive pacing to reduce the cardiac output. Further endografts are placed as necessary with the required overlap between endografts. Angiographic imaging is then used to ensure correct positioning and that adequate proximal and distal seal is achieved.

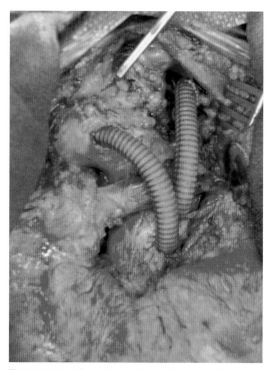

Figure 14.4 • Operative photograph of ascending aorta to innominate and left common carotid. Surgery performed to create an adequate landing zone in a patient with a very proximal thoracic aneurysm.

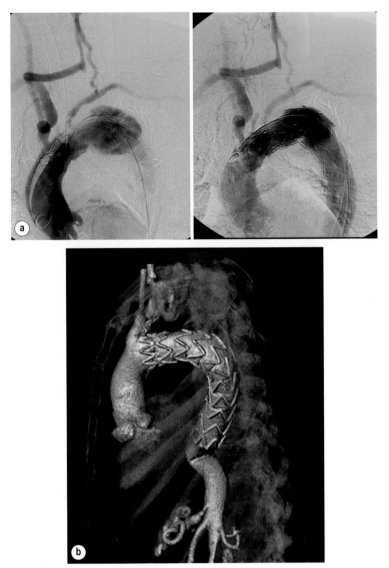

Figure 14.5 • Angiogram demonstrating a large thoracic aneurysm with the landing zone involving the left common carotid artery. To enable endovascular aneurysm repair a right-to-left common carotid bypass has been performed with ligation of the proximal left carotid artery.

Neurological complications following endovascular thoracic procedures

Neurological complications after TEVAR are not uncommon and are related to disturbance of flow in supra-aortic trunks or in the supply to the spinal cord. Stroke and paraplegia have devastating consequences for patients and both are associated with a significant reduction in mid-term survival.[16] No independent precipitating factor of paraplegia has been identified, although coexisting infrarenal aortic pathology or previous abdominal aortic repair may reduce the collateral network supplying the spinal cord.[17] To protect against this, some centres advocate prophylactic drainage of cerebrospinal fluid (CSF) whilst others adopt a selective approach. If signs of spinal cord ischaemia occur then cord perfusion pressure must be increased by reducing CSF pressure (target 10–12 mmHg) via the use of a spinal drain and ensuring a mean arterial pressure of 90–100 mmHg with the use of fluid boluses and inotropes.[11] Controversy has surrounded the management of the left subclavian artery during thoracic endografting. Early experience suggested that it was reasonable to cover the origin of the subclavian artery where necessary to achieve stent-graft seal. Patients with a left internal mammary artery (LIMA) bypass graft or with a dominant left vertebral artery comprised a group where left subclavian revascularisation was considered mandatory. However, in most cases coverage of the left subclavian artery did not appear to be associated with upper limb claudication or other complications. However, it is now generally recommended by consensus guidelines to perform left subclavian revascularisation in an elective situation where possible. Revascularisation can be performed with low morbidity and has been shown to reduce the risk of posterior circulation stroke and also, perhaps, paraplegia in some series, but this is not a consistent finding.[16,18,19]

Outcome of treatment

Results of open repair in centres of excellence have generally been good, with less consistent results reported by smaller institutions. Focus in the last decade has been on comparing the outcome of open and endovascular repair. The GORE TAG trial recruited 140 patients to undergo implantation of the GORE TAG (W.L. Gore & Associates, Flagstaff, Ariz, USA) device, retrospectively comparing outcomes with 94 patients undergoing repair of aneurysms in the descending or distal arch of the thoracic aorta. The 30-day mortality rate was 2.1% in the TEVAR group versus 11.7% in the open repair group.[20] The VALOR trial recruited 195 patients who had the Talent thoracic endograft (Medtronic, Santa-Rosa, CA, USA) implanted. An OSR control arm of 189 patients were matched retrospectively as a control group.[21] As with the TAG device, a lower 30-day mortality was noted in the TEVAR groups when compared to the OSR group (2% vs 8%), and there were approximately half the number of major adverse events. The Cook TX2 pivotal trial recruited 160 patients to undergo treatment with the Cook TX2 thoracic endograft (Cook, Bloomington, USA), with 70 historical open surgical controls.[22] The rate of perioperative adverse events was low in both groups, but there was a significantly lower rate of severe morbidity in the TEVAR group. The MOTHER registry included 670 patients who underwent TEVAR for aneurysmal disease from five Medtronic device specific trials (including VALOR I) and a single institution reported an early death rate of 5%.[2] Despite the protection that repair confers against aortic rupture, patients treated with TEVAR experience a high level of all-cause mortality that is often not related to the primary treated condition.

This can be seen in comparisons with matched control groups of the same age and gender who do not have aneurysmal disease.[23] The MOTHER registry reported a 5-year survival rate of 56%, with most patients dying of cardiovascular causes or malignancy.[2] The Medicare and HES studies study showed a similarly poor rate of survival, with many patients dying of cardiovascular or respiratory disease.[3,24] Appropriate patient selection is vital in maximising mortality benefits from TEVAR.[25]

Recommendations for practice

Endovascular repair of thoracic aortic aneurysms is now first-line therapy for most thoracic aneurysms. The exceptions to this would be in patients with unfavourable anatomy in whom there is a likelihood of poor long-term durability, and elderly frail patients with a poor predicted life expectancy in whom the prevention of aneurysm-related death would not improve their overall survival.[15,25] The endovascular management of patients with connective tissue disease is controversial. These patients are usually younger and fitter than patients with degenerative aneurysms and often have good outcomes from conventional surgery and poorer results from TEVAR.[26] As a result, the routine use of TEVAR in patients with connective tissue disorders is not recommended.

Thoraco-abdominal aortic aneurysms (TAAAs)

Classification and aetiology

Thoracic aneurysms that involve the visceral segment of the abdominal aorta are traditionally described as thoraco-abdominal aneurysms and are classified according to the extent of the aneurysmal disease (see **Fig. 14.6** for a description of the Crawford classification). The aetiology of thoraco-abdominal aneurysms differs from infrarenal aneurysms, with medial degenerative disease and chronic dissection being particularly prevalent.[27] As with thoracic aortic aneurysm, connective tissue disorders are a strong risk factor for the development of TAAAs.

Incidence, clinical presentation and indications for treatment

The incidence of TAAA is poorly studied, but is thought to be 5–10 per 100 000 per year. Relatively more patients with TAAAs are symptomatic than patients

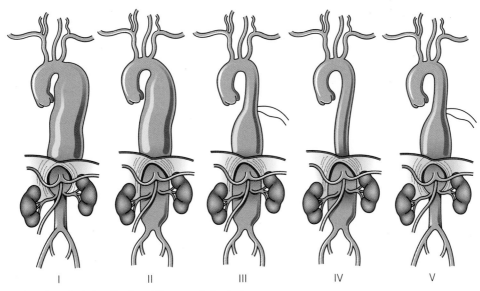

Figure 14.6 • Crawford classification of thoraco-abdominal aneurysms.

with other aortic aneurysms. The presence of back pain is particularly common, and this symptom may precede aortic rupture or intramural dissection. The rationale for treatment of TAAAs largely derives from a natural history study from Crawford and DeNatale, who reported a series of 94 patients unsuitable for surgery.[28] After 24 months' follow-up, only 24% of these patients were alive, which contrasted with the 59% 5-year survival of a concurrent cohort of patients who underwent operative repair. On the basis of these results, it was concluded that patients with significant thoraco-abdominal aneurysms should have an operative repair unless precluded by coexistent medical conditions. The advent of fenestrated and branched stent-graft systems has meant that many patients can now be treated by endovascular means. Despite being minimally invasive this is a technically demanding procedure, and there is a relatively higher risk of morbidity and mortality in comparison with 'standard' infrarenal EVAR.

Technique of surgical repair

Before any surgery can be considered, detailed imaging of the aorta must be obtained and examined using multiplanar reconstruction software. The physiological reserve of the patient should be comprehensively assessed and should include cardiac stress testing.

A left thoracotomy is performed for extent of I–III aneurysms, although it is possible to repair some type IV aneurysms via a totally abdominal approach. The abdominal aorta is usually exposed by left medial visceral rotation and the diaphragm is partially divided with a circumferential incision preferred to preserve nerve supply. After the dissection has been completed the aneurysm is clamped at its proximal and distal extents, and an arteriotomy made in the lateral aneurysm wall. It is important that the arteriotomy is sited away from the visceral origins in the abdominal portion of the aneurysm. The proximal anastomosis is performed with a completely transected aorta to prevent aorto-oesophageal fistula. If possible, the proximal anastomosis is fashioned to include adjacent intercostal or visceral arteries, whilst any remaining intercostal arteries are directly reimplanted into the graft or revascularised by separate jump grafts. The visceral arteries are then directly anastomosed into elliptical openings in the graft, utilising an inclusion technique. If possible, the coeliac, superior mesenteric and right renal arteries are taken on one patch; anastomosing the distal graft to the aortic bifurcation or iliac arteries completes the reconstruction (**Fig. 14.7**). During thoraco-abdominal aneurysm repair, prolonged visceral ischaemia is the main cause of postoperative renal dysfunction and can also contribute to multiple organ failure. To reduce the severity of organ hypoperfusion, partial left heart bypass with a centrifugal pump may be utilised to drain blood from the left atrium or upper pulmonary vein, and return it via the femoral artery or aorta. This facilitates renal and visceral perfusion whilst the proximal anastomosis is fashioned as long as the distal aortic clamp remains proximal to the visceral vessels.[29] During the abdominal

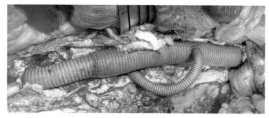

Figure 14.7 • Operative picture of completed reconstruction of a TAAA. The visceral patch has been reinforced with Teflon pledgets. A separate graft has been anastomosed to a large intercostal.

part of the aneurysm repair, the coeliac trunk, superior mesenteric artery and both renal arteries can be selectively perfused with catheters that are connected to the left heart bypass. Paraplegia may complicate thoraco-abdominal aneurysm repair in up to 20% of cases and is increased in more proximal aneurysms, with lengthy clamp time, renal impairment, advanced age and emergency presentations. Paraplegia results from damage to the spinal cord due to a combination of division of spinal cord arteries, prolonged spinal cord ischaemia during aortic clamping, reperfusion injury and postoperative hypotension. Maintenance of spinal cord blood supply may be achieved by reimplantation of patent intercostal arteries and by distal aortic perfusion. CSF pressure increases during aortic clamping, and CSF drainage has been advocated to reduce paraplegia.[29] A functional approach to the problem of neurological deficit aims at intraoperative monitoring of the spinal cord function. Somatosensory-evoked potentials are widely used to detect spinal cord ischaemia during aortic cross-clamping and to identify vessels critical to spinal cord blood supply, which may then be perfused and reimplanted. An alternative approach is to use motor-evoked potentials, which have been reported to improve paraplegia rates.[30] This technique involves stimulating the brain with electrical currents and monitoring the resulting signals in peripheral muscles. If these are damped perioperatively then measures may be taken to improve spinal perfusion.

Results of surgical repair of thoraco-abdominal aneurysms

The mortality and morbidity rates following conventional repair of TAAAs are still significant, with specialised centres reporting mortality rates of 5–16%, with paraplegia rates of 4–11%.[31,32] However, these excellent results are not representative of outcomes outside of these centres, with national/community mortality rates exceeding 20% at 30 days and 30% at 1 year.[33]

Endovascular repair of thoraco-abdominal aortic aneurysms

Advances in stent-graft technology (**Fig. 14.8**) have allowed the manufacture of stent-grafts with fenestration (FEVAR) or branches (BEVAR) to treat thoraco-abdominal aneurysm. These seal above and below the diseased segment of aorta in a similar fashion to standard endografts, but allow visceral branch perfusion via the placement of bridging stents between the main body of the stent-graft into the ostia of visceral vessels. Fenestrated stent-grafts are customised for each individual patient and require a period of weeks to months from ordering to being ready to use. Stent-graft systems with preformed branches can be used 'off the shelf' provided the necessary ancillary components are available. Anatomical suitability is important, and access problems, aortic tortuosity and target vessel morphology are some of the main reasons that patients are not suitable for this kind of repair. Initially the application of this technology was limited, and the number of patients receiving this kind of repair was low and confined to a small number of super-specialised units. The results of these procedures have improved as technology and perioperative care have developed, and now many centres are beginning to offer this as first-line therapy, often with the exception of young patients or those with a connective tissue disease. Both FEVAR and BEVAR require the partial deployment of an endograft in the visceral aorta through which the fenestrations or branches are cannulated. This is performed via access from the groin or the upper limb, and once secure access is obtained the device can be fully deployed and the visceral stents can be advanced into position. When these are in position the graft can be completed with a bifurcated section if necessary and a final angiographic run obtained to check that the aneurysm has been sealed and the visceral vessels are patent.

Results of endovascular repair of TAAA

Excellent early results have been reported in selected groups of patients treated at centres of excellence, although it is unclear to what extent these results are generalisable.[34] The largest modern institutional series reported the results of 354 procedures with a perioperative mortality of 3.5–7%.[35] As with open repair, paraplegia remains a serious problem and

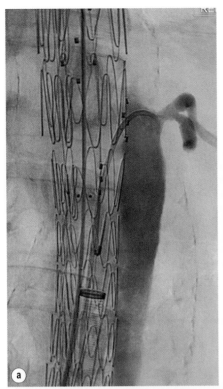

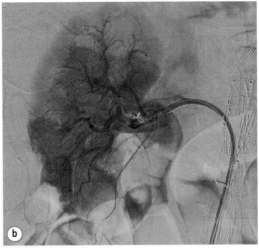

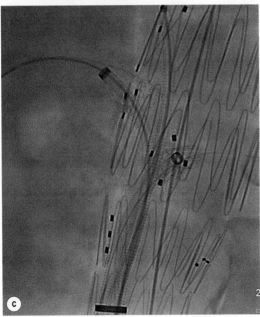

Figure 14.8 • Intraoperative images of a fenestrated endograft being placed for a type IV thoraco-abdominal aneurysm: **(a)** shows a catheter being placed through the left renal fenestration and some contrast being injected prior to cannulation of the vessel; **(b)** shows a sheath advanced into the right renal artery with an angiogram to confirm correct positioning before the deployment of bridging stents; **(c)** shows stents deployed in both renal arteries.

complicated up to 4% of procedures. Long-term durability appeared to be good, with target vessel patency of 96% at mid-term follow-up, although reinterventions were reported in 19% for a variety of reasons. Longer-term all-cause mortality remains a concern, with this series reporting 57% freedom from mortality.

Hybrid visceral revascularisation and endovascular repair of thoraco-abdominal aortic aneurysms

A combination of open surgical and endovascular strategies has been suggested to reduce surgical insult by removing the need for thoracotomy and aortic cross-clamping, whilst reducing the duration of visceral and renal ischaemia. There are fewer technical considerations than for complex endovascular solutions as all that is required is sufficient length of proximal and distal landing zones in non-diseased or replaced aorta. In addition, visceral vessels must be able to be accessed for bypass from a healthy donor site, such as the iliac system. Most often a transperitoneal retrograde visceral revascularisation is used to allow an adequate distal landing zone for placement of an endovascular stent-graft that extends from the thoracic to the distal abdominal aorta or iliac vessels. This approach may be combined with supra-aortic debranching to create a very proximal landing zone (**Fig. 14.9**). A collaborative paper reporting outcomes of 107 consecutive cases across three units described a 15% mortality and 8.4% permanent paraplegia rate in all-comers.[36] Superficially, these results do not appear

to show a significant advantage over conventional surgery, but these patients tended to be older, have more comorbidity, and a higher proportion of type II and III aneurysms than comparable open series.

Recommendations for practice

Endovascular techniques have evolved significantly in recent years, and many centres would preferentially offer minimally invasive surgery as first-line therapy for patients with thoraco-abdominal aneurysms. Open surgery is recommended for younger, fitter patients and those with connective tissue disorders, due to proven durability in these cases. Improvements in the delivery of FEVAR and BEVAR have rendered hybrid techniques less attractive in recent years. Most would now recommend them only in urgent cases unsuitable for an off-the-shelf branched device or for more extensive open surgery.

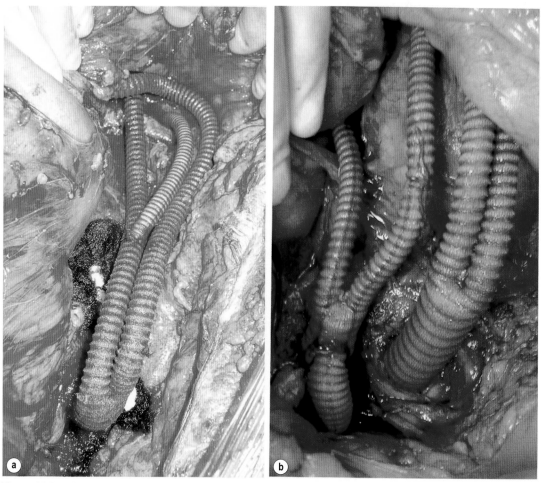

Figure 14.9 • Operative pictures of two patients undergoing retrograde visceral revascularisation. Many different graft configurations are possible, with varying numbers of vessels requiring revascularisation.

Thoracic dissection and acute aortic syndrome

Pathology, classification and clinical presentations

The acute aortic syndromes are a group of conditions affecting the thoracic aorta that cause patients to present to hospital with chest pain and encompasses three main pathological entities: aortic dissection (**Fig. 14.10a,b**), intramural haematoma (IMH; **Fig. 14.11**) and penetrating aortic ulcers

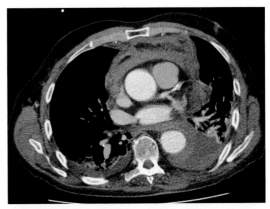

Figure 14.11 • Axial CT appearance of intramural haematoma. There is a relatively high-density crescentic rim of fresh blood in the wall of the aorta.

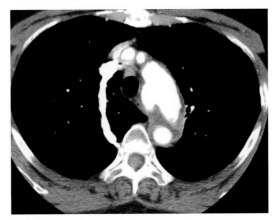

Figure 14.12 • Axial CT appearance of penetrating aortic ulcer.

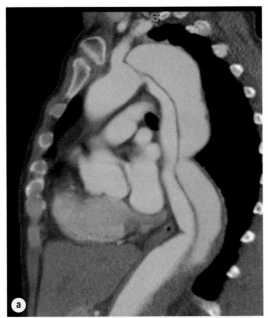

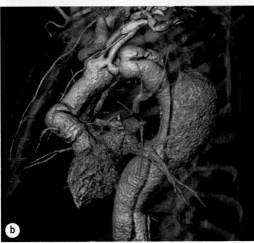

Figure 14.10 • **(a)** Sagittal reconstruction showing the classic appearance of a type B aortic dissection. **(b)** A three-dimensional reconstruction of the same pathology.

(PAUs; **Fig. 14.12**).[37] All three conditions may coexist, and both IMH and penetrating ulcer may instigate a classical aortic dissection.

Aortic dissection is defined as a tear in the intima of the aorta that allows blood to form a pathological plane of cleavage between itself and the adventitia by disrupting the media. These two new channels are referred to as the true and false lumens. Typically the pressure within the false lumen is higher than the true lumen, as the outflow is usually a small re-entry tear. This leads to compression of the true lumen, which can result in malperfusion of the viscera or limbs, or rupture of the false lumen. Such branch vessel malperfusion may be described as 'dynamic', due to a mobile dissection flap intermittently 'shuttering' the ostia of vessels during systole, or static due to a relatively fixed flap (**Fig. 14.13**).

IMH is defined as clotted blood in the intramural space without an obvious intimal tear. This is thought to result from rupture of medial vasa vasora, and

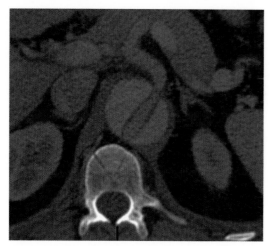

Figure 14.13 • Patient with a type B thoracic aortic dissection showing compression of the true lumen causing malperfusion of the coeliac artery and therefore visceral ischaemia.

is often regarded as a precursor to dissection. IMH accounts for up to 5–15% of acute aortic syndromes and has a prognosis similar to classical aortic dissection.[38] PAU results from focal ulceration of an atherosclerotic plaque into the media, and may be associated with haematoma within the aortic wall. Penetrating ulcers have a poorer prognosis than classical dissection, with higher rates of aortic rupture, but make up only 5% of acute aortic syndrome presentations. PAU is considered to be a disease of the intima, in comparison with dissection and IMH, which are considered to be diseases of the media.

Aortic dissections are classified by site, chronicity and presentation. The most crucial classification involves the site of dissection. Under the commonly used Stanford classification, type A dissection involves the ascending aorta whereas type B dissection originates distal to the left subclavian artery. The DeBakey system is also used to classify site. DeBakey I dissections extend from the ascending aorta into the descending, DeBakey II involve only the ascending aorta and DeBakey III originate from beyond the left subclavian artery (IIIa do not extend below the diaphragm whereas IIIb do). Dissections are termed acute when they are less than 2 weeks after the onset of symptoms, and are chronic after this period. Many now recognise a third, subacute phase between 2 and 12 weeks which may have significance in terms of the predicted response to endovascular treatment.[39] In addition, dissections may be complicated or uncomplicated. Complicated aortic dissections exhibit clinical or imaging findings such as impending or frank rupture, malperfusion, persistent pain and refractory hypertension. A recent expert consensus suggested a more comprehensive

way of classifying dissection using the mnemonic 'DISSECT', which stands for Duration of disease, Size of the aorta, Segmental Extent, Clinical complications and Thrombus within the lumen.[40]

Acute aortic syndromes often present with the sudden onset of sharp tearing or stabbing chest pain, which radiates to the neck and back. Pain is absent in 10% of patients, and asymptomatic presentation is more common in diabetics.[41] Acute rupture or malperfusion may lead to collapse and death, neurological deficits, symptomatic limb ischaemia, or visceral ischaemia. Hypotension is seen in patients with rupture or critical malperfusion, but hypertension is often present. Chronic dissection is often asymptomatic but can cause back pain or chronic visceral ischaemia. Consensus guidelines from the American Heart Association place high-risk features into three categories.[42] High-risk predisposing conditions include aortic instrumentation, Marfan's syndrome or thoracic aortic aneurysmal disease. High-risk pain features include an abrupt onset of ripping, tearing, or stabbing pain in the chest, back, or abdomen. High-risk features of the examination include discrepancy in limb perfusion, focal neurological signs, a new murmur of aortic regurgitation and circulatory shock. Urgent imaging should be undertaken if clinical suspicion of aortic dissection is sufficient based on the presence of these features.[43]

Investigation of suspected acute aortic syndrome

Axial imaging to visualise the whole aorta must be undertaken if a diagnosis of acute aortic syndrome is suspected. Serum D-dimer levels can be raised, and concentrations above 500 ng/mL are often present in patients with acute dissection, although this has a relatively low specificity.[44] Multidetector computed tomography angiography (CTA) is the preferred investigation and a meta-analysis of 1139 patients with aortic dissection found that CTA had a sensitivity of 100%, specificity of 98% and a diagnostic odds ratio of 6.5. The disadvantages of computed tomography angiography are the need to use potentially nephrotoxic contrast media, exposure to ionising radiation, and inability to assess functional aortic insufficiency. This technique is limited due to inability to visualise the descending aorta, although aortic valve insufficiency and pericardial tamponade can be diagnosed effectively. Transoesophageal echocardiography can visualise the entire thoracic aorta and despite the requirement for oesophageal intubation, can be performed at the bedside.[45] Transoesophageal echocardiography can also be an adjunct to endovascular repair due to the ability to see devices within the aortic lumen. Magnetic resonance angiography has a high sensitivity and specificity when used to diagnose aortic dissection. Gadolinium contrast agents are less nephrotoxic than iodinated substances used for computed tomography angiography and there is no associated ionising radiation. Disadvantages include its limited use in patients with claustrophobia or metal devices, although it can be used in those with nitinol aortic stent grafts. Long acquisition times and limited availability reduce its usefulness in the emergency setting, for which computed tomography angiography is ideal. The use of newer 'four-dimensional' cine MRI techniques may offer the potential for dynamic assessment of aortic dissection to determine the nature of blood flow within the true and false lumen. This information may be used to determine which patients are likely to benefit from earlier treatment due to an increased risk of subsequent aortic expansion.[7]

Initial management of acute aortic dissection

Management of aortic dissection involves rapid pharmacological control of blood pressure and left ventricular ejection velocity. The short-term goal of management is to resuscitate the patient and arrange definitive investigations to confirm the diagnosis. Persistent hypertension should be managed with intravenous beta-blockade using an agent such as labetalol to reduce aortic wall shear stress in the arch. A target heart rate of 60–80 beats/min. and systolic blood pressure of 100–120 mmHg should be the aim, taking into account the patient's normal blood pressure. Glyceryl trinitrate should be avoided as the reduction in diastolic blood pressure it causes may lead to a widened pulse pressure and a reflex tachycardia, which increases aortic wall shear stress. Invasive cardiovascular monitoring will be required and transfer of the patient to a level II or III environment in a sufficiently experienced cardiovascular centre is mandatory. Whilst maintaining a low blood pressure is ideal, it is important to ensure adequate organ perfusion by monitoring urine output, neurological status checks and checking peripheral perfusion. Regular arterial blood–gas analysis and examination for trends in markers of tissue perfusion may provide clues that malperfusion is developing. Type A dissection has a 1% mortality per hour from aortic rupture, aortic regurgitation, pericardial tamponade or coronary ischaemia and is treated by emergency surgical graft repair of the ascending aorta, with or without aortic valve replacement.[46]

After the acute phase, the management of type B dissections is initially medical in those with acute uncomplicated presentations, with intervention reserved for those exhibiting signs of complications. Intravenous agents can be replaced by oral antihypertensives, and European, American and Japanese guidelines advocate beta-blockers with a target blood pressure of <130 mmHg, with the addition of vasodilators in refractory cases.[47] For many years this was thought to be adequate treatment in the longer term, but recent studies have shown a high rate of failure of medical treatment in the mid-term.[48,49] Open surgical repair was the mainstay of treatment for acute complicated dissection for many years, but is associated with high levels of mortality and morbidity as it is highly invasive. With mortality rates as high as 30% reported in multinational registry data, endovascular repair is now seen as an attractive alternative.[50]

Endovascular management of complicated acute type B thoracic dissection

Endovascular therapy is now the first-line treatment for complicated type B thoracic dissections due to superior perioperative results compared with open surgery.[2] The aim of treatment is to cover the primary entry tear with an endovascular stent-graft, depressurising the false lumen and allowing expansion of the true lumen. In the acute phase this reduces the probability of aortic rupture and alleviates dynamic branch vessel occlusion by allowing preferential perfusion of the true lumen (**Fig. 14.14**). If there is residual static branch vessel occlusion this may be treated by secondary stent placement. In the longer term this promotes aortic remodelling, which is defined as the restoration of normal anatomy occurring with thrombosis and regression of the false lumen over time. The operative technique is similar to that described above for thoracic aneurysms. The proximal stent-graft is deployed in non-dissected aorta, usually in Ishimaru zone 2 or 3. Graft oversizing is limited to 10% and balloon dilatation should be avoided where possible. Some recommend avoiding stents with proximal bare stents, although the evidence for this conflicting. These measures are designed to reduce the risk of retrograde dissection, and careful deployment of the proximal stent-graft is necessary to avoid this.[51] A long length of aortic coverage is generally recommended to promote remodelling, although there is limited evidence to support this approach. A shorter length of aortic coverage may seal the primary tear but will rely on distal aortic remodelling to reduce perfusion in the distal aorta. A longer endograft promotes a greater degree of

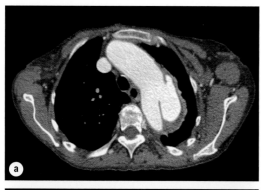

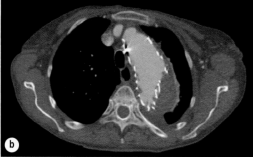

Figure 14.14 • Patient with a subacute type B dissection who underwent treatment by endovascular stent-grafting. The first picture shows the preoperative appearance and the second shows complete remodelling of the false lumen following repair.

false lumen thrombosis by direct compression, but may increase the risk of paraplegia. A combination of a short covered stent to seal the primary tear and a long uncovered stent which pins back the false lumen has been described with some encouraging results.[52] In addition, other endovascular techniques including visceral stenting or percutaneous fenestration may be required to treat malperfusion.

The early results of TEVAR of complicated type B dissections are significantly better than for open repair, with combined registry data suggesting a mortality rate of 13%, a stroke rate of 6% and a paraplegia rate of 2%.[2,53]

Early management of uncomplicated type B dissection

Given the relatively high rate of failure of medical management observed at mid-term follow-up, it has been suggested that patients with uncomplicated acute type B dissections might benefit from TEVAR in preventing acute and long-term complications. The rationale is that promoting aortic remodelling prevents the progressive degenerative changes that lead to late aortic events. The INSTEAD-XL trial randomised 140 patients with a diagnosis of uncomplicated type B dissection a median of 3.5 weeks after diagnosis to be treated either by TEVAR and best medical therapy (72 patients) or by best medical therapy alone (68 patients).[48] In the intervention group, the peri-procedural mortality and morbidity was low, with two deaths, two serious intra-procedural technical complications and three serious neurological complications. A total of 14 patients were crossed-over from best medical therapy to the intervention group, with five of these performed as an emergency and four requiring open repair. Although the risk of mid-term all-cause death was similar in both groups (11.1% vs 19.3%), aortic specific mortality was lower (6.9% vs 19.3%) and later disease progression was less frequent in the TEVAR group (27% vs 46.1%). These results in conjunction with other registry data have prompted some to suggest that uncomplicated type B dissection should be treated with early TEVAR in the subacute phase. The rationale for this is that the aorta has stabilised enough to reduce the risks associated with treating acute dissection, such as retrograde type A dissection, but still retains enough plasticity to allow remodelling of the aorta to take place. This remains a point of controversy and there is no conclusive evidence to support this viewpoint although many experts advocate this approach.

Careful morphological studies and long-term follow-up will be required to define which subgroup of patients are at risk from late events and therefore may benefit from early TEVAR for uncomplicated disease. Many risk factors such as false lumen diameter of over 22 mm, entry tear located on the lesser curve of the aortic arch and partially thrombosed false lumen have been suggested, but at present none has been satisfactorily validated in any kind of model.[54]

Treatment of chronic type B dissections

Uncomplicated chronic type B dissection is preferably managed conservatively, with regular surveillance scanning performed on an annual basis. Most published guidelines recommend the use of beta-blockers for blood pressure control, and findings from the International Registry of Aortic Dissection (IRAD) support this by demonstrating a reduction in mortality. Calcium channel blockers were also shown to reduce mortality specifically in patients with type B dissection,[47] although there is no consensus algorithm for management of hypertension in patients with dissection. Despite medical management, many patients develop aortic dilatation that may eventually require intervention. Generally, patients are considered for surgery when the aorta measures over 5.5 cm, or when the false lumen measures over 4 cm. Open surgical repair has the perceived benefit of completely replacing the diseased segment of aorta, therefore reducing the need for re-intervention in the future, but even modern series from specialised centres report high levels of debilitating perioperative adverse events.[55] Endovascular treatment can be performed with a relatively low morbidity and mortality in comparison with open surgical repair, and protects against aortic-related death in the mid-term,[56,57] although there remain some concerns regarding long-term durability due to the relatively high rate of aortic re-intervention rates observed in the MOTHER registry.[2] This is thought to be due to the tendency of the dissection flap to become relatively fixed and immobile, and therefore resistant to remodelling. The success of TEVAR for chronic dissection is dependent on maximising the chances of aortic remodelling, and there is some evidence to suggest that certain factors relating to the repair may influence this.

A longer length of aortic coverage seems to be preferable in chronic dissections, allowing a greater proportion of false lumen to be directly compressed as well as covering the main entry tear and any minor fenestrations in the descending thoracic aorta.[58] Despite this, high rates of false lumen thrombosis were achieved in the INSTEAD trial where only a single stent-graft was used in 83% of patients.[48] There are limited data regarding which type of endovascular device is most suited to treating aortic dissection and how to correctly plan endovascular repair. Most stent-graft systems are primarily designed to treat thoracic aortic aneurysms, and their indications for use reflect this. There is evidence to suggest that proximal and distal oversizing of endografts should be less aggressive to avoid unnecessarily excessive radial force, which has been associated with damage to the aortic wall and retrograde dissection.[51]

According to existing published current definitions, the cut-off point at which a dissection becomes 'chronic' varies, with some using 14 days from presentation and others using 90. There is no upper limit, however, and some studies group patients who are 2 weeks from presentation with those who presented up to 15 years previously.[59] The INSTEAD trial intervention arm recruited patients at a median of 3.5 weeks after the diagnosis, meaning many would be categorised as subacute dissections. This partially explains why a 90.6% total false lumen thrombosis at 5 years was achieved in a group of patients with chronic dissection. Another study that treated patients at a mean of 100 weeks post diagnosis only achieved false lumen thrombosis in 39% at 3-year follow-up.[60] This further supports the idea of a subacute group which may exist for up to a year in some cases.[39]

Management of intramural haematoma and penetrating aortic ulcer

Management of these conditions closely resembles that of dissection in both the acute and chronic phase. There is a relative paucity of data to direct therapy in comparison with aortic dissection, and the most recent consensus guidelines for management incorporated mostly institutional series combined with expert panel opinion.[38] Medical management of both conditions appears safe in the early phase unless there is haemodynamic instability, persistent pain, signs of impending rupture or progressive peri-aortic haemorrhage. Patients must then undergo surveillance to look for increase in diameter to over 55 mm or a yearly increase of >5 mm. In both conditions, endovascular treatment is preferable to open surgery given the superior perioperative and 3-year mortality reported in existing series.

Recommendations for practice

TEVAR is now considered to be the gold standard for complicated acute type B thoracic dissections and other acute aortic syndromes. Some patients with uncomplicated disease appear to benefit from early TEVAR although it is difficult at present to define which group this is. The indications for treatment and best interventional approach to chronic dissection, IMH and PAU require further study and refinement.

Traumatic aortic injury (TAI)

After head injury, TAI is the second commonest cause of death in patients following blunt injury: 15–30% of deaths from blunt trauma have aortic transection at post-mortem. The mechanism of injury is usually caused by deceleration, creating shear forces at the aortic isthmus, where the relatively mobile arch joins the fixed descending aorta (**Fig. 14.15**). There is a spectrum of degree of injury to the aorta ranging from intimal haemorrhage through to complete transection (grade I: intimal tear; grade II: intramural haematoma; grade III: pseudoaneurysm; grade IV: rupture). The surgical approach to treatment has changed considerably in the last decade. Previously, it was thought that emergency repair was mandatory because of the belief that there was a high risk of early rupture (79% within 24 hours) in immediate survivors, although procedural mortality rates of this approach were in excess of 30%. Pharmacological lowering of blood pressure and reduction in systolic ejection dynamics facilitate stabilisation of patients and the opportunity for delayed repair. Therefore surgery may be delayed

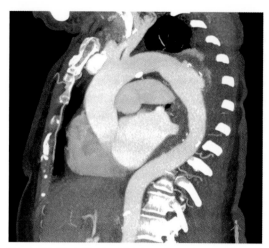

Figure 14.15 • Blunt aortic injury shown in a patient with an unfolded arch in the classical location. In this case there is a grade III injury with pseudoaneurysm formation.

for use in the thoracic aorta, such as abdominal endograft limbs.

Nevertheless, at the very least endografting can act as a temporary measure to prevent rupture until the patient is well enough to undergo definitive surgical repair. In the future, we may expect to see the development of endografts specifically designed to treat aortic trauma.

Recommendations for practice

TEVAR is the gold standard for treatment of TAI irrespective of the age of the patient, providing it is technically possible. In selected cases serial imaging and conservative management is acceptable, but for more severe injury it should be performed within 24 hours.

Aorto-oesophageal and aortopulmonary fistula

Aorto-oesophageal fistula is a rare and highly lethal condition. Open surgical treatment is complicated by difficult access to the aorta, which is often surrounded by adhesions in the mediastinum, and the need for high thoracic aortic cross-clamping. TEVAR is therefore an attractive option, but concern exists regarding the risk of endograft infection. Most patients present with haematemasis and many have signs of hypovolaemic shock and sepsis. Causes of this condition include prior aortic surgery, malignant and benign disease of the oesophagus, primary pathology of the aorta and ingestion of foreign bodies. The perioperative mortality rate for emergent open repair ranges from 45% to 55%, whereas a recent systematic review showed that for patients undergoing TEVAR this was 28%. Despite this, late infection rate was 15% in patients treated with TEVAR, and this led to death in a significant number of these patients.[65] In patients where a staged endovascular and open approach was taken, infection was less likely to be the cause of death and overall mortality at a mean of 6 months' follow-up was reduced. There is insufficient evidence to firmly recommend one treatment strategy for all, but it would appear that TEVAR is effective in preventing exsanguination but should probably be combined with open surgery after a suitable interval of targeted antibiotic therapy. Aortopulmonary fistula is rare and generally described after TEVAR, with cases caused by primary aortic pathology being very rarely described.[66] The mechanism of development is thought to be compression by the aneurysm sac and endoleak formation, and most patients develop clinical and radiological signs of pulmonary haemorrhage at presentation. Mortality was 61% over a 10-year period of study in a European-wide registry, although this was significantly better in patients fit for radical surgery (63% vs 21% survival at 2 years).

until the immediate threat to life from other injuries is controlled.[62] In many cases of low-grade injury, conservative management is now considered to be safe, and in those where intervention is necessary TEVAR is now the mainstay of treatment for TAI.[61,62] It can be performed rapidly via percutaneous access under local anaesthetic and as a result causes very little in terms of additional morbidity to patients who often have multisystem injuries. Due to the focal nature of the injury, only a short length of aorta requires covering with an endograft. The perioperative results reported in the literature are extremely good, and recently some institutional case series have suggested that longer-term durability is satisfactory.[63] Perioperative mortality across the available literature is reported to be 8% versus 19% for open repair, with lower rates of spinal cord injury.[61] The main disadvantage to TEVAR for TAI is that most devices are designed to treat dilated aortas with degenerative aneurysms or dissection. TAI occurs in a relatively young population with smaller aortas, more angulated aortic arches and smaller access vessels. Device conformability has improved over time which has allowed greater confidence when placing them in cases of TAI, and has reduced the risk of so-called 'birdbeaking' (where the aortic stent-graft does not conform to angulated aortic arch, seen especially in younger people, and the flow of the aorta conforms to the outer aspect of the stent-graft) resulting in endograft collapse and pseudocoarctation.[64] In addition, there is a lack of availability of small-calibre endografts. The smallest endograft is 22 mm, which limits the smallest size of aorta that can be stented to 18–19 mm. This may cause problems in young patients, and in some cases operators may resort to the use of smaller endografts not designed

Key points

- There are no prospective randomised controlled trials to guide practice with regard to diseases of the thoracic aorta, and current practice is driven by data from case series, registries, device-specific trials and consensus documents.
- It would appear from these data that endovascular repair is now the first-line treatment for thoracic aneurysms, type B dissections, PAU, IMH and traumatic aortic injury.
- Thoraco-abdominal aneurysm repair remains a technical challenge, with a relatively high mortality and morbidity rate regardless of treatment modalities employed. Open surgery has traditionally been considered as the first-line therapy for fitter patients, with low predicted mortality. Recent advances in technology and surgical practice have meant that branched and fenestrated endovascular repair is now the treatment of choice in many centres.
- The results of endovascular therapy in patients with connective tissue disorders are equivocal and open surgery should be considered preferable in this patient group.
- Aorto-oesophageal and aortopulmonary fistula are rare conditions that often occur secondary to previous aortic surgery. TEVAR may be a bridge to definitive treatment but radical surgery is associated with the best outcome if performed at a suitable interval.

🌐 Full references available at **http://expertconsult.inkling.com**

15

Disorders of the renal and mesenteric circulation

Indrani Sen
Ramesh K. Tripathi
Martin Björck

Renal vascular disease

Vascular involvement of the renal vessels involves a multitude of conditions and aetiopathologies; the treatment options for these are equally broad and evolve constantly. We present here a brief review of the traditional understanding of these diseases and the current evidence available in the management of a few specific conditions.

Renal artery disease

Atherosclerotic renal artery stenosis is the commonest symptomatic renal vascular pathology in the Western world. The renal arteries may also be affected in many other conditions, like aneurysmal disease, vasculitis, fibromuscular dysplasia (FMD), trauma and congenital hypoplasia.

Atherosclerotic renovascular disease

Prevalence

Atherosclerotic renal disease is symptomatic in about 7% of elderly Americans, the incidence increasing with age. The prevalence of asymptomatic disease is higher, with autopsy studies showing renal vascular disease in over 40% of those aged 75 years or older. Atherosclerotic renal vascular disease (ARVD) and renal artery stenosis (RAS) are terms used interchangeably; however, the former may be a better term as a high-grade stenosis of the renal artery may not be present in all patients. ARVD is thus a manifestation of generalised atherosclerotic disease; concomitant disease in coronary, carotid and peripheral vascular fields is present in 15–45%. The correlation of ARVD and end-stage renal disease is complex and causality may be difficult to determine in this patient group: Selective use of renal revascularisation also shows inconsistent associations with cardiovascular outcomes, renal replacement therapy and death.[1]

Definitions

ARVD occurs with between 50% and 75% renal artery diameter loss as diagnosed on conventional angiography (gold standard); however, lesions less than 50% may also be associated with significant (15 mmHg) pressure gradients.[2]

Pathophysiology

A haemodynamically significant RAS will lead to a reduction in renal artery perfusion pressure and thus potentially an impairment of renal function simply due to a hydraulic effect, but only in a minority of patients. More commonly, there is a compensatory rise in renin and angiotensin levels in the post-stenotic kidney, constricting the post-glomerular efferent arteriole, which in turn helps to support glomerular capillary hydraulic pressure and filtration rate (Table 15.1). As glomerular perfusion in these patients is critically dependent upon angiotensin II, the risk of developing acute renal failure is significant, especially if the stenosis is bilateral or affects a solitary functioning kidney.

Studies in large cohorts of patients with ARVD have shown that there is often poor correlation between

Table 15.1 • Pathogenesis of renovascular hypertension

Pathogenetic pathway progression	Stage of renovascular hypertension	Response to intervention
Renal artery occlusion Ischaemia Renin release Secondary increase in BP Conversion of angiotensin I to angiotensin II Severe vasoconstriction Aldosterone release (sodium and water retention)	Renin–angiotensin-dependent phase Salt retention phase	Responds to correction of renal artery stenosis/occlusion
? Functioning contralateral kidney Pressure diuresis / Previous volume retention / Hypertension Absence of pressure diuresis / Volume retention / Stimulus for renal renin production reduced / Renal renin levels fall / Renal parenchymal/vascular injury / Persistent hypertension	Renin–angiotensin-independent phase	Does not respond to correction of obstructions

the degree of anatomical atheromatous stenosis, glomerular filtration rate (GFR) and overall renal function.[3,4] Patients with unilateral ARVD can have GFRs that range from normal to stage 5 kidney disease. Nuclear studies in patients with unilateral stenosis reveal that GFR may be the same or even lower in the non-stenotic kidney. This lack of correlation between the severity of renal ischaemic injury and kidney function may explain why renal function often fails to improve significantly after revascularisation despite restoration of renal artery patency. It should also be noted that 1–5% of patients with hypertension are diagnosed to have a significant RAS.

Patients with severe aortic atheroma undergoing arterial surgical or angiographic procedures, thrombolysis or anticoagulation are at risk of developing renal dysfunction secondary to cholesterol emboli.

Clinical presentation

The clinical index of suspicion remains essential in determining an appropriate diagnostic and therapeutic strategy in ARVD. Specific clinical pointers include:

- hypertension; hypertensive crises;
- renal impairment;
- concominant cardiovascular disease;
- ACE-induced acute renal impairment;
- 'flash' pulmonary oedema;
- vascular bruit, pulse deficit.

Diagnosis[5,6]

Laboratory findings other than plasma renin levels are non-specific; their major role is in ruling out other conditions like Conn's syndrome or a pheochromocytoma.

Duplex scanning is a good initial diagnostic tool; however, problems with operator dependency and body habitus can hinder this. Significant lesions can be identified by measurement of peak systolic velocity in the main renal artery and its branches, along with end diastolic velocity, parenchymal Doppler signals, the presence of post-stenotic turbulence, nature of waveforms, measurement of acceleration times, resistivity index, renal size and the ratio of renal artery to aortic peak systolic velocity. Assessment protocols differ between institutions and a standardisation would be clinically useful.

Computed tomography angiography (CTA; **Fig. 15.1a**) provides information about the aorta and visceral vessels, neighbouring organs to exclude secondary causes or fibromuscular dysplasia and is of particular value in patients under consideration for open or endovascular revascularisation. The drawback of CTA is the risk of contrast nephropathy in a patient cohort that is already at risk for renal impairment.

An alternative is magnetic resonance imaging (Fig.15.1b), but this requires long scan times with comparatively poor image quality. The risk of nephrogenic systemic sclerosis in RAS is significant; gadolinium should be avoided in patients with a glomerular filtration rate of less than $15\,mL/min$ per $1.73\,m^2$. Other advances like fusion or cone beam technology may become clinically useful in the future. CO_2 angiography also has a limited role in those in whom both MRI and CTA are contraindicated.

Functional studies such as captopril renography and selective renal vein renin sampling have a role in the detection of ARVD, with the potential to predict a blood pressure response to revascularisation or to document the functional significance of RAS.

Management

Medical management is twofold: to promote modification of atherosclerotic risk factors (aspirin, lipid-lowering drugs, cessation of smoking, glycaemic control) and targeted management for hypertension. Involvement of a nephrologist at an early stage is often necessary as sudden drastic blood pressure reduction may be harmful. All imaging should be done with adequate hydration; the use of other renal protective agents (NAC) is described but not universally accepted.

Renal revascularisation

Surgical treatment

A range of surgical options are available to treat renal artery disease (Box 15.1). Endarterectomy and bypass grafting are the two main surgical options for revascularisation. Current guidelines recommend surgery in patients with ARVD who have indications for revascularisation and have multiple small renal arteries or require aortic reconstruction near the renal arteries for other indications (e.g. aneurysm, severe aorto-iliac occlusive disease). The site of the lesion is also important, and if extra-anatomical bypass is considered, the condition of the donor visceral vessels must be optimal. In patients with renal artery occlusion, renal biopsy (performed either preoperatively or perioperatively) can indicate whether the kidney is viable and functionally salvageable on the basis of collateral

Box 15.1 • Options for surgical revascularisation

Aortic graft and renal bypass
Aortorenal bypass
Aortorenal endarterectomy and patchplasty
Extra-anatomical bypass
Extracorporeal bench surgery

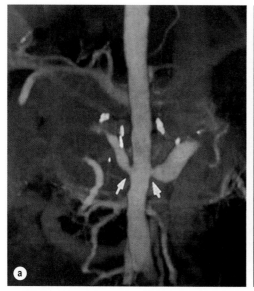
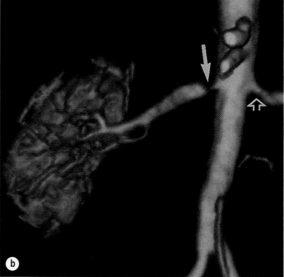

Figure 15.1 • Bilateral renal artery stenosis. **(a)** CT; **(b)** MRA.

vessels. However, this is not without risk of bleeding and potentially the loss of the kidney.

Nephrectomy is the oldest surgical procedure used in the treatment of ARVD, although rarely performed nowadays. In the presence of a normal contralateral kidney, it remains an option if the affected kidney measures less than 8 cm. In this situation measurement of renal vein renin levels is of value, with nephrectomy being indicated when the ratio of renal vein renins is greater than 1.5.

In the presence of aortic aneurysmal disease affecting the renal ostium, aortic graft and renal bypass may be indicated, particularly if the aneurysm is not suited to endovascular aortic repair (EVAR). Surgical options include a 6–8-mm limb of Dacron or polytetrafluoroethylene (PTFE) graft sutured onto the aortic graft with an end-to-end renal anastomosis and then bypass onto the affected renal artery in either an end-to-end (usually easiest) or end-to-side manner. Where bilateral RAS is present, an inverted bifurcated Dacron graft is preferred. When the pattern of aneurysm disease dictates that a suprarenal clamp is required for open surgery, transaortic endarterectomy may be performed. The ostial lesion is then carefully endarterectomised and the procedure is completed with patch closure. Five-year patency in large centres can reach 90%.

Extra-anatomical bypass grafting is an attractive option for patients with unilateral RAS in the absence of significant aortic disease. Access is obtained via a subcostal incision, without the need for aortic cross-clamp or extensive dissection, and revascularisation is achieved using inflow from either the hepatic or splenic artery. An interposition saphenous vein graft may be used where there is insufficient arterial calibre and length for an end-to-end anastomosis. The inferior vena cava, the right renal vein and often the left renal vein must be fully mobilised. On the left side, the splenic artery is dissected from its midpoint from the pancreas. Splenectomy can be avoided, as there is a rich collateral supply and perfusion via the short gastric arteries. The Cleveland Clinic reports 175 extra-anatomical bypass procedures over a 12-year period, with 2.9% operative mortality. Graft patency reached 96%,[7–9] renal function improved in 40%[10–14] and hypertension was improved or cured in three-quarters of the series.[10–13]

Aortorenal bypass (**Fig. 15.2**) can be carried out using the long saphenous vein, PTFE, Dacron or rarely the internal iliac artery. The infrarenal aorta is preferred as an inflow site if it is relatively disease-free. If not, then a 'rooftop' incision is necessary in order to expose the aorta above the coeliac axis. The thoracic aorta can also be used as an inflow site. Where multiple small anastomoses are required, extracorporeal or bench surgery is performed for patients with disease affecting renal artery branches. Removal of the kidney, cooling and preservation as

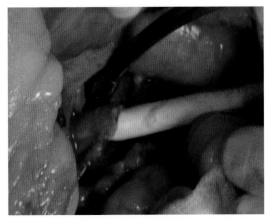

Figure 15.2 • Aortorenal bypass with PTFE graft.

in renal transplantation surgery will allow multiple microvascular anastomoses to be performed before autotransplantation takes place. The internal iliac artery is commonly used for direct end-to-end anastomosis. The Cleveland Clinic again has the largest reported series of autotransplantation, with excellent long-term results.[14]

Surgical revascularisation is considered to be a high-risk option when compared to less invasive treatment methods. Results vary, with cure or improvement of hypertension and renal failure noted in 63–91% and 33–91%, respectively. Primary patency rates of 93–97% and mortality rates of 2–8% are reported.[10–16] These morbidity and mortality rates have set the standards against which other treatment modalities can be compared. There have been no large trials to date comparing the outcomes of stenting with surgical revascularisation in ARVD. In young, fit patients surgery may be preferred as it is cost-effective and the long-term restenosis rate is reported to be 3–4%. The management of ARVD can be complex and certainly requires a multidisciplinary approach to maximise the therapeutic potential for each individual patient. Societal recommendations and guidelines form an effective template for evidence-based management of ARVD[17–19] (Boxes 15.2–15.5).

Endovascular treatment

Percutaneous transluminal renal angioplasty and stenting (PTRAS) is the current standard for renal revascularisation (**Fig. 15.3a,b**). Following initial reports of preventing renal vascular recoil in animal models by the use of stents, de Ven et al. demonstrated better patency with the use of stents compared to angioplasty in isolation. In a meta-analysis by Weinberg et al.,[20] the results of five studies (HERCULES, SOAR, RENAISSANCE, RESTORE, ASPIRE) in patients with uncontrolled

Box 15.2 • Recommendations and guidelines for revascularisation

Percutaneous revascularisation is recommended in patients with haemodynamically significant AVRD and any of the following:[17–19]

Evidence class I
- Recurrent congestive heart failure or sudden unexplained pulmonary oedema

Evidence class II
- Unstable angina (class IIa)
- Accelerated, resistant, or malignant hypertension or hypertension with unexplained unilateral small kidney and intolerance to medication (class IIa)
- Asymptomatic bilateral or single functioning kidney; however, this treatment is clinically unproven in asymptomatic unilateral haemodynamically significant AVRD in a viable kidney (class IIb)

Box 15.3 • Recommendations for percutaneous revascularisation

Percutaneous revascularisation is *reasonable* for patients with:[17–19]
- Progressive chronic kidney disease (CKD) and bilateral renal artery stenosis (RAS)
- RAS to a single functioning kidney
- Unilateral RAS with chronic renal insufficiency[17]

Class I recommendation
- Renal stent placement recommended for ostial ARVD
- Balloon angioplasty with bailout stent placement recommended for fibromuscular dysplasia lesions, if necessary

Box 15.4 • Contraindications for renal artery stenting

Patients with any of the following are typically *not good* candidates for renal artery stenting:[17]
- Mild or moderate stenoses (less than 70%)
- Long-standing loss of blood flow
- Complete occlusion of the renal artery

Box 15.5 • Indications for surgical revascularisation

Class I recommendation[32]
- Atherosclerotic RAS
- Multiple small renal arteries
- Early primary branching of the main renal artery
- Fibromuscular dysplasia, especially complex disease or macroaneurysms

blood pressure, renal dysfunction and/or failed angioplasty and hypertension undergoing renal artery stent revascularisation were combined. Both the systolic and diastolic blood pressure were significantly lower at 9 months with an elevated baseline SBP (>150 mmHg) being predictive of lowering of blood pressure in response to stenting. There are no robust data on the utility of drug-eluting balloons or stents in the renal circulation.

Revascularisation versus medical therapy

A review by Raman et al.[21] reports the results of management strategies for atherosclerotic RAS from 1993 to 16 March 2016. Fifteen comparative studies with a total of 4006 patients were identified; seven were randomised controlled trials (RCTs) and eight were non-randomised, comparative studies (NRCSs). Trial designs, interventions, endpoints, outcomes, follow-up and reporting were very variable. The ASTRAL, CORAL, STAR, RASCAD, NITER and RADAR trials remain the major trials on this topic to date. The meta-analysis demonstrated a low possibility of improvement of kidney function, with no difference in blood pressure change, subsequent mortality, progression to need for renal replacement therapy, cardiovascular events and adverse events. However, the authors note that most of these studies exclude patients with high-grade lesions, presenting with acute decompensation. Patients with ARVD are at an overall threefold risk of cardiovascular and all-cause mortality to age-matched controls; the challenge remains in identifying the patient subset in ARVD who, if managed interventionally, will have improvement in renal function and mortality. Current evidence can justify intervention in patients with progressive, but not severe, chronic renal insufficiency and systolic hypertension with global high-grade stenosis, ARVD and rapidly declining kidney function or flash pulmonary oedema. It also has a role in the management of congestive heart failure. Efforts at developing predictors of clinical benefit from intervention (including high blood oxygen level-dependent MRI, brain natriuretic peptide levels) are under investigation but cannot yet be utilised generally.

Renal stenting during treatment of aortic aneurysmal disease

Advances in the endovascular treatment of aortic aneurysms with surgeon modified/fenestrated or branched devices have created a subgroup of patients who undergo renal intervention when grafts cross the renal artery. Adjunctive renal stenting may be needed to salvage inadvertent coverage (**Fig. 15.4a,b**) or as a planned procedure when suprarenal fixation or endovascular repair of a thoracoabdominal aneurysm or dissection is planned. Stent placement in these patients may be more challenging due to complex anatomy, technical risks and risk of atheroembolisation leading to a higher complication rate and reports of late decline in GFR.[22,23] Occurrence of secondary intimal hyperplasia in such patients and the need for

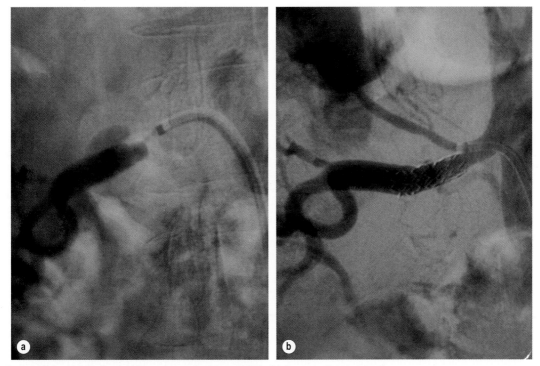

Figure 15.3 • **(a)** Right renal artery stenosis due to ARVD. **(b)** Post renal artery stenting.

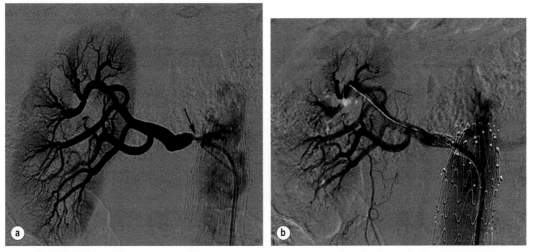

Figure 15.4 • **(a)** Renal artery stenosis following endovascular aortic repair. **(b)** Adjunctive renal stenting performed to salvage as a planned procedure.

subsequent intervention is also an area that requires further study.

Renal artery denervation

Renal artery denervation (RDN) is an endovascular procedure for the treatment of resistant hypertension. This condition is thought to involve overactivity of the afferent and efferent sympathetic nerves that run in the adventitia of the renal arteries, the nerves running closest in the distal renal arteries and renal artery branches. Radical nephrectomy and surgical sympathectomy have been associated with the normalisation of blood pressure in patients with end-stage renal disease (ESRD) and hypertension. It has also been established that increased renal sympathetic nerve activity has an important role in the development of essential hypertension. Following positioning of a sheath within the renal artery, a probe is positioned with its tip in contact with the inner luminal surface of the vessel. Radiofrequency energy is then applied to disrupt the nerve fibres running in the renal artery adventitia. The procedure is repeated at several points in both arteries to interrupt the neurogenic signals thought to be involved in the maintenance of sympathetic overactivity and, hence, resistant hypertension.

In 2010, the Symplicity HTN-2 study demonstrated for the first time in humans that endovascular renal denervation is a safe and effective technique to reduce blood pressure in patients with resistant hypertension.[24] A total of 106 patients with uncontrolled blood pressure (systolic >160 mmHg) and taking at least three antihypertensive agents were randomised to renal denervation plus best medical therapy or best medical therapy alone. At 6 months the group receiving renal denervation showed a significantly reduced blood pressure measurement. The larger Symplicity HTN-3 study included a total of 535 patients from 88 sites in the United States but this did not reveal a significant effect on systolic blood pressure reduction. Pooled data from SYMPLICITY HTN-3 and the Global SYMPLICITY Registry revealed that reduction in blood pressure among patients with isolated systolic hypertension was less pronounced than the reduction in patients with combined systolic–diastolic hypertension.[25,26] Thus, this trial paradoxically did not provide the definitive proof in support of RDN that was expected. However, the results have been analysed in detail and have generated further insight into the location of the perirenal sympathetics and there is still a need for further trials in this area.

Other renal vascular disorders

Renal artery aneurysm

Renal artery aneurysms[27] are rare and their natural history is poorly studied. The annual growth rate is estimated to be 0.6 mm a year; the rupture rate being 3–5%, with a mortality of <10%. Treatment indications are the presence of clinical symptoms, thromboembolism, refractory hypertension, size >2 cm, female in reproductive age, dissection or rupture. Open, endovascular and robotic repair are reported with primary patency rates of 75–100%, reintervention rates of 0–22% and overall mortality of 1%.

Renal trauma

Renal trauma[28] can be penetrating or blunt; concomitant renovascular injury is usually severe (American Association for the Surgery of Trauma grade 4 or 5) and associated with other injuries. Management options tend to be conservative unless complications occur; nephrectomy, open vascular repair, angioembolisation and endovascular repair have all been reported. The latter should not delay the management of other life-threatening injuries. Results of vascular salvage depend on the ischaemia time of less than 3 hours and the suitability of anticoagulation. The role of revascularisation is limited.

Fibromuscular dysplasia

Fibromuscular dysplasia (FMD)[29,30] is a non-inflammatory, non-atherosclerotic disorder that may be observed in almost any arterial bed and can lead to arterial stenosis. Five different types are recognised and usually affect younger patients, with a female predominance, involving the distal main artery and/or the intrarenal branches. Rarely, FMD may be complicated by an aneurysm. Patients may be asymptomatic but the most usual presentation is hypertension. Hypertension is commonly treated successfully with medication, but RAS and renal dysfunction may progress in up to one-third of patients. Occlusion and complete loss of renal function is exceptional. Magnetic resonance angiography (MRA) can detect FMD in the proximal vessels, but is less sensitive for visualising the second- and third-order branches. The diagnosis will usually require conventional digital subtraction angiography and selective views may be necessary to detect subtle branch lesions. When treating FMD, the results of percutaneous angioplasty (PTA) are good (**Fig. 15.5a,b**), with 10-year cumulative patency rates of 87% and up to 50% of patients cured of their hypertension. The remainder often have a reduced drug burden and improved blood pressure control. Stenting is usually reserved for suboptimal PTA.[17–19]

Post-transplant renal artery stenosis

Post-transplant RAS[31] is another area that is being recognised to need further study. A meta-analysis by Ngo et al. included 32 studies with 884 interventions reporting the results of post-transplant stenosis managed with angioplasty or stenting. The overall patency rates were 42–100% with technical success in 90% but the diagnostic and reporting criteria were very heterogeneous and need further study.

Mid-aortic syndrome

Mid-aortic syndrome[32,33] can be congenital or acquired secondary to neurofibromatosis or Takayasu's disease and may present with severe/resistant hypertension in a younger patient group. This group may require operative management with an emerging role of endovascular management. Concomitant medical management of systemic disease is crucial.

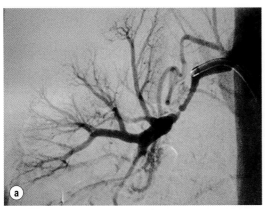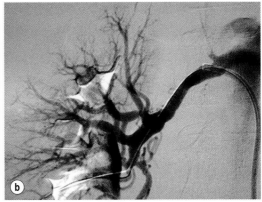

Figure 15.5 • (a) Renal artery stenosis due to fibromuscular dysplasia. **(b)** Good result post percutaneous angioplasty.

Mesenteric vascular disease

The mesenteric arteries and veins are affected by a number of diseases. In the clinical situation it is not always obvious if the ischaemia is acute or chronic, or acute-on-chronic. It is also not always clear whether the main disease is arterial or venous, nor if it is a result of embolus from the heart, local thrombosis due to atherosclerosis, an underlying aneurysm or a dissection.

✔✔ The difficulties in diagnosis provided the rationale behind the 2017 European Society of Vascular Surgery (ESVS) guidelines on the 'Management of the diseases of the mesenteric arteries and veins' which cover all of these pathologies.[34] These clinical practice guidelines give 64 recommendations regarding diagnosis and treatment of the different clinical scenarios that are most commonly encountered.

Acute thromboembolic occlusion of the superior mesenteric artery

This condition is more common than expected, and in most epidemiological studies embolism is more common than primary thrombosis.[3] Without a high grade of clinical suspicion and targeted diagnostic tests, many patients are diagnosed too late, when the entire bowel is gangrenous and the patient beyond salvage. The classical clinical triad associated with acute embolic occlusion of the superior mesenteric artery (SMA) consists of: (1) acute severe abdominal pain without signs of peritonitis ('pain out of proportion'); (2) bowel emptying, most often both diarrhoea and vomiting; and (3) a source of embolus, most often atrial fibrillation or acute myocardial infarction.

Although a normal D-dimer can exclude the diagnosis,[3,35] it is not specific and in fact there is no specific laboratory test to detect acute mesenteric ischaemia (AMI).

✔✔ Lactate is effectively metabolised in the liver, explaining why it is elevated only late. It becomes diagnostic when the bowel is gangrenous and the patient has become septic and hypotensive,[3] explaining why the ESVS guidelines[34] issued a strong recommendation not to use lactate to diagnose this condition early. Modern CT angiography is the mainstay investigation to diagnose an occlusion of the SMA, but it should be performed in all three phases and with thin slices over the SMA in the arterial phase.

✔ When treatment is discussed, one controversial issue is whether revascularisation should be performed before or after bowel resection (when needed). There are no RCTs but cohort data suggest that revascularisation should be performed prior to bowel resection.[3,36]

Another controversial issue is whether open or endovascular revascularisation is the preferred approach. Here the data suggest that endovascular techniques are associated with better outcomes if the occlusion is thrombotic, but with an embolic occlusion, open or endovascular surgery have similar outcomes.[37,38]

There is consensus regarding the need for second-look laparotomy, completion control (with angiography or flow measurements) and antibiotic treatment. The damage control strategy, first developed in trauma patients, should also be considered when treating patients with AMI, and this may be the explanation why treatment of a thrombotic occlusion with open surgery is less successful than with stenting. An alternative when antegrade stenting through the aorta is difficult, and in particular if there is also contamination due to bowel gangrene, is the retrograde open mesenteric stenting (ROMS),[39] when the SMA is punctured through laparotomy.

A case example of how the damage control concept can be applied to a patient with AMI is illustrated in **Fig. 15.6**. The case involved an 85-year-old man who was admitted with atrial fibrillation and 2 days of abdominal pain. He had a slightly elevated troponin level, was thought to have a myocardial infarction, and was admitted to the cardiology unit. Twelve hours later the diagnosis was questioned and CTA showed an embolus in the SMA (**Fig. 15.6a**). The patient had no peritonitis, but severe abdominal pain, and was taken to the hybrid operating room. An aspiration embolectomy was performed with a stiff 6-Fr introducer (**Fig. 15.6b**), and the final angiography showed an almost complete revascularisation of the branches (**Fig. 15.6c**). The procedure was performed under local anaesthesia and the patient experienced an almost complete and immediate relief of his abdominal pain, which prevented the need for an exploratory laparotomy. After 3 days of surveillance at the hospital, and initiation of warfarin treatment, the patient returned to his home. This case illustrates the potential benefit of endovascular therapy in these often elderly and frail patients.

Mesenteric ischaemia

Chronic mesenteric ischaemia

The typical clinical presentation of chronic mesenteric ischaemia (CMI) is postprandial pain, weight loss and diarrhoea. The typical patient is a female smoker around the age of 60. In contrast to the patient with malignant disease, the patient's appetite is not affected. The patient refrains from eating, or eats very small meals, for fear of the pain that comes after the meal. The clinical history is the key to the diagnosis.

The patient usually has known cardiovascular disease, and has often undergone multiple examinations for abdominal pain. One of the main problems is how to diagnose the condition, since asymptomatic stenosis and even occlusion of one of the mesenteric arteries is quite common, explained by the collateral network that is well developed in most people (**Fig. 15.7**). Duplex ultrasound is the recommended screening examination, when CMI is expected (in contrast to AMI when it is not recommended due to the risk of false-negative findings), and has the advantage of also including physiological evaluation of stenoses.[40]

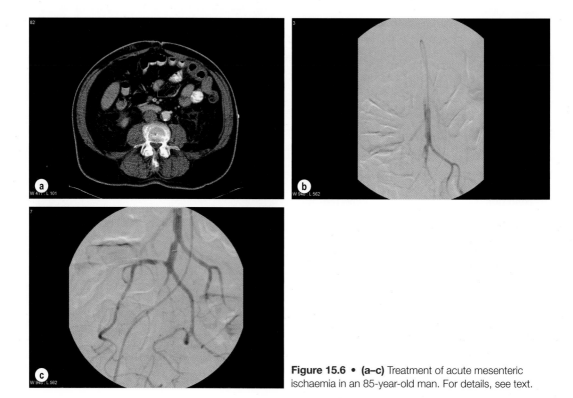

Figure 15.6 • (a–c) Treatment of acute mesenteric ischaemia in an 85-year-old man. For details, see text.

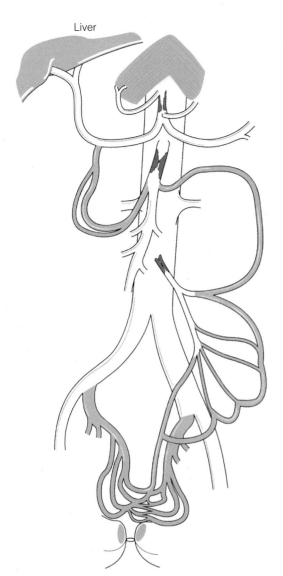

Liver

Figure 15.7 • Collateral network of the mesenteric arteries.

treatment should not be delayed, since there is a risk of developing acute-on-chronic ischaemia with bowel gangrene. Whether the patient with severe CMI should be given parenteral nutritional support prior to surgery is controversial. Data suggest that this is not advisable, since the delay may result in worsening ischaemia, and the ESVS mesenteric guidelines issue a strong recommendation not to delay treatment in this clinical scenario.[34]

When it is decided to treat the patient, a number of alternatives and controversial issues need to be addressed. Many vascular centres would consider endovascular treatment as the first option, but risk factors for failure of endovascular treatment must be considered. These include anatomical factors such as severe eccentric calcification, flush occlusions and long lesions that extend into the middle segment of the SMA. In these cases, stenting may still be possible, but is not optimal since the risks of restenosis and of perioperative complications are increased. The superior long-term results of open surgery should be balanced against a possible early benefit of endovascular intervention with regard to lower immediate mortality and morbidity.[34]

There are two other situations when an open arterial reconstruction may be preferred: after failed endovascular treatment and in young patients, often with non-atherosclerotic disease such as vasculitis or mid-aortic syndrome. A special case is also the median arcuate ligament syndrome (MALS), when the coeliac trunk is compressed by muscular fibres from the diaphragm. In this situation primary stenting is contraindicated, but can sometimes be necessary and successful after prior open surgical release.[34,41]

Balloon angioplasty has been replaced by primary stenting in most centres because of the increased risk of elastic recoil and restenosis. The lesions are most often ostial, a result of atherosclerosis of the aortic wall. However, there are no RCTs comparing different treatment modalities, making the evidence base weak.

Another controversial issue is whether a bare-metal stent or a covered stent graft should be used.

✅✅ If a single vessel is affected, the diagnosis of CMI is less likely and careful examination for alternative causes is warranted.[34]

If two or three of the mesenteric arteries are affected, and no other explanation has been identified despite extensive gastroenterological examinations, CMI should be considered the cause of the symptoms. Before treatment, the anatomy of occlusions and stenosis needs to be mapped. CTA is most often used for mapping the disease prior to any intervention, although MRA is an alternative.

If there is severe CMI (defined as significant weight loss, diarrhoea and/or continuous pain)

✅✅ The SMA has multiple branches, some of which may be sacrificed with a covered stent, which should be balanced against the fact that data suggest that restenosis is less common after having used a stent graft. This was shown in a large retrospective study on 225 patients,[42] and a Dutch RCT is ongoing.

Another debated issue is whether one or multiple vessels should be revascularised in the case of multivessel disease, and if the SMA or the coeliac trunk should be treated. The literature shows retrospective studies with diverging results: some have shown no significant advantage of two-vessel stenting, others have reported better long-term results after two-vessel revascularisation.[34] Given the lack of proven benefit of the more extensive procedure, most centres would focus on the SMA, and treat only that vessel.

In the postoperative management it is obvious that secondary prophylaxis and risk factor management should be performed, including antiplatelet therapy, smoking cessation and statins. CMI is a life-threatening disease, and the patient benefits from a multidisciplinary approach. Since both diagnosis and treatment are rather complex, and these patients are not common, the patient should ideally be referred to a specialist centre that can offer a multidisciplinary team, as well as both open and endovascular treatment.[34] Most patients do benefit from a routine follow-up to assess the clinical outcome, but it has not been shown that routine imaging adds benefit to the patient. An asymptomatic patient probably does not require any imaging.

Acute mesenteric venous thrombosis

Acute venous thrombosis of the superior mesenteric vein is the most common cause of acute venous ischaemia, also called mesenteric venous thrombosis (MVT). MVT is less common than AMI by a factor of seven.[43] The condition is underdiagnosed, due to rather diffuse symptoms, and a less acute onset compared to AMI. It can also be overdiagnosed due to the fact that many patients with abdominal symptoms undergo abdominal CT investigations. Incidentally reported MVT was reported to be present in approximately 2% in one large post-mortem study.[44] This explains the great variations in incidence estimates, but a recent Finnish population-based study estimated it to be 0.5/100 000 inhabitants/year.[45] When bowel gangrene develops, its extension is usually less than in cases caused by arterial occlusion. Typically, the middle part of the small bowel is affected, and it is associated with oedema and ascites. The oedematous mesentery makes it technically demanding to perform both anastomosis and stoma.

When MVT is diagnosed, underlying prothrombotic conditions should be considered, since they may also need to be treated. Considering Virchow's triad is a systematic approach, including damage to the vessel wall, reduced flow and/or a pro-coagulant blood. The most common underlying risk factors are venous thromboembolism (often inherited monogenetic disorders) and obesity,[34,43] but malignant disease, undiagnosed portal hypertension, intra-abdominal infections or injury during surgery should also be considered.

✔✔ Anticoagulation with heparin is first-line therapy.[34]

Most patients can be managed without laparotomy or bowel resection, but especially during the first days this possibility needs to be considered. Bowel gangrene can develop late, however. The ischaemic injury is a product of the duration and the depth of ischaemia. This means that a low-grade ischaemic condition, such as MVT, can result in bowel gangrene after 1–2 weeks. Until resolution of abdominal pain, the risk of gangrene prevails.

This is the background to why unfractionated heparin is the best initial treatment, since it can be reversed more quickly, if a need for bowel resection develops. Later, low-molecular-weight heparin (LMWH) may be used. The strong anti-inflammatory effect of heparin is also an important therapeutic principle that explains why it is so effective in most cases.

In approximately 5% of cases heparin treatment is not successful: the abdominal pain continues and the general status of the patient deteriorates.[34] In this situation, catheter-delivered thrombolysis may be considered. Direct puncture of the liver and delivering the thrombolytic agent (usually rTPA) directly to the superior mesenteric vein is associated with a rather high risk of bleeding complications, and since the outflow through the liver is compromised, significant clearance of the thrombus is seldom achieved. A solution is to puncture the jugular vein, perform a transjugular intrahepatic portosystemic shunt (TIPS) and through that perform mechanical aspiration thrombectomy and direct thrombolysis.[46] This approach has the advantages of both reducing the bleeding risk and improving the outflow. The TIPS will usually thrombose spontaneously after some time.

After the acute episode it is important to investigate whether there is an underlying condition explaining the MVT. In patients with reversible causes (e.g. trauma, infection, or pancreatitis), anticoagulation for 3–6 months is recommended in the ESVS guidelines.[34] Lifelong anticoagulation is recommended in case of proven thrombophilia, recurrent venous thrombosis or when progression or recurrence of thrombosis would have severe clinical consequences, such as in a patient with short bowel.

Non-occlusive mesenteric ischaemia

The term non-occlusive mesenteric ischaemia (NOMI) was first used by Ende in 1958.[47] In critically ill patients with low cardiac output, multiple interventions are often performed to save the life, but as a side-effect the intestinal circulation may suffer.[48] The vasoconstriction can be caused by vasoactive drugs (in particular vasopressors, but also cocaine or crack-cocaine among drug addicts), as well as secondary to resuscitation leading to the abdominal compartment syndrome.[49] Other patients at risk are those with hypovolaemia during renal replacement therapy or after burn injury, as well as those who have undergone cardiac surgery.[34]

As in most cases of mesenteric ischaemia, clinical suspicion is the key to a timely diagnosis. In one study on patients who died from NOMI, 40% had a stenosis at the origin of the SMA.[50] Dilating and stenting such a stenosis may be life-saving, as well as placing a catheter for selective intra-arterial administration of vasodilators into the SMA. For this reason the ESVS guidelines[34] recommend that a patient with life-threatening NOMI should be taken to a hybrid operating room, or an operating room with a C-arm, where both endovascular interventions and laparotomy (if necessary) can be performed.

Key points

Renal disease

- ARVD usually presents with hypertension, chronic renal failure, acute renal failure or pulmonary oedema. However, it is often asymptomatic and should be considered in patients with extrarenal vascular disease.
- Angioplasty (PTA) is the procedure of choice for non-atheromatous lesions.
- The improvement of blood pressure control in non-atheromatous lesions is good to excellent following PTA.
- Stents have a higher technical success and patency rate compared with PTA in atheromatous ostial lesions.
- Surgery gives the lowest restenosis rates but should be reserved for stent failures or young fit patients.
- Improvement of blood pressure control in atheromatous lesions following stenting is marginal but may reduce the drug burden.
- There is currently no consensus on the role of stenting in ARVD for hypertension or renal insufficiency. Further trials are under way.
- Societal guidelines form an effective template for evidence-based management of ARVD (see Boxes 15.2–15.5).

Mesenteric vascular disease

- Patient history and clinical suspicion are important for diagnosing all kinds of mesenteric ischaemia.
- Laboratory examinations are not helpful in diagnosing acute mesenteric ischaemia (AMI).
- Triphasic CT angiography is the most important imaging in AMI.
- Endovascular surgery is associated with better survival if an acute occlusion of the superior mesenteric artery (SMA) is thrombotic.
- An embolic occlusion can be treated with similar results with both techniques.
- Most patients with AMI will need bowel resection, but that should take place after revascularisation.
- Second-look laparotomy, completion control and antibiotics are recommended after revascularisation for AMI.
- If a single vessel is affected, the diagnosis of chronic mesenteric ischaemia (CMI) is less likely and careful examination for alternative causes is warranted.
- In CMI the superior long-term results of open surgery should be balanced against a possible early benefit of endovascular intervention.
- Primary stenting of the SMA is recommended in CMI.
- Heparin treatment is first-line therapy in patients with venous mesenteric ischaemia.

Key references

17. Parikh SA, Shishehbor MH, Gray BH, et al. SCAI expert consensus statement for renal artery stenting appropriate use. Catheter Cardiovasc Interv 2014;84(7):1163–71. PMID: 25138644.

18. Anderson JL, Halperin JL, Albert NM, et al. Management of patients with peripheral artery disease (compilation of 2005 and 2011 ACCF/ AHA guideline recommendations): a report of the American College of Cardiology Foundation/ American Heart Association Task Force on Practice Guidelines. Circulation 2013;127(13): 1425–43. PMID: 23457117.

19. Tendera M, Aboyans V, et al. ESC Guidelines on the diagnosis and treatment of peripheral artery diseases. Document covering atherosclerotic disease of extracranial carotid and vertebral, mesenteric, renal, upper and lower extremity arteries: the Task Force on the Diagnosis and Treatment of Peripheral Artery Diseases of the European Society of Cardiology (ESC). Eur Heart J 2011;32(22):2851–906. PMID: 21873417.

34. Björck M, Koelemay M, Acosta S, et al. Management of the diseases of the mesenteric arteries and veins. Clinical practice guidelines of the European Society of Vascular Surgery (ESVS). Eur J Vasc Endovasc Surg 2017;53:460–510. PMID: 28359440.

42. Oderich GS, Erdoes LS, Lesar C, et al. Comparison of covered stents versus bare metal stents for treatment of chronic atherosclerotic mesenteric arterial disease. J Vasc Surg 2013;58(5):1316–23. PMID: 23827340.

48. Bjorck M, Wanhainen A. Nonocclusive mesenteric hypoperfusion syndromes: recognition and treatment. Semin Vasc Surg 2010;23(1):54–64. PMID: 20298950.

16

Central venous and dialysis access

Peter W.G. Brown
David C. Mitchell

Introduction

Access to the venous circulation is an almost universal requirement in hospitalised patients for intravenous fluid administration or blood transfusion. This is most commonly achieved with an indwelling peripheral intravenous cannula but central venous access may be required for pressure monitoring, intravenous nutrition, haemodialysis, haemofiltration or the administration of cytotoxic drugs.

For acute haemodialysis, central venous catheters (CVCs) are the mainstay of access and provide high dialysis flows (>300 mL/min) but have high complication rates and are less suitable for chronic use. For long-term haemodialysis, an arteriovenous fistula (AVF) or graft (AVG) can provide a sufficiently high dialyser flow (>300 mL/min) to allow dialysis via two needles inserted into the efferent vein or the graft itself.

Central venous access

Indications

In addition to central venous pressure monitoring, CVCs can be used to infuse large volumes of irritant solutions, such as antibiotics, blood products, parenteral nutrition and chemotherapeutic agents, particularly if required over long periods. In an emergency, CVCs allow the rapid administration of large volumes of fluid if peripheral access cannot be achieved. Other indications include haemodialysis and plasmapheresis. Implantable injection ports, 'portacaths' (e.g. Bardport, Passport, Infuse-a-Port

or MediPort), may be used for chemotherapy or long-term administration of other drugs.[1] One has also been developed for haemodialysis (Lifesite).[2]

Methods

CVCs are generally inserted under local anaesthetic through the internal jugular, subclavian or femoral veins, preferably using ultrasound guidance, by the Slinger technique.[3] If short-term access is required a multi-lumen catheter is inserted into the internal jugular vein so that the tip lies in the superior vena cava. For long-term access a catheter with an attached Dacron cuff is placed in a subcutaneous tunnel (e.g. Hickman line) for fixation and to act as a barrier to infection.

Implantable access ports are usually inserted into the jugular or subclavian vein in the operating theatre and tunnelled so that the port lies over the anterior chest wall. They contain a diaphragm that may be accessed repeatedly using a special side-hole needle. Central vein access can also be achieved using a peripheral intravenous central catheter inserted in the antecubital or long saphenous vein. These are relatively small but widely used in neonates, as an alternative to umbilical vein catheters.

Complications

Air embolus can be avoided by ensuring a head-down position during insertion.

✅✅ Accurate placement under ultrasound guidance will reduce the incidence of arterial puncture, haematoma, haemothorax and pneumothorax.[4]

The long-term complications of infection and thrombosis are dealt with below.

Temporary dialysis access

Renal replacement therapy may be accomplished by renal transplantation or peritoneal dialysis but most patients require at least a period of haemodialysis. About 75% of patients are known to have deteriorating renal function at least 90 days before dialysis is required so that permanent haemodialysis access can be created in advance. Unfortunately, this opportunity is frequently missed in UK practice, with less than a third of patients starting haemodialysis with definitive access.[5] Over 87% of patients start haemodialysis on a CVC if presenting late, with most still using the same modality 3 months after onset of dialysis. Referral to a surgeon before commencing dialysis leads to 70% of patients having an AVF, whereas 90% will start dialysis on a CVC if not seen by the surgical team prior to the onset of dialysis.[5] Dialysis is required for hyperkalaemia or when symptoms of weight loss, nausea, vomiting, anorexia or itching occur, usually at a serum creatinine level of 500–1500 mmol/L.

For patients presenting as an emergency with end-stage renal disease (ESRD) without prior access, haemodialysis can start using a double-lumen CVC whilst awaiting a permanent AVF. However, CVCs have a high risk of infection,[6] cause central venous stenosis or thrombosis[7] compromising further access in the upper limbs, and have a higher mortality than AVFs,[8] so should not be used long term except where other options have been exhausted.

✅ Temporary (non-tunnelled) catheters are used in patients who require short-term dialysis for transient renal failure or who present acutely with ESRD. They are also indicated after failure of a permanent access, whilst awaiting maturation of a new AVF. Tunnelled catheters are preferred if dialysis is required for more than 2 weeks or for permanent access when the creation of an AVF or AVG is contraindicated or technically impossible.

The subcutaneous tunnel may reduce the rate of infection, but this has not been proven in a randomised trial.[9]

Methods

Temporary femoral vein catheters are useful for acute dialysis but have a higher rate of infection than internal jugular CVCs[10] and should be replaced by a tunnelled (preferably jugular) venous catheter at the earliest opportunity. A median survival of 166 days has been reported for tunnelled femoral CVCs.[11]

The right internal jugular vein (IJV) is preferred as this provides the most direct route to the superior vena cava (SVC) and right atrium (RA). The left IJV has a greater complication rate because the catheter has to traverse two 90° bends to reach the RA. The subclavian route is discouraged because of the high incidence of subclavian vein stenosis and thrombosis that compromises future access in the ipsilateral arm. When other routes have been exhausted, tunnelled catheters can be placed in the femoral vein or even the inferior vena cava (IVC) via a transhepatic or translumbar approach.

The catheter tip is usually placed at the SVC/RA junction. Atrial placement minimises recirculation and reduces the risk of migration on standing,[12] but may cause arrhythmias.

✅✅ The preferred site for a CVC is the right IJV. CVCs should be inserted under fluoroscopic or ultrasound guidance, without which there is a malposition rate of 29%.[13]

Complications of CVCs

Insertion
The complications related to catheter insertion are the same as for other CVCs described above and can be reduced by ultrasound guidance and a micro-puncture technique.

Catheter dysfunction
Catheter dysfunction occurs when an adequate extracorporeal blood flow of 300 mL/min cannot be achieved. Early dysfunction is usually caused by malposition or kinking and is corrected by repositioning. Later dysfunction is primarily due to thrombosis or fibrin sheath formation. Rarely, tip migration demands repositioning with a snare or exchanging over a wire.

Catheter-locking solutions
Catheter patency can be maintained between dialysis sessions using a catheter-locking solution. The standard procedure has been heparin instillation (1000–10 000 u/mL) into the catheter lumen in a volume sufficient to fill to the lumen tip. There is a risk of heparin loss due to diffusion into the bloodstream and unintentional systemic anticoagulation. Low-dose heparin (1000–2500 u/mL) seems as effective as high-dose.[14] Trisodium citrate, which also has antibacterial properties, is also an effective catheter lock but there are no randomised trials versus heparin.[15]

A recent randomised study compared 225 patients on haemodialysis who had a central venous catheter using a locking regime of heparin 5000 u/mL or recombinant tissue plasminogen activator (rTPA) 1 mg in each lumen. The rate of catheter malfunction in the heparin group (34.8%) was significantly worse than in the patients assigned to rTPA and the risk of bacteraemia was three times higher than in the heparin group.[16]

Catheter lumen thrombosis

Catheter thrombosis is the most common cause of poor long-term function.[17] Prophylactic warfarin can be effective at reducing thrombosis[18] but there are no randomised data comparing international normalised ratio (INR) ranges and controls. There is a risk of bleeding and a need for regular monitoring.

Catheter malfunction due to thrombus can be treated by lytic agents such as rTPA or urokinase.

rTPA may be superior to urokinase but this has not been proven in a randomised trial. Urokinase has been withdrawn in the USA due to safety concerns.

Poor flow can be treated by a post-dialysis lock or intra-dialysis lytic infusion. Both are effective but again there are no randomised trial data to guide clinical practice.

Lytic agents are also used for the treatment of catheter thrombosis. An instillation of rTPA 1 mg/mL for 30 minutes restored or maintained a flow rate of greater than 300 mL/min without line reversals in 36 of 50 (72%) patients, with a second instillation restoring patency for a further four patients (80%). The majority of patients required further thrombolysis or radiological intervention in the 4-month follow-up period.[19]

The optimal dwell times for lytic agents have yet to be determined. rTPA infusions are effective even when there is an associated fibrin sheath.[20]

Tenecteplase is a new lytic agent with increased fibrin specificity, greater resistance to plasminogen activator inhibitor 1 and a relatively long half-life. A randomised study showed a 1-hour dwell of 2 mg of tenecteplase more effective than placebo in restoring flow in dysfunctional haemodialysis catheters.[21] An extended dwell improves treatment success.[22]

Central vein thrombosis

Mural thrombus is commonly seen in the SVC and RA with central venous catheters. If it compromises venous return, facial and arm oedema results. Central vein thrombus can be identified by magnetic resonance or conventional venography. Infusion of a fibrinolytic agent is usually successful, although organised thrombus may require angioplasty and stenting.

Fibrin sheaths

Fibrin sheaths cause up to 43% of catheter dysfunction.[23] Contrast injection through the dialysis line may show a filling defect near the catheter tip or retrograde flow along the external surface of the catheter (**Fig. 16.1**). This may be treated by infusing a

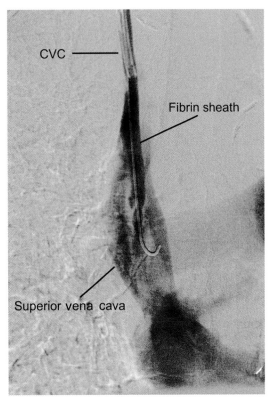

Figure 16.1 • A venogram showing fibrin sheath around a partially withdrawn central venous catheter.

fibrinolytic agent over 6 hours, mechanical stripping using a snare from the femoral vein, or catheter exchange over a guidewire.

Stripping has a high technical success rate but the fibrin sheath frequently recurs. In a randomised trial there was no significant difference in additional patency between percutaneous stripping or urokinase.[24] In another randomised trial 4-month catheter patency was significantly better after catheter exchange than percutaneous stripping.[25]

If the catheter is exchanged over a guidewire, the sheath must be mechanically disrupted or the new catheter will be reinserted down the existing sheath. There are no controlled trials comparing all three techniques.

Catheter-related infection

Catheter-related infection is a major cause of morbidity and mortality and is related to the duration of placement. Gram-positive bacteria are the usual cause[26] and resistant organisms such as methicillin-resistant *Staphylococcus aureus* (MRSA) are increasing. Catheter-associated sepsis can result in infective endocarditis, osteomyelitis, septic arthritis, epidural abscesses and death. Infection spreads either through the lumen of the catheter or along the outside from the exit site. An associated biofilm reduces the effectiveness of antibiotics.

Infections in non-tunnelled catheters should be treated by catheter removal and systemic antibiotics. In tunnelled catheters 90% of exit-site infections respond to oral antibiotics but intravenous antibiotics and catheter removal may be necessary for more serious tunnel infections. Systemic infections associated with tunnelled catheters can be treated initially with antibiotics but catheter removal is usually required. A new catheter should be inserted at a different site when the systemic sepsis has settled. Catheter exchange over a guidewire is controversial but there is some evidence that infection-free survival is similar to that after removal and delayed replacement.[27]

The cornerstone of prevention is scrupulous asepsis with regular exit-site inspection and dressing changes. Chlorhexidine and alcohol 70% provide superior asepsis to povidone–iodine 10% as an exit-site cleaning solution.[28] Mupirocin ointment is also effective,[29] but may increase colonisation by fungi and multiresistant organisms. Antibiotic-coated catheters reduce line sepsis in intensive care patients[30] and temporary dialysis catheters[31] but there is no evidence of benefit for long-term dialysis as the antibiotic is washed off over time. Bismuth has been demonstrated to have antibiofilm and antibiotic properties. A recent randomised clinical trial of bismuth-coated non-tunnelled dialysis catheters in 77 patients showed a reduction in catheter colonisation compared with non-coated catheters.[32] There is also recent evidence that bacterial growth can be reduced by altering catheter surface irregularities.[33] Antibiotic catheter locks have also been used and are effective at reducing catheter infections but there is a danger of antibiotic resistance. Antibiotic heparin and citrate heparin locks are superior to heparin alone but there are no randomised trials comparing antibiotic and citrate locks.[34]

Permanent dialysis access

✔ An AVF should be constructed 16–24 weeks before the anticipated need for dialysis, when the creatinine clearance falls to 25 mL/min or the serum creatinine level rises above 400 μmol/L (4 mg/dL) to allow time for maturation or revision in the event of failure.[35–38]

Whereas CVCs are usually introduced on the ward or in the radiology department, peripheral arteriovenous (AV) access procedures require an operating theatre. However, most can be performed under local anaesthetic, often as day cases.

✔ Dedicated access operating lists are an enormous advantage and one such list is required per week for every 120 patients on dialysis to prevent unacceptable waiting times and prolonged CVC usage.[5,38] Service organisation should include provision for regular interventional radiology lists to support such a service.[36,37]

Access planning

✔ In patients with chronic renal failure it is essential that the cephalic and antecubital veins of both arms be reserved for dialysis access. Intravenous cannulae for other purposes should only be inserted into the back of the hand or the small veins on the anterior surface of the wrist, except in emergencies. A CVC, AVF or AVG should only be used for dialysis.[35–38]

An AVF should be created as distally as possible to preserve sites for future access. The non-dominant arm is preferred to allow greater freedom on dialysis or to facilitate self-cannulation for home dialysis patients. When upper limb access sites are exhausted the lower limbs may be used.[35–38] Autogenous AVFs are preferable to prosthetic AVGs as they have higher patency,[39] lower infection rates, require fewer revisions[40] and are associated with a slightly lower mortality, especially in diabetics.[8,41]

Whereas a side-to-side radiocephalic AVF was originally described,[42] an end-to-side configuration is now preferred as there is less risk of peripheral venous hypertension. Some advocate an end-to-end anastomosis for distal radiocephalic AVFs, provided there is a good ulnar pulse, to reduce the small incidence of steal.[43] Autogenous AVFs require a period of maturation to allow arterialisation of the venous outflow whereas AVGs can be needled directly as soon as the wounds have healed.

Preoperative assessment

✔ In many centres, patients proceed directly to primary AVF formation if there is a satisfactory radial pulse and suitable forearm veins. Opinion is divided on the need for preoperative imaging: the latest US National Kidney Foundation – Dialysis Outcomes Quality Initiative (NKF-KDOQI) clinical guidelines now recommend routine duplex imaging in all patients,[44] whereas the Vascular Access Society recommends a selective approach.[36]

There is an increasing trend for preoperative imaging to reduce primary failure, non-maturation and unnecessary surgery.[35–38,44] This remains untested by clinical trial.

Venography is advisable if central vein stenosis is suspected. In complex cases with unclear venous anatomy, particularly predialysis patients in whom iodinated contrast could exacerbate renal failure, duplex ultrasound or magnetic resonance imaging may be preferable in the first instance. Angiography or arterial duplex is recommended if arterial pulses are diminished.

Duplex ultrasound

Preoperative duplex ultrasound is particularly useful for obese patients with impalpable superficial veins or following previous access failure, but cannot assess central vein patency. In studies from the USA, where AVGs are more frequently used than in Europe, routine preoperative ultrasound significantly increased the prevalence, reduced early failure rate and increased primary patency of autogenous AVFs compared with historical controls.[45-47] Prosthetic AV access reconstruction and access complications also decreased significantly. In another study duplex mapping changed the proposed procedure in a third of patients and almost doubled the proportion of AVFs constructed.[48] However, in a British study, duplex scanning rarely added any useful information except in those patients with poor vessels on clinical examination, when the proposed procedure was altered in 50%. This suggests that patients with good pulses and clinically adequate veins may proceed to surgery safely without preoperative ultrasound mapping.[49]

A radial artery luminal diameter of less than 1.6 mm is associated with early fistula failure[50] and a minimum diameter of 2 mm is now usually advised.[36,38,44] Above this threshold there seems to be no correlation between arterial diameter or flow and fistula success.

Venous diameter is an important determinant of outcome. In prospective studies, mean cephalic vein diameters are significantly smaller in non-functioning AVFs. Minimum venous diameters (with a tourniquet) of 2–2.5 mm have been advised for AVFs and 3.5–4.0 mm for synthetic grafts.[36,38,44]

Venous distensibility is another important predictor of success. Veins were found to dilate 48% with a tourniquet in successful fistulas compared with only 12% in fistulas that subsequently failed.[51]

Venography

✅ For many years, contrast venography was the gold standard and has the advantage of providing a venous map. It is mandatory in patients with prior ipsilateral central vein catheterisation, collateral vein development, oedema or arm swelling, indicating possible central vein obstruction.[36,38] Construction of a peripheral fistula in these patients can cause massive arm swelling. Previous radiotherapy to the shoulder area (e.g. for breast carcinoma) is a further indication for preoperative venography.

Iodinated contrast may precipitate acute renal failure and is relatively contraindicated in predialysis patients. Duplex ultrasound is an alternative but is poor for assessing central vein stenosis. Contrast-enhanced magnetic resonance venography is promising, as the small volume of paramagnetic contrast agent used does not compromise renal function, but there have been concerns about the rare complication of nephrogenic systemic fibrosis. Imaging is likely to improve significantly with new pulse sequences and blood pool contrast agents.

Carbon dioxide venography is not nephrotoxic and is widely used in France but requires a costly injector, causes local pain during injection, can overestimate the degree of venous stenosis and occasionally cause acute right heart failure.

Primary access

The snuffbox AVF is the most distal access possible and gives the longest length of vein for needling. It is possible in about 50% of patients and, in the event of failure, a wrist AVF can still be performed in half of the cases[52] (**Fig. 16.2**).

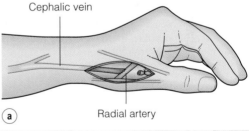

Cephalic vein

Radial artery

(a)

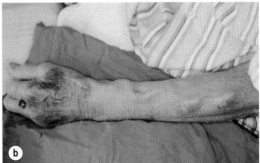

(b)

Figure 16.2 • The snuffbox arteriovenous fistula. **(a)** Diagram showing position of anastomosis. **(b)** A mature snuffbox fistula showing the long length of available vein for needling.

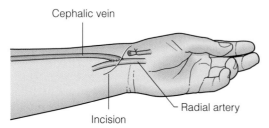

Figure 16.3 • The radiocephalic arteriovenous fistula at the wrist.

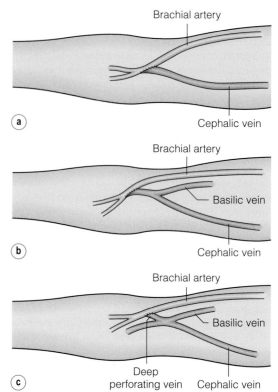

Figure 16.4 • Configurations of the brachiocephalic arteriovenous fistula at the antecubital fossa. **(a)** Direct anastomosis between the cephalic vein and brachial artery. **(b)** Anastomosis including both median basilic and cephalic veins. **(c)** Gracz fistula between the deep perforating vein and the brachial artery.

The wrist radiocephalic AVF (**Fig. 16.3**) was the first to be described[42] and remains the standard access in most units. It has a low complication rate and gives a good length of available vein. Patencies of 65% at 1 year are usual.[53] If a wrist AVF fails, further forearm radiocephalic fistulas can often be created more proximally. In obese patients the vein may remain difficult to needle so that it may be advisable to excise the subcutaneous fat overlying the vein through one or more transverse incisions.

The brachiocephalic AVF is the next option, which can be performed in a variety of configurations (**Fig. 16.4**), and gives excellent flows at the expense of a greater incidence of steal (see below). To avoid this, some authors advocate anastomosing the cephalic vein to the radial artery 2 cm beyond its origin instead of the brachial artery itself.[54]

The ulnobasilic AVF is often possible after a failed brachial fistula but is more difficult to needle and seems to have a poorer patency than other upper limb AVFs.[55]

When the options are limited by venous thrombosis or arterial disease an ulnocephalic or radiobasilic fistula may be possible in the forearm, but these require more extensive mobilisation and subcutaneous tunnelling of the vein across the forearm.[56]

Secondary and tertiary access

When the cephalic vein is thrombosed, an antecubital brachiobasilic AVF may be possible but this leaves only a short length of vein for needling. Therefore the basilic vein is usually mobilised and rerouted superficially over the biceps muscle either in a single procedure or in a second stage after the vein has arterialised (the basilic vein transposition; **Fig. 16.5**).[57]

When an autogenous AVF cannot be performed, a prosthetic graft (AVG) can be used. A variety of graft materials are available, but polytetrafluoroethylene (PTFE) is the most popular. The graft can be used for needling after 2 weeks, and may be used sooner though this can be associated with perigraft haematoma formation. Prosthetic grafts have a higher rate of infection compared to AVF. Thrombosis is also more common than in AVF

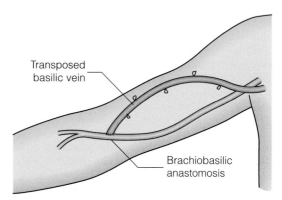

Figure 16.5 • The basilic vein transposition arteriovenous fistula.

and is usually due to intimal hyperplasia, at or just beyond the venous anastomosis. A wider graft,[58] a vein cuff[59] or an expansion of the venous end of the graft (Venoflo)[60] may reduce this and provide better patency. It is widely recognised that revision rates for grafts approach 80% annually compared to about 15% for AVF.

Biological grafts such as bovine mesenteric vein and bovine ureter are preferred in some units as they have greater resistance to infection, but they are prone to aneurysm formation.[61] A forearm AVG either in a looped or straight configuration allows a basilic vein transposition to be performed if it fails, but has a poorer patency than the latter,[62] so which should be performed first is a matter of debate. A brachio-axillary AVG is the next option (**Fig. 16.6**).

Lower limb access is less popular but may be the only option when the SVC or both subclavian veins are occluded. An AVF at the ankle between the greater saphenous vein (GSV) and the posterior tibial artery is rarely possible because of underlying arterial disease. The GSV can be anastomosed to the popliteal artery above the knee or used as a subcutaneous loop from the femoral artery in the groin, but these are more difficult to needle. Transpositon of the GSV in the thigh is less popular as it is more difficult to needle, but has fewer infective complications than synthetic thigh loop grafts.[63] The superficial femoral vein can be used in the same configurations (or transposed to the forearm) and gives an excellent fistula at the expense of a high incidence of steal.

In desperate cases, a variety of possibilities exist: axillofemoral, axillo-axillary, ilio-iliac or even aorto-IVC AVGs can be used. Where there are no available veins the RA can be used as an outflow. Alternatively an arterio-arterial graft, usually in the axillary position, is possible but risks distal embolisation to the arm.[64] Occlusion of arterial interposition grafts may precipitate acute limb ischaemia.

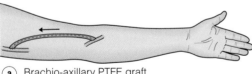

(a) Brachio-axillary PTFE graft

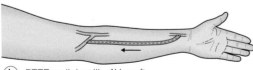

(b) PTFE radiobasilic AV graft

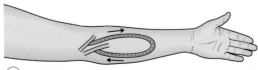

(c) PTFE forearm loop

Figure 16.6 • Popular configurations for upper limb arteriovenous grafts: straight **(a,b)** and looped **(c)** brachio-axillary forearm grafts.

Factors affecting access patency

The following factors are known to affect access patency:

- **Vessel size.** Small arteries and veins have higher initial failure rates, more frequent failure to mature and poorer long-term patency.[50]
- **Fistula flow rate.** The flow rate the day after surgery correlates inversely with the risk of thrombosis, although intraoperative flow rates are less reliable.[50] The hyperaemic response of brachial artery blood flow is a strong predictor of access patency and maturation, presumably by detecting proximal arterial stenoses.[65]
- **Mode of presentation.** Patients presenting acutely with renal failure have poorer AVF patency, which may be linked to the need for temporary access via a central venous catheter.[66]
- **Anastomotic method.** Non-penetrating vascular clips, which give an interrupted anastomosis with excellent endothelial apposition and less bleeding, are quicker and have improved patencies compared with sutured anastomoses in randomised trials.[67,68]
- **Access position.** More proximal AVFs have improved patency[68] but leave fewer options for access in the event of failure.
- **Gender.** Patency of AVFs is poorer in women than men.[52,66,69,70]
- **Diabetes.** There is conflicting evidence as to whether diabetes is an adverse factor, with some authors suggesting that AVF patency is poorer[68] whereas others have found no effect.[52,71,72]
- **Age.** In a meta-analysis, access patency was found to be worse in the elderly.[73] Wrist fistulas may perform as well as more proximal AVF.[74]
- **Obesity.** Veins are more difficult to cannulate in obese patients, which may account for poorer patency reported by some authors.[75]
- **Smoking.** Smoking reduces AVF patency.[76]
- **Drugs.** Antiplatelet agents such as aspirin and dipyridamole prolong fistula survival and are used routinely.[77–79] A combination of aspirin and clopidogrel increased haemorrhagic complications without influencing patency in prosthetic AVGs in one study,[80] but clopidogrel alone significantly prolonged graft survival in another.[81] Warfarin reduces AVF thrombosis in patients with hypercoagulable states,[82] but routine use is best avoided because of the risk of haemorrhage. Surprisingly, warfarin was associated with poorer

patency in the Dialysis Outcomes and Practice Patterns Study (DOPPS), but this may reflect its use in patients with a history of fistula thrombosis or known thrombotic disorders.[79] Calcium channel blockers are associated with improved primary patency.[79] Angiotensin-converting enzyme inhibitors did not affect primary patency in one study[83] but were associated with improved secondary patency in DOPPS.[78] Fish oil reduced AVF thrombosis in one randomised trial.[8,84] Erythropoietin does not reduce and may increase patency, at least in AVGs.[85,86]

- **Thrombotic tendencies and vasculitis.** Increased fibrinogen and vasculitis predispose to access thrombosis.[87]

Access failure

Failure to mature

About 10% of AVFs remain patent but never achieve an adequate flow for dialysis. A duplex scan may reveal a proximal arterial or a venous stenosis, treatable by angioplasty or surgery. Otherwise a more proximal fistula will be required.

Stenosis and thrombosis

Early thrombosis may result from technical error, unrecognised pre-existing arterial stenoses or thrombophlebitis in the outflow vein, usually from previous intravenous cannulation. Late failure can result from hypotension, dehydration and hypercoagulable states, 'blowout' after traumatic needling or inappropriate use for intravenous infusions, but the most common cause is juxta-anastomotic venous intimal hyperplasia in AVG. In AVF failure may result from perianastomotic stenosis, but in long-standing AVF used for dialysis, mid-fistula stenosis between needling sites is also common.

> ✅ Percutaneous angioplasty of stenoses in AVFs and AVGs preserves veins and may prevent access thrombosis. Stenting is controversial but probably offers little extra advantage. Endovascular thrombolysis or thrombectomy of occluded AV accesses is effective provided that any underlying stenosis is dilated.[35–38]

Prevention of access failure

To prevent damage, careful needling and the avoidance of inappropriate use of AVFs are essential. Attempts to prevent intimal hyperplasia pharmacologically (e.g. with drug-eluting wraps), or external stenting, have yet to lead to routine clinical application.[88,89]

Access surveillance

AVFs and AVGs may suddenly occlude without prior warning, resulting in hospitalisation and the need for a CVC. Most of these will have unrecognised stenoses due to intimal hyperplasia. Detection by routine surveillance and treatment of such stenoses can prevent thrombosis and allow continuous use of the access.

Impending failure may be indicated by the loss of a palpable thrill, needling difficulties or a reduction in dialysis efficiency (e.g. reduced Kt/V (the volume cleared of urea/distribution volume), a reduced urea reduction ratio at each dialysis, a rising predialysis serum potassium or evidence of recirculation through the dialysis machine). Such monitoring is useful but does not identify all failing fistulas.

> ✅ Access surveillance is controversial but there is increasing evidence that access flow monitoring can identify stenoses in AVFs and AVGs and allow endovascular treatment to prevent access failure.

A variety of surveillance methods using static (with the pump turned off) or dynamic (at a standard pump speed) venous pressure measurements during dialysis have been proposed but are unreliable because the direction of any pressure change depends on whether the venous needle is upstream or downstream of the stenosis. Flow measurements are usually performed by an indicator dilution technique (e.g. ultrasound dilution).[90,91] A low flow (<500 mL/min) is a strong predictor of impending thrombosis in AVGs and is better than dynamic venous pressure.[92–94] The change in graft flow over time is a better predictor than a single value[95] and a 25% drop has been proposed as the trigger for further imaging and intervention.

Detection of stenoses is worthwhile, as intervention-free survival is better for grafts after pre-emptive angioplasty than after thrombectomy and angioplasty,[96] and vascular access flow monitoring reduces access morbidity and costs.[97] Reducing hospitalisation is an important element of providing high-quality care for patients.[98]

Surveillance using flow measurements also reduced thrombosis rates in AVFs in non-randomised[97,99] and randomised studies.[100] Others have failed to show improvement with surveillance but have been criticised on grounds of inadequate sensitivity[101] or inadequate angioplasty of detected stenoses.[102] Duplex surveillance also reduces thrombosis rates,[103] hospitalisation and CVC usage[104] in AVFs and AVGs.

Access salvage

AVF stenosis

In radiocephalic fistulas, most stenoses occur close to the AV anastomosis (**Fig. 16.7**), with the remainder more proximally in the vein. In upper arm AVFs they also occur at the cephalic/subclavian vein junction.

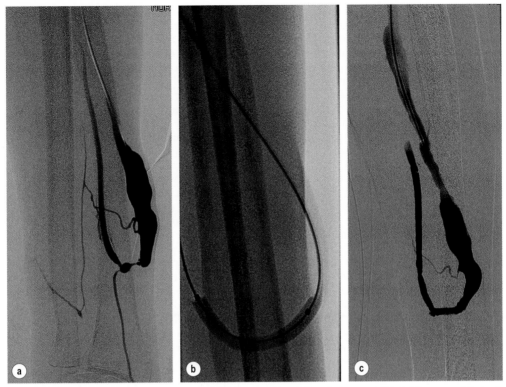

Figure 16.7 • Fistulogram showing a stenosis adjacent to a radiocephalic arteriovenous fistula **(a)** successfully treated by angioplasty **(b,c)**.

Intervention is indicated for stenoses greater than 50% associated with flow reduction, compromised dialysis or arm oedema. Fistulography is usually performed through the draining vein, reserving brachial artery puncture for inflow and anastomotic lesions. The venous run-off and central veins should also be demonstrated.

Primary angioplasty is indicated for upper forearm and upper arm significant stenoses, with technical success rates of over 90% and 1-year primary patency of 51% for forearm and 35% for upper arm fistulas.[105] Secondary patencies of over 80% can be achieved but more frequent interventions are needed in the upper arm. Stents have not been shown to offer an advantage.

Stenoses in the upper arm cephalic vein (cephalic arch) are a common cause of failure in patients with brachiocephalic fistulas. These lesions respond poorly to angioplasty as they are resistant to dilatation, develop early restenosis and have high vein rupture rates. Primary patencies at 6 months and 1 year after angioplasty are 42% and 23%, respectively.[106] A small randomised trial of stent grafts versus bare-metal stents for the management of cephalic arch stenosis showed a 6-month primary patency of 81.8% for stent grafts and 39.1% for bare-metal stents.[107] There have been no randomised

studies comparing angioplasty and stent placement. There is a danger of stent migration into the subclavian vein that could jeopardise future access in the whole ipsilateral limb. Surgical revision with cephalic vein transposition to the basilic or axillary veins can be considered if angioplasty fails, although this may be technically difficult in an extensively needled AVF. If recurrent stenoses are angioplastied in patients who have undergone surgical revision, secondary patency rates of 92% at 1 year can be achieved.[108]

If endovascular intervention fails, stenoses can also be repaired surgically using a vein or prosthetic patch. Alternatively, inserting a short PTFE graft segment appears to be as good as an autogenous patch.[109] Stenoses adjacent to a distal AVF are best treated by creating a more proximal fistula, which may have better patency than angioplasty.[110]

AVG stenosis

The most common cause for AVG dysfunction is a stenosis at or near the venous anastomosis. Indications for intervention are similar to those for AVFs, with similar high technical success rates. Restenosis is a greater problem and leads to poor primary patency rates of 23–44% at 1 year,[111] but 1-year secondary patencies of 92% can be achieved by repeated angioplasty.[105] Intragraft stenoses from excessive ingrowth of fibrous tissue through cannulation defects can be treated similarly, but may require surgical curettage or segmental replacement.

When angioplasty fails repeatedly, bare-metal stents can be considered but their primary patency is generally no better than angioplasty. There is an emerging role for covered stents in the treatment of angioplasty rupture and poor results from simple angioplasty. In one randomised trial, adding a covered stent after AVG angioplasty increased the 6-month patency from 23% to 51%.[112] However, there were similar access-assisted and cumulative patency rates at 6 months in both groups, and it remains unclear whether the high cost of stent grafts can justify their routine use.[113] There are no published randomised trials on the use of drug-eluting stents.

Unassisted graft survival after thrombectomy and angioplasty is significantly worse than after elective angioplasty of patent grafts. Graft survival after thrombectomy and angioplasty may also be improved by stent implantation,[114] but there are no prospective controlled data.

There is no evidence favouring surgical revision over endovascular repair, but revisional surgery by segmental replacement or a jump graft to bypass a venous outflow stenosis may be required for recurrent stenoses. A pragmatic approach of reserving surgery for resistant or rapidly recurring stenosis will minimise unnecessary surgical intervention.

AVF and AVG thrombosis

Percutaneous declotting of AVGs is well established and effective, but AVFs are also being increasingly referred for radiological salvage. A thrombosed access should be declotted as soon as possible, preferably within 48 hours, and the underlying stenosis treated by angioplasty (with or without stenting). Available techniques include thrombolysis, thromboaspiration and mechanical thrombectomy. None seems superior but the expertise and experience of the operator are paramount.

Thrombus in an AVF causes phlebitis. Keeping the inflammatory response to a minimum is a key component of successful intervention. Whilst AVG can be declotted up to several weeks after thrombosis, most AVF require intervention within 24–48 hours for success. The amount of thrombus can vary significantly. In some AVFs only a short segment of vein thromboses because a side-branch just proximal to a perianastomotic stenosis maintains patency. These can usually be treated by simple angioplasty. In others the large volume of thrombus in an aneurysmal draining vein has a risk of a significant pulmonary embolus unless it is aggressively aspirated or a mechanical clot-removing device is used.

Technical success is reported as 73–90%, with widely differing 1-year primary and secondary patencies of 9–70% and 44–93%, respectively.[115] Patencies are higher in the forearm than upper arm. There are no randomised trials of percutaneous intervention versus surgery for AVFs. Primary endovascular intervention has the advantage of preserving veins for needling, but surgical revision or a new AVF is often necessary.

AVGs thrombose more frequently than AVFs but are well suited to percutaneous intervention. Radiological declotting is less invasive than surgery and allows accurate treatment of the underlying cause, which is nearly always a venous outflow stenosis. No single device or declotting technique has been shown to be superior, and the success of treatment of the underlying stenosis seems to be the only predictive value for graft patency.[116] Thrombolysis or mechanical thrombectomy have clinical success rates of 74–94% but 6-month primary patencies are only 18–39%.[117] However, with repeated intervention secondary patency rates of up to 83% have been reported.[118] Whilst there has been no prospective randomised multicentre trial, a meta-analysis found surgical intervention to have higher primary patency than endovascular intervention.[119] In many centres endovascular declotting is preferred because of its low morbidity, reserving surgical revision for technical failures or repeated thromboses.[117]

The most common complication of endovascular declotting is distal arterial embolisation, which occurs in 1–9% of cases.[117] Others include vessel rupture (2–4%) and non-puncture site bleeding (2–3%). All methods of declotting, especially mechanical techniques, cause venous embolisation, but this is usually asymptomatic because of the small volume of thrombus displaced.

Surgical thrombectomy is usually easy if the access has failed recently. Any underlying stenosis must be corrected by bypass or patch angioplasty at the same time. If surgery is delayed for 10 days or more it may be best to abandon it and create a new access at another site.

Other access complications

Infection

Infection is the commonest cause of hospital admission and mortality in dialysis patients. It is most frequent in patients with CVCs and commoner in patients with AVGs than AVFs. The most frequent organism is *Staphylococcus aureus*. Bacteraemia or septicaemia may lead to endocarditis, mycotic aneurysms and septic arthritis.

Local needle-site infections may be controlled with antibiotics in the early stages but can lead to

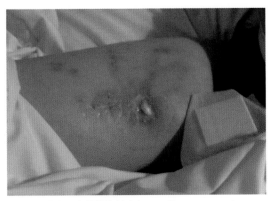

Figure 16.8 • A PTFE thigh loop with an exposed segment.

Table 16.1 • The stages of access steal syndrome

Stage	Clinical features
I	Pale/cyanosed and/or cold hand without pain
II	Pain on exercise and/or dialysis
III	Rest pain
IV	Ulcer/necrosis/gangrene

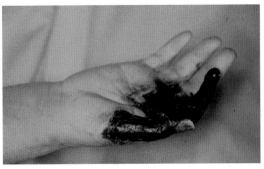

Figure 16.9 • Severe steal with digital gangrene after a brachial arteriovenous fistula.

uncontrollable haemorrhage in autogenous fistulas, requiring emergency ligation or bypass of the infected area. AVGs with chronic needle-site infections or exposed segments (**Fig. 16.8**) may be salvaged by local excision and bypass of the area with appropriate antibiotic cover, but when the whole graft is infected it requires total excision. A further graft may be inserted once the wounds have healed.

Haemorrhage

Traumatic cannulation leads to localised haematomas. Prosthetic grafts can be destroyed by repeated punctures in the same area. This may necessitate local graft replacement.

Steal

An AVF tends to reduce digital arterial pressures[120] by lowering the peripheral resistance and may cause ischaemia (high-flow steal). The presence of a proximal arterial stenosis will amplify the reduction in finger pressures on AVF creation by limiting the increase in inflow (low-flow steal).

> ✓✓ Mild steal symptoms, such as coldness, pain, cramps, diminished sensation or reduced grip strength, are common in patients with AVFs. At least one symptom is present in 80% of brachial AVFs, 50% of those with forearm AV loops and 40% of radiocephalic AVFs,[121] but clinically significant steal with rest pain or tissue loss occurs in only 1–8% of patients.

Four grades of steal are recognised (Table 16.1). Grades 1 and 2 can usually be managed conservatively, but grades 3 and 4 require surgical intervention.

Predisposing factors include proximal AVF, diabetes mellitus, cardiac ischaemia, peripheral vascular disease[122,123] and low preoperative finger pressures.[120] Steal is the most likely cause of unilateral hand or finger ischaemia occurring after AVF creation (**Fig. 16.9**).

The clinical diagnosis can be made by a clear history of steal associated with the finding of an absent radial pulse that returns when the fistula is occluded. If in doubt, the diagnosis is confirmed by a digital pressure of 60 mmHg or less, with a significant increase on AVF occlusion.[124] A digital:brachial pressure index of less than 0.4 is also associated with steal. A duplex scan will demonstrate any proximal stenosis, quantify AVF flow and show reversed flow in the artery distal to the AVF (although this is not diagnostic). Fistulography is rarely required.

Steal syndrome should be treated promptly to avoid permanent neurological sequelae. These rarely recover completely if allowed to persist for any length of time.

AVF ligation cures steal syndrome and may be the sensible course of action in severe cases with rapid onset. Clinicians should undertake this only if they are confident that alternative access can be safely provided. As the majority of patients have similar arterial and venous pathologies in all of their limbs, attempting new access in the contralateral limb may simply reproduce steal in a new site. Steal syndrome associated with arterial inflow stenosis can usually be corrected by angioplasty or bypass. There are a variety of treatment options for steal with evidence of proximal arterial disease. At the wrist, radial arterial ligation distal to the fistula to prevent reversed flow is usually successful in those AVFs with an intact ulnar artery and palmar arch.

Distal arterial ligation may also be sufficient in brachial AVFs but intraoperative monitoring with finger or needle pressures is essential as in most cases finger pressures rarely improve sufficiently. In these cases a bypass from the proximal brachial (at least 8 cm proximal to the AV fistula anastomosis) or the axillary artery to the brachial artery distal to the ligature increases the distal pressure enough to relieve symptoms in most cases. This is the so-called DRIL (distal revascularisation interval ligation) procedure[125] (**Fig. 16.10**).

Another technique to prevent distal reversed flow is 'proximalisation of the arterial inflow' in which a brachial AVF or AVG is taken down and a prosthetic graft is led from the axillary or proximal brachial artery and anastomosed to the outflow vein or the arterial end of the AVG[126] (**Fig. 16.11**). This preserves fistula flow but transfers the inflow to a larger, high-flow artery capable of adapting to the reduction in peripheral resistance without distal flow reversal. This may be useful in patients where a diseased run-off might compromise the distal revascularisation of a DRIL procedure.

An alternative flow-reduction method is the 'extension procedure',[127] which is also known as the 'revision using distal inflow' (RUDI),[128] in which the cephalic vein or AVG is detached from its origin on the brachial artery and extended

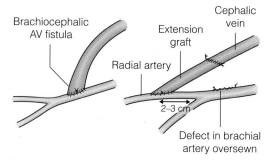

Figure 16.12 • The extension procedure.

onto the radial artery 2–3 cm from its origin using a vein or prosthetic graft. This narrows the inflow and permits hand perfusion through the ulnar artery (**Fig. 16.12**). The choice of procedure depends on experience and personal preference, but the DRIL procedure is currently the most popular.

Fistula flow can be reduced by narrowing the outflow vein ('banding'), but achieving the appropriate degree of stenosis is difficult. It is not uncommon to either narrow the outflow sufficiently to cause thrombosis, or to fail to reduce flow and relieve the steal. However, in a recent report the degree of stenosis was successfully controlled by tightening a polyester band in stages whilst monitoring the flow rate, digital pressures and subclavian venous oxygen saturation.[129] In another report banding was accomplished by a spindle-like suture and a PTFE strip during intraoperative flow monitoring.[130]

Carpal tunnel syndrome

The incidence of carpal tunnel syndrome is increased by the presence of an AVF, possibly owing to mild oedema due to venous hypertension.[131]

Cardiac failure

High-output cardiac failure is a rare complication, occurring occasionally with proximal AVFs with fistula flows in excess of 1.5 litres per minute. Bramham's sign (slowing of the heart rate on AVF compression) confirms the diagnosis. Treatment is either by fistula ligation or flow reduction by the extension procedure or controlled banding.[129]

Venous hypertension and central vein obstruction

Venous hypertension with oedema, venous collateral formation, or ulceration and tissue loss can occur with side-to-side AVFs but is more commonly associated with central venous obstruction (**Fig. 16.13**). If venous hypertension occurs with a side-to-side AVF, ligation of the distal vein draining the AVF is easy to perform and usually curative.

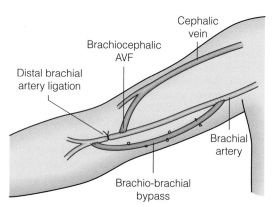

Figure 16.10 • The DRIL (distal revascularisation interval ligation) procedure.

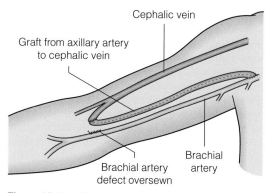

Figure 16.11 • Proximalisation of the arterial inflow.

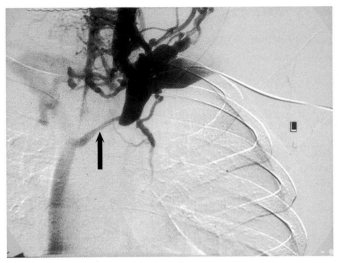

Figure 16.13 • Venogram showing an innominate vein stenosis.

An AVF distal to a central obstruction is likely to exacerbate venous hypertension and may precipitate symptoms. Treatment of central vein obstruction by endovascular means or, as a last resort, surgical bypass will preserve the AVF, but sometimes the access must be ligated and created elsewhere, usually in the lower limb.

Subclavian stenosis or thrombosis is usually caused by a previous subclavian CVC. IJV catheters are now preferred but there is still a significant incidence of innominate and SVC stenosis (**Fig. 16.13**) or thrombosis. Endovascular treatment of these lesions is ideal, but simple angioplasty has a disappointing primary patency rate at 1 year of less than 40% in most studies.[7] Primary assisted or secondary patency rates are more encouraging at 35–97%.[132] Stents have a major role and can either be routinely placed at the initial intervention or reserved for early and frequent restenosis. There are no randomised trials versus angioplasty. There is no evidence at present advocating covered stents.

Surgical bypass gave a similar primary patency rate (70–80%) at 1 year to primary angioplasty and stenting in one study,[133] but has significant morbidity and mortality. Isolated subclavian vein occlusions may be repaired surgically by direct patch angioplasty, an axillo-jugular venous bypass or the jugular turndown operation.

SVC obstruction is best treated endovascularly, often requiring stent insertion to achieve patency. The symptomatic relief for the patient is immediate. Surgical bypass is a major undertaking with significant morbidity and should be regarded as a last resort in younger patients. Surgical incisions in an engorged neck can be associated with significant venous bleeding.

Aneurysm

The AVF outflow vein usually hypertrophies but sometimes reaches aneurysmal proportions (**Fig. 16.14**). In general, such aneurysms can be observed, as rupture is rare. Indications for intervention are rapid or persistent enlargement, skin breakdown with or without bleeding and patient request. The psychological effects of large and unsightly access in younger patients should not be underestimated. Surgical aneurysmorrhaphy can significantly reduce the bulk of AVF whilst excising damaged skin and preserving the AVF for use. In AVF with multiple aneurysms, the author's preference is for sequential aneurysmorrhaphy allowing continued use of the unoperated segment of the AVF while healing occurs.

There is debate as to whether mesh wrapping of the aneurysmorrhaphy is required, but this has not been formally tested.[134,135]

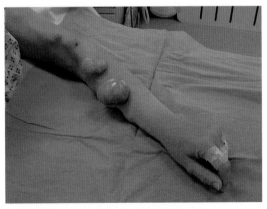

Figure 16.14 • An aneurysmal wrist arteriovenous fistula.

There is interest in the use of covered stents for exclusion of pseudoaneurysms, but this has not been formally tested in a clinical trial.

Cannulation

Cannulation of AVFs should be performed by adequately trained staff under strict aseptic conditions. A new autologous AVF is usually rested for 6 weeks before needling, to allow the vein wall to thicken, although early cannulation did not appear to be a risk factor in the DOPPS.[136] There may be cultural differences, with a tendency to earlier needling in Japan. An experienced dialysis nurse should always perform the first cannulation. Prosthetic grafts are needled directly and are usable for dialysis after 2 weeks.

There are three major strategies:

- The buttonhole technique, where the same site is needled at each dialysis, which is less painful and causes less aneurysm formation but is less suitable for grafts because it can cause local graft destruction.

- Area puncture, where the vein or graft is needled over a specific area for each of the withdrawal and reinfusion sites, results in venous dilatation over an area but can also cause stenoses between aneurysmal sections.
- The rope-ladder technique, where needles are inserted for each dialysis by moving along the vein or graft in a sequential pattern. This is probably most suitable for AVGs as the damage of repeated needling is distributed over a larger area and delays the need for revision.

Access in children

The small calibre of the vessels has discouraged many surgeons from constructing AVFs in small children. Alternative methods such as continuous ambulatory peritoneal dialysis (CAPD) are therefore preferred in many units, but when haemodialysis is unavoidable CVCs are commonly used. However, excellent results of radiocephalic or brachial AVFs constructed by microsurgery in small children have been reported from experienced units.[137]

Key points

- The veins of the dorsum of the hand should be the preferred site for intravenous cannulation. The cephalic and antecubital veins should be reserved for dialysis access in patients with renal failure.
- The right IJV is the preferred site for central venous cannulation, which should be performed under ultrasound control.
- The use of CVCs for acute or short-term dialysis should be minimised because of the risks of septic complications, central venous thrombosis and a higher mortality than AVFs.
- Tunnelled CVCs should be used for dialysis if required for longer than 2 weeks but should only be used long term when an AVF or AVG cannot be constructed.
- Permanent vascular access should, wherever possible, be constructed 16–24 weeks before the anticipated need for dialysis.
- For permanent dialysis access an autogenous AVF should be constructed as distally as possible, preferably in the non-dominant arm.
- AVGs should be used only when the construction of an autogenous AVF is not possible.

Full references available at **http://expertconsult. inkling.com**

Key references

13. Mallory DL, McGee WT, Shawker TH, et al. Ultrasound improves the success rate of internal jugular vein cannulation: a prospective, randomised trial. Chest 1990;98:157–60. PMID: 2193776.

In this prospective randomised trial ultrasound was shown to increase the success rate and reduce the complications of internal jugular cannulation.

39. Huber TS, Carter JW, Carter RL, et al. Patency of autogenous and polytetrafluoroethylene upper extremity arteriovenous hemodialysis accesses: a systematic review. J Vasc Surg 2003;38:1005–11. PMID: 14603208.

A review and meta-analysis comparing 34 non-randomised studies of upper limb AV access showing a significantly better primary patency for autogenous AV fistulas at 6 months (72%) and

18 months (51%) than PTFE AV grafts (58% and 33%, respectively).

40. Hodges TC, Fillinger MF, Zwolak RM, et al. Longitudinal comparison of dialysis access methods: factors for failure. J Vasc Surg 1997;26:1009–19. PMID: 9423717.

A large retrospective single-centre study showing similar secondary patency for autogenous and prosthetic access but a much higher revision rate for AV grafts.

41. Astor BC, Eustace JA, Powe NR, et al. Type of vascular access and survival among incident hemodialysis patients: the Choices for Healthy Outcomes in Caring for ESRD (CHOICE) Study. J Am Soc Nephrol 2005;16:1449–55. PMID: 15788468.

A large non-randomised multicentre study on the outcome of different forms of AV access, showing a relative mortality for central venous catheters of 1.5 and prosthetic access 1.2 in comparison with autogenous AV fistulas.

17

Varicose veins

Manjit S. Gohel

Introduction

Varicose veins are extremely common and the management of venous disease is a major cause of healthcare expense in the UK National Health Service (NHS) and worldwide.[1,2] The impact of venous disease on patient quality of life is widely accepted.[3,4] In view of the wide range of clinical presentations, a variety of clinical teams may be involved in the management of patients with venous disease and associated complications, including vascular surgeons, dermatologists, plastic surgeons, primary care teams and other specialists. A widespread appreciation of the growing prevalence and importance of chronic venous disease has driven a wave of research and innovation in venous diagnostics and treatment modalities.

Optimal patient management involves a detailed holistic patient assessment, evaluation of patient expectations and minimally invasive, multimodal therapy to address underlying haemodynamic abnormalities and reduce venous hypertension.

Pathophysiology

Normal venous function

The venous system returns deoxygenated blood from the capillary beds to the right atrium via low-pressure, high-volume venous channels. Flow towards the heart is maintained by unidirectional valves throughout, predominantly the peripheral venous system and muscle pumps located in the calf and foot, which contract during ambulation and promote venous flow. Retrograde flow (away from the heart) is termed venous incompetence or reflux and is usually due to damage to the venous valves.

Chronic venous hypertension

The underlying cause of venous disease is chronic venous hypertension. Persistent high venous pressure causes pathophysiological changes leading to the clinical manifestations of chronic venous disease. A common cause is superficial venous reflux secondary to vein valve incompetence, but other factors contributing to chronic venous hypertension may include deep venous reflux, venous outflow obstruction (post-thrombotic, non-thrombotic or extrinsic compression), calf muscle pump failure (usually due to ankle stiffness or poor calf muscle bulk), dependency or patient obesity.[5] The clinical consequences of venous reflux depend not only on the severity of reflux, but also on other factors contributing to venous hypertension (**Fig. 17.1**) and the effectiveness of measures that reduce venous hypertension (elevation, compression, calf muscle pump activity). The traditional dogma that venous skin changes and ulceration are due to deep venous disease has been disproved in recent years; anatomical studies have clearly demonstrated that patients with chronic venous ulceration often have superficial reflux only.[6]

Varicose veins

Varicose veins are usually due to superficial venous reflux affecting the great saphenous vein (GSV) (**Fig. 17.2**), small saphenous vein (SSV), accessory

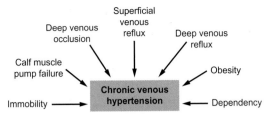

Figure 17.1 • Factors contributing to chronic venous hypertension.

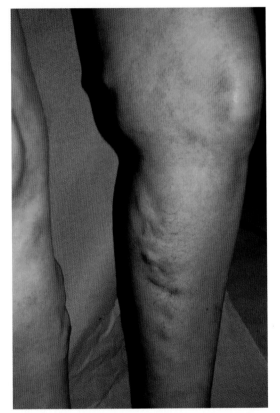

Figure 17.2 • Typical varicose veins secondary to reflux in the great saphenous vein (CEAP C2).

have merits and proponents, the development of varicose veins is likely to be multifactorial.[9]

Epidemiology and natural history

The incidence of venous disease in the population has been evaluated by several large European population studies.[10-13] These observational studies have demonstrated that most adults have reticular or thread veins, whereas varicose veins or more severe stages of venous disease (CEAP C2–C6, see Box 17.1) are present in 25–40% of the population. Venous disease is more common in highly industrialised rather than less industrialised countries, possibly due to differences in lifestyle and activity. Interestingly, deep reflux was more common in men, whereas superficial reflux had a higher incidence in women.[11,14] Overall, the incidence of venous disease was similar in males and females, which is contrary to most clinical studies, where a female preponderance of 3–4:1 is commonly reported. This discrepancy may reflect

Box 17.1 • CEAP classification

Clinical classification
C0: no visible or palpable signs of venous disease
C1: telangiectasias or reticular veins
C2: varicose veins
C3: oedema
C4a: pigmentation or eczema
C4b: lipodermatosclerosis or atrophie blanche
C5: healed venous ulcer
C6: active venous ulcer
S: symptomatic, including ache, pain, tightness, skin
    irritation, heaviness and muscle cramps, and other
    complaints attributable to venous dysfunction
A: asymptomatic

Aetiological classification
Ec: congenital
Ep: primary
Es: secondary (post-thrombotic)
En: no venous cause identified

Anatomical classification
As: superficial veins
Ap: perforator veins
Ad: deep veins
An: no venous location identified

Pathophysiological classification
Pr: reflux
Po: obstruction
Pr,o: reflux and obstruction
Pn: no venous pathophysiology identifiable

saphenous or non-truncal veins. Whether the valve failure is a primary phenomenon or secondary to vein wall dilatation has been debated for decades.[7] Two theories have been proposed to explain the development of superficial venous reflux leading to varicose veins. The 'descending theory' was popularised by Trendelenburg in the 19th century and suggests that superficial venous incompetence begins at the saphenous junctions and progresses distally. The 'ascending theory' advocates the proximal progression of distal venous incompetence and is supported by the observation that superficial venous incompetence often occurs with a competent saphenous junction.[8] Although both explanations gender differences in symptoms experienced, or in the threshold to seek medical advice. The prevalence of chronic venous ulceration (CEAP C6) is 0.3–1.0% and venous skin changes (CEAP C4–C5) were present in 5–10%. Although the progression of venous disease is poorly understood, between 3% and 7% of patients with venous skin changes (CEAP C4) are thought to progress to venous ulceration per annum. In general, the greater the patient age, the higher the prevalence and the more advanced the chronic venous disease.[12]

Clinical presentation

Patients with venous disease may seek medical help for a variety of reasons. In the Edinburgh Vein Study, patients reported an inconsistent and gender-dependent association between lower limb 'venous' symptoms (heaviness/tension, feeling of swelling, aching, restless leg, cramps, itching, tingling) and the presence and severity of thread, reticular or varicose veins. Clinical experience also suggests that there is little concordance between the size and extent of varicose veins and the severity of presenting symptoms. However, venous symptoms correlate with severity of venous reflux on duplex imaging.[15] The CEAP classification was devised in 1994, revised in 2004, and offers a useful and widely used tool to describe a patient using Clinical, aEtiological, Anatomical and Pathophysiological criteria (Box 17.1).[16] The clinical component of the CEAP classification is often used in isolation. It should be noted that the CEAP classification is a descriptive tool and is not intended for monitoring progression of disease or response to treatment. Other recognised scoring systems include the venous clinical severity score (VCSS) and venous disability score (VDS).[17] In recent years, there has also been a growing interest in patient reported outcomes and quality-of-life scores, which are likely to be most useful for evaluating success after venous interventions.[18]

Thread veins and reticular veins (CEAP C1)

These small, superficial veins may be highly visible and can cause cosmetic concern (**Fig. 17.3**) or symptoms. Thread veins (also known as spider veins, telangiectasia, venous flare) are <1 mm, whereas veins of 1–3 mm are termed reticular veins. Superficial, tortuous veins >3 mm are considered varicose veins. Patients with thread or reticular veins may find them unsightly and request treatment. Although not usually funded by state healthcare systems, these veins can be effectively treated using injection sclerotherapy or laser techniques.

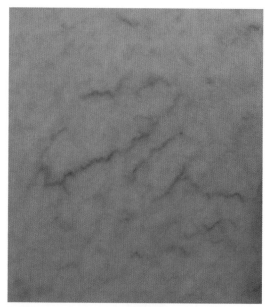

Figure 17.3 • Typical reticular and thread veins.

In general, significant underlying superficial reflux should be addressed before treating thread veins.

Varicose veins (CEAP C2)

Varicose veins are superficial, dilated and tortuous veins usually caused by superficial venous reflux (see Fig. 17.2). They are usually seen below the knee, but are also common in the thigh, with the precise location depending on the anatomical distribution of the underlying venous reflux. Most varicose veins are due to an incompetent GSV, although SSV reflux is the cause in around 20% of patients. Up to a quarter of patients have had previous varicose vein intervention, with the new veins either truly recurrent veins, residual veins not treated in the previous intervention or de novo varicose veins arising in a new distribution. Some patients may have varicose veins due to an incompetent perforating vein, refluxing pelvic/abdominal or other, unnamed, veins. It should be noted that in thin patients, or those with an athletic physique, superficial veins may be very prominent. However, these veins are usually straight and physiological, rather than abnormal.

Oedema and skin changes (CEAP C3–C4)

Venous oedema occurs secondary to increased hydrostatic pressure from chronic venous hypertension. The lymphatic system is unable to adequately drain the excessive interstitial fluid produced. This usually occurs around the ankle, but may involve the foot and leg. Symptoms are often worse after prolonged standing, towards the end of the day. Isolated oedema due to venous disease is unusual, in the absence of other signs of venous disease. Non-venous causes of oedema, including lymphoedema and cardiac failure, should be considered and may coexist with venous disease.

Chronic venous hypertension is associated with a number of skin changes (**Fig. 17.4**), including:

- **Venous eczema (also known as 'venous stasis dermatitis').** Itchy, dry and scaly skin is a common early skin change due to venous hypertension. As with most venous skin changes, eczema often occurs on the medial aspect of the lower leg (the 'medial gaiter area'). While symptoms may be improved with topical creams, eczema is likely to persist or deteriorate unless the underlying causes of venous hypertension are addressed.
- **Haemosiderinosis and skin pigmentation.** Chronic venous hypertension may lead to extravasation of red blood cells, resulting in pigmentation due to haemosiderin deposition in the subcutaneous tissues. There may be an associated inflammatory response, which can mimic cellulitis (see section on Lipodermatosclerosis below). Once the inflammation has settled, pigmentation is usually permanent, despite subsequent venous treatment.
- **Lipodermatosclerosis.** Chronic venous hypertension and inflammation may result in fibrosis and thickening of the skin and subcutaneous fat in the lower leg, with the classic 'inverted champagne bottle' appearance. Acute inflammation due to venous

hypertension may be referred to as 'acute lipodermatosclerosis'. As with haemosiderinosis, chronic skin and subcutaneous changes are generally considered irreversible. The primary aim of venous treatment is usually to reduce symptoms, improve patient quality of life and prevent disease progression.

- **Corona phlebectatica.** Also referred to as 'malleolar flare' or 'ankle flare', this refers to a leash of prominent intradermal veins, located around the medial malleolus. The skin is often fragile and patients may progress to venous ulceration.
- **Atrophie blanche.** Literally translated as 'white atrophy', this refers to a pale, smooth scarring, often associated with telangiectasia, that may occur at the site of previous ulceration. Patients with atrophie blanche have a high risk of developing venous ulceration.

Chronic venous ulceration: healed or active (CEAP C5–C6)

Venous ulceration is the commonest cause of leg ulceration and is considered the worst extreme in the spectrum of chronic venous disorders. Venous ulcers are distressing for patients, expensive to manage and challenging to treat. The estimated prevalence is 0.3–1% of the adult population in Western countries, with an increased prevalence in patients >65 years.[19] A chronic venous ulcer may be defined as a full-thickness defect of the skin, occurring primarily due to chronic venous hypertension, of >4 weeks' duration, but where there are clear signs of venous hypertension, treatment should not be delayed. The medial aspect of the lower leg (the medial gaitor area) is the most common location and other signs of chronic venous hypertension are frequently present, helping to differentiate chronic venous ulcers from other causes of leg ulceration. Ulcers are usually superficial and although a healthy granulating base is commonly seen, healing times are generally protracted, with the median healing duration of 4–6 months. As venous ulcers often affect elderly and frail patients, other factors contributing to poor wound healing (medication, comorbidity, poor nutrition) are frequently present in addition to chronic venous hypertension.

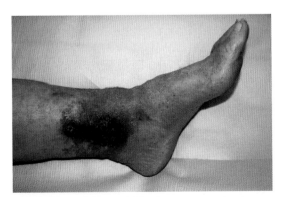

Figure 17.4 • Advanced skin changes secondary to chronic venous hypertension.

✔ Varicose veins are part of a spectrum of venous disease caused by chronic venous hypertension.

Clinical assessment

History

When assessing patients with venous disease, a detailed history of the presenting symptoms should be recorded and potential non-vascular causes should be excluded (particularly orthopaedic, spinal and arterial disorders). It is important to describe the impact of symptoms on patient quality of life as the decision to treat, choice of treatment modality and funding approval may all be guided by these considerations. Cosmetic appearance is a common concern and should always be a consideration when planning intervention, although this is rarely enough to justify treatment in state-funded healthcare systems. Other common symptoms include heaviness, aching, itching, swelling, restless legs, cramping or 'tingling'. The correlation between the size of veins and the severity of symptoms reported by the patient is often poor. Those involved in the management of patients with varicose veins should consider that this patient group accounts for a significant proportion of medicolegal claims in surgical specialties.[20] Discontent after treatment is often due to recurrent/residual varicose veins or neurological symptoms.

Patients should be asked specifically about the following:

- history of deep vein thrombosis (DVT);
- history of thrombophilia or major risk factors for previous DVT;
- use of oestrogen-containing medications (combined oral contraceptive pill, hormone replacement therapy) or tamoxifen;
- details of previous venous interventions (open or endovenous).

Patient examination

Patients should be evaluated in the standing position to allow filling of varicosities. Most of the required clinical information can be elucidated from inspection alone. Both legs should be examined, in addition to the groins and lower abdomen. The following features should be specifically assessed and documented:

- distribution and extent of varicosities (the examiner should specifically document the presence of a saphenovarix and other particularly large or troublesome varicosities);
- presence of skin changes of chronic venous disease (oedema, pigmentation, lipodermatosclerosis, ulceration);

- arterial status (pulses, or ankle–brachial pressure index);
- scars and evidence of previous venous interventions;
- other factors potentially contributing to venous hypertension (immobility, obesity, ankle stiffness, poor calf muscle bulk);
- general patient status and suitability for an intervention (fitness, mobility).

It should be noted that the association between clinical signs of venous disease and the presence of reflux is notoriously poor. Chronic venous skin changes and ulceration may be present without visible varicose veins. Nevertheless, where chronic venous hypertension is evident, appropriate venous investigations should be performed to detect treatable superficial reflux or deep venous disease.

Hand-held Doppler and other bedside tests

The accuracy and widespread availability of colour venous duplex scanning has meant that hand-held Doppler assessment of veins should not be used to guide venous interventions. Other bedside tests, such as the Trendelenburg test or tourniquet test, are well described in clinical textbooks, but rarely utilised in routine practice.

Venous investigations

The primary goal of venous investigations is to identify treatable superficial and deep venous disease, although in some atypical cases investigations may help to make the diagnosis of venous disease. A wide range of tests are available, but clinicians should adopt a pragmatic, step-wise approach starting with cheap, non-invasive investigations and avoiding radiation where possible.

Colour duplex ultrasound scanning

Colour duplex ultrasound scanning (DUS) is undoubtedly the first-line and gold standard investigation for patients with venous disease.[21] In appropriately trained hands, use of this non-invasive imaging modality can accurately identify the presence of reflux or occlusion in deep or superficial veins and confirm or refute the presence of arterial disease. Increasing availability and reducing cost of duplex machines has meant that appropriately trained vascular surgeons are able to perform scans in the outpatient clinic and during interventions to improve outcomes. Routine duplex

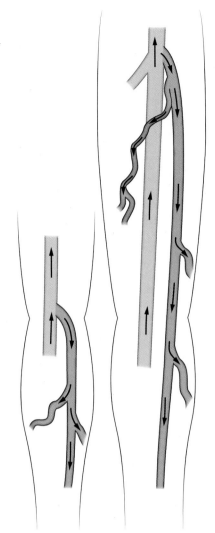

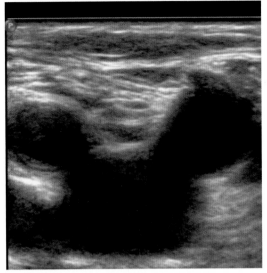

Figure 17.6 • Duplex ultrasound image demonstrating the typical 'Mickey Mouse' appearance of the common femoral artery (*left*), common femoral vein (*middle*) and great saphenous vein (*right*).

- accurate evaluation of recurrent varicose veins;
- identification of anatomical variants.

There is good justification for the use of DUS post-intervention as a tool for quality control and prognostication. However, economic considerations have meant that routine follow-up with DUS after superficial venous intervention is uncommon in the UK.

> ✅ All patients being considered for superficial venous intervention should undergo colour venous duplex imaging.

Other venous investigations

While DUS is often the only investigation needed to plan intervention for varicose veins, other diagnostic modalities may be useful in specific circumstances.

Transvaginal ultrasound.
In some female patients, transvaginal ultrasound may supplement conventional DUS and provide additional information about the presence of reflux in pelvic veins.[23] Currently, this has a limited role as the technique is highly user-dependent, more invasive than conventional DUS and, most importantly, the clinical significance of pelvic or ovarian vein reflux is unclear.

Computerised tomography or magnetic resonance venography
Cross-sectional imaging techniques can accurately visualise iliac veins, the inferior vena cava and may help identify sources of pelvic vein incompence.

Figure 17.5 • Example of report from colour duplex scan for patient with varicose veins. Reflux is present in the GSV and SSV arising from saphenofemoral and saphenopopliteal junctions.

imaging prior to venous intervention should be considered mandatory.[22]

DUS is increasingly considered an almost routine extension of the clinical examination (**Fig. 17.5**) and modern vascular training programmes include specific duplex ultrasound components. For the assessment of venous disease, specific advantages include:

- accurate evaluation of pattern of superficial reflux (including incompetent perforating veins) (**Fig. 17.6**);
- identification of deep venous disease;
- assessment of suitability of superficial veins for endovenous intervention and assistance in identifying the best modality for treatment (see 'Treatment' section);

Diagnostic venography (or phlebography)

Traditional diagnostic venography for the assessment of superficial veins has virtually no role in modern clinical practice. However, venography to assess deep veins is increasingly utilised for patients with deep venous outflow obstruction and may be a useful investigation for complex patients with mixed superficial and deep venous disease.

Haemodynamic assessments

Numerous tools are available to assess haemodynamic venous function in the leg. Ambulatory venous pressure (AVP) monitoring is considered the gold standard, but is invasive and generally limited to research use. Potential clinical benefits of digital photo-plethysmography, air plethysmography and other minimally invasive assessments of venous hypertension have been reported, but these techniques are rarely used in routine practice.

Intravascular ultrasound (IVUS)

IVUS is an excellent tool for the evaluation of venous outflow obstruction and is commonly used to guide deep venous stenting procedures.[24] IVUS may be helpful in some complex cases with mixed deep and superficial disease, but there is no role in the assessment of superficial veins.

Treatment

With dramatic recent advances in the treatment of venous disease, a wide range of modalities are now available and an individualised management strategy should be considered for each patient. This may involve using multiple treatment modalities and/or more than one treatment episode. For patients with bilateral varicose veins, opinion varies regarding the optimal approach (one-stage or multistage intervention). Patient preference should be considered and the treatment strategy adapted accordingly.

The CEAP classification is commonly used as a tool for rationing treatment and identifying which patients may get the greatest benefits. This approach is likely to be suboptimal, as CEAP is a descriptive tool only and significant quality-of-life improvements are seen after superficial venous intervention in patients with all classes of venous disease.

✔ The CEAP classification is an important descriptive tool for patients with venous disease.

Conservative options, medications and compression

Even in an era of minimally invasive interventions, conservative measures or compression may be the most appropriate therapy in some patients, particularly those unsuitable for or unwilling to undergo a procedure. Specific groups where conservative therapy or compression may be preferred include:

- pregnant patients;
- elderly patients with significant comorbidity;
- patients with mild symptoms, or symptoms that may not be due to venous disease;
- patients unwilling to accept the risks of surgical or endovenous interventions.

Conservative options

Conservative measures such as weight loss, limb elevation and reduced periods of standing may improve symptoms, but may be difficult to achieve for patients in full-time employment or those with young families.

Venoactive drugs and pharmacotherapy

Several venoactive drugs have been studied in patients with chronic venous disease.[25] Commonly studied medications include micronised purified flavonoid fraction and suledoxide, with some promising clinical results. However, these drugs are not available in the UK or North America. Small studies have suggested potential benefits with rutins and horse chestnut seed extract, although their use is limited.

Compression stockings and garments

Compression therapy has been used for the treatment of venous disease for centuries and remains the mainstay of management for patients with venous ulceration.[26,27] For patients with healed venous ulceration (CEAP C5), the use of elastic compression stockings has been shown to reduce the risk of recurrent ulceration. For patients with CEAP C2–C4 disease, stockings are prescribed frequently, but the evidence for benefit is less clear.

✔✔ Compression therapy is the mainstay of treatment for patients with chronic venous ulcers and may reduce symptoms of varicose veins in other patients.

Potential benefits of compression therapy include:

- improvement of venous symptoms and patient quality of life;
- prevention or slowing of disease progression;
- aiding clinical assessment in patients where there may be uncertainty about the extent to which the symptoms are attributable to venous disease;
- concealment of visible varicosities.

Compression stockings may be classified by the sub-bandage pressure applied at the ankle. Using the British Standard system for classification, class I stockings apply 14–17 mmHg, class II 18–24 mmHg and class III 25–35 mmHg. In practice, patients are often unable to tolerate stockings greater than class I and many patients find class III stockings practically impossible to don. Before commencing compression therapy, arterial disease should be excluded (by clinical assessment ± ankle–brachial pressure index measurement). Great care should be taken to fit stockings correctly and to avoid rolling down of the stocking, as this may cause pressure damage to the skin or create a tourniquet effect.

Patient compliance remains a major problem with compression stockings, as they may be itchy, hot (particularly in summer months) and difficult to put on and take off, despite the availability of applicator devices. Moreover, any benefit from compression stockings only exists while they are worn and they need to be replaced regularly. Studies have suggested that compliance may be as low as 50% overall and probably much lower with class III stockings.[28] There have been recent advances in compression therapy, with the availability of Velcro-based compression garments, which may be easier to wear and promote more patient independence in managing their compression.[29]

In a systematic review and meta-analysis assessing the efficacy of compression stockings, the paucity of high-quality evidence was highlighted.[28] Although many prospective studies were identified, there was significant heterogeneity in patient populations, type of compression and outcome measures evaluated. The authors concluded that wearing compression stockings improved patient symptoms, although selection bias could be a confounding factor. Compression was also found to reduce oedema, but the suggestion that wearing compression can slow the progression or reduce recurrence after intervention was not supported by the published literature.

Principles of endovenous and surgical interventions

In patients with significant symptomatic superficial reflux, the underlying principle of intervention is to remove or obliterate the incompetent superficial venous channel. A confusing range of modalities are now available to achieve this goal and choice of treatment modality is often based on personal experience. Before undertaking any superficial venous intervention, the clinician should have strong evidence that the superficial reflux is significantly contributing to symptoms of venous hypertension. Consequently, the treatment of patients with mixed superficial and deep venous reflux presents a challenge. In general, these patients can be safely treated with superficial venous intervention and some studies have shown that the refluxing deep veins may even become competent after superficial venous intervention (possibly because the incompetent venous reservoir is removed).[30]

However, the level of expected benefit is difficult to predict, as residual deep venous reflux may cause significant ongoing venous hypertension. A trial of compression stockings (which generally compress superficial veins only) may be a useful test in these circumstances and tourniquet tests using haemodynamic evaluation (digital photoplethysmography) have also been proposed.[31] The treatment of superficial veins in patients with venous outflow obstruction is usually not advisable, as these channels may be contributing to venous drainage, even if incompetent.

Informed consent

Varicose vein interventions are notorious for the relatively high number of medicolegal claims following procedures.[20] In this context, the process of informed consent is worthy of specific mention. Patients should be specifically warned of common complications such as bruising and paraesthesia. They should also understand that veins may (and often do) recur and that DVT or nerve pain are recognised risks. Other, modality-specific risks should also be explained (see below), both verbally and using written information. In patients with visible varicosities, they should appreciate that some residual veins may be present and their legs will not be cosmetically perfect. Information leaflets should be used, specific consent forms may be useful and discussions with the patient should be clearly documented in the medical records. Patient distress and complaint after intervention is commonly driven by a disappointing clinical outcome from intervention. Therefore, the patient's expectations from treatment should be clarified before intervention and ideally match those of the treating clinician.

✔ Varicose vein treatments are a common cause of medicolegal claims. The patient's expectations from intervention should match those of the surgeon.

Endovenous thermal ablation

Largely driven by an appreciation of the slow recovery and suboptimal outcomes after traditional varicose vein operations, and patient desire for less invasive interventions, there has been an explosion of endovenous procedures in the last 15 years. Walk-in walk-out interventions, performed using only local anaesthesia, are feasible and expected. Perceived potential advantages of these procedures include:

- avoidance of the risks of general anaesthesia;
- improved early morbidity (no groin dissection or stripping) with earlier return to normal activity/work;

- ability to perform procedures in modified outpatient or 'office-based' settings (with the associated cost savings);
- lower risk of complications such as nerve injury, bruising and recurrence.

Despite the drive towards endovenous treatments, surgical stripping operations are still common and critics of endovenous ablation would highlight potential disadvantages, including:

- expense of the generators, endovenous catheters and consumable items;
- learning curve associated with the new procedure;
- some patients may be unsuitable (tortuous or superficial veins);
- lack of long-term follow-up data.

In view of the similarities between endovenous laser ablation (EVLA) and radiofrequency ablation (RFA) procedures, and the tendency to combine the techniques in many of the published guidelines, both are described in this section.

Setting and anaesthesia

Both EVLA and RFA are ideal for outpatient or 'office-based' therapy as procedures can be performed using only 'tumescent' anaesthesia. This refers to a very dilute mixture of local anaesthesia (0.1% lidocaine) with epinephrine (1:2 000 000), which is injected under ultrasound guidance to surround the truncal vein to be ablated. The use of sodium bicarbonate to neutralise the mixture may reduce the pain during tumescent injections. The anaesthetic allows the ablation to be performed without pain, but also provides a heat buffer to protect surrounding nerves, tissues and skin. Initially, procedures were commonly performed in operating theatres. However, with a growing appreciation of the potential cost savings[32] by liberating operating theatre capacity, many centres in the UK now have suitable outpatient treatment rooms.

Technique

Accurate, colour venous duplex assessment is essential to plan and perform endovenous ablation procedures.[21] Suitability for treatment should be evaluated using duplex, ideally by the specialist performing the procedure (see **Fig. 17.5**). Although specific eligibility criteria vary between clinicians, veins should be straight, >3 mm in diameter and in the saphenous fascia, or deep enough to be >1 cm from the skin after infiltration of tumescent anaesthesia. The patient should be positioned in the supine position for GSV ablation and prone for SSV procedures. The stages of the procedure are summarised below:

- With the patient in the reverse Trendelenburg position, the vein to be treated is cannulated

under ultrasound guidance, using a Seldinger technique. The site of cannulation should ideally be at the distal point of reflux. A sheath appropriate to the catheter to be used can then be inserted (**Fig. 17.7**).

- The endovenous ablation catheter is positioned 2 cm from the saphenofemoral (SFJ) or saphenopopliteal (SPJ) junctions under ultrasound guidance. The bed is tilted to move the patient to the Trendelenburg position.
- Tumescent anaesthesia is injected around the vein under ultrasound guidance, with the aim of creating a 'halo' of infiltration surrounding the circumference of the vein to be ablated (**Fig. 17.8**). Care should be taken to infiltrate between the proximal GSV and CFV and to ensure that the vein is at least 1 cm from the skin. Tumescent injection may be facilitated by using local anaesthetic cream (to reduce the pain of injection) and an injection pump. Volumes of tumescent anaesthesia injected may vary between patients and practitioners, but are typically around 75–100 mL per 10 cm of vein.
- The technique and speed of thermal ablation will depend on the catheter used. This may be a slow pull-back technique, or segmental ablation. With experience, it is common to adapt the ablation depending on anatomical factors (such as the size and depth of the vein).
- After ablation, access site haemostasis is secured with direct pressure and patency of the deep vein should be verified with duplex and documented.

✅ During endovenous thermal ablation procedures, the vein should be cannulated at the distal point of reflux.

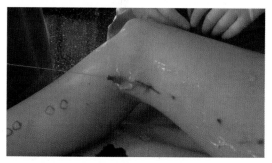

Figure 17.7 • Cannulation of GSV in distal thigh under ultrasound guidance, using Seldinger technique.

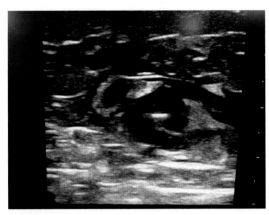

Figure 17.8 • Duplex image demonstrating 'halo' of tumescent anaesthesia around truncal vein to be ablated.

Endovenous laser ablation (EVLA)

Endovenous ablation using laser was first described in 2001.[33] The laser fibre is slowly withdrawn at a steady pace while delivering energy within the vein. The temperatures exceed 1000°C and although the precise mechanism of action is not fully understood, diffuse thermal damage to the intima has been observed. Initial fibres were forward-firing and utilised laser wavelengths of 810 or 980 nm. Recent advances have included a 1470-nm laser (thought to better target water and therefore the vein wall) and radial-firing fibres (better targeting of the vein wall, reducing the risk of vein wall perforations and pain). Using the early laser fibres, a dose of >60 joules/cm is thought to be necessary to ensure vein closure. The dose required may be less for radial fibres. One disadvantage is that EVLA procedures must be performed in an appropriate clinical area complying with laser safety regulations and protective goggles must be worn during periods of activation.

Radiofrequency ablation (RFA)

RFA also involves the delivery of thermal energy to the vein wall, derived from an electrical current.[34] A bipolar catheter is used to generate temperatures of 85–120°C and an inbuilt feedback mechanism can assess the quality of vein wall contact, which is required for effective energy delivery. Several RFA catheters are available and can be broadly classified into continuous pull-back or segmental ablation systems. Using the latter, the heating element is activated and the fibre is left in contact with the vein, for a standard period, before withdrawing to the next segment to be treated. Most systems offer some feedback mechanism (either auditory or visual) to confirm energy delivery to the tissues. Histological studies have demonstrated a homogeneous thermal ablation to the vein wall.

Other modalities for thermal ablation

Endovenous steam and microwave ablation techniques have been proposed as alternative thermal ablation modalities by some authors. While clinical and technical outcomes have been reasonable in some reported studies, uptake has been very limited. While there are two, well-established thermal ablation modalities in widespread use (EVLA and RFA), it may be difficult to make the case to advocate a less tested thermal modality, such as steam.

Complications

In general, the rate of complications after endovenous interventions is low. Many of the complications after EVLA and RFA are comparable to those seen after traditional surgery and other modalities.

1. Bleeding/bruising: In general, the incidence of early complications is significantly lower after endovenous procedures in comparison to traditional surgery. Significant discomfort or bruising is uncommon, but is probably more likely after EVLA than RFA. Pain using the newer radial laser fibres may be reduced compared to the older fibres.

2. Thromboembolic events: The incidence of DVT after RFA and EVLA is very low (<1%). However, a tongue of thrombus is sometimes seen at the SFJ or SPJ at the level of or protruding into the deep vein. This phenomenon has been termed endovenous heat-induced thrombosis (EHIT) and four classes have been described:[35]
   • Class 1: thrombus to the level of the deep vein, without protrusion;
   • Class 2: protrusion into the deep system, with <50% luminal occlusion;
   • Class 3: protrusion into the deep system, with >50% luminal occlusion;
   • Class 4: protrusion into the deep system, with total deep venous occlusion.

3. Skin burns: Thermal injury to the skin is a complication unique to endovenous thermal ablation modalities. This usually occurs after ablating a superficial vein after inadequate tumescent anaesthesia. This may result in an area of pigmentation, although frank ulceration may also occur. This complication may be more common when treating extrafascial saphenous veins.

4. Phlebitis: Phlebitis can occur after any venous intervention. After endovenous thermal ablation, phlebitis is most frequently seen in varicosities, where flow may have diminished after ablation of the truncal vein.

5. Nerve injury: Although less common than in traditional surgery, areas of abnormal sensation are common after endovenous ablation. This is often an area of paraesthesia over the ablated truncal vein. Thermal injury to saphenous, sural or other nerves may occur, although the generous and accurate use of tumescence should reduce this risk. An added advantage of treating the awake patient is that they are likely to feel pain when an EVLA or RFA catheter is near a nerve. Most areas of abnormal sensation recover with conservative management.

Ultrasound-guided foam sclerotherapy (UGFS)

Sclerotherapy is a type of chemical ablation, where the sclerosant acts on the vein wall to induce fibrosis and closure of the lumen.[36] Three broad categories of endovenous sclerosant are available: detergent (sodium tetradecyl sulphate [STS], polidocanol), osmotic (hypertonic saline, used in Europe and the USA), chemical irritant (chromated glycerine). In the UK, STS and polidocanol are in popular use, although the latter is unlicensed. In general, larger veins require a stronger concentration of sclerosant. The conversion of liquid sclerosant into foam by mixing it with air or carbon dioxide (Tessari method) has gained popularity in recent years. This approach has the advantage of increasing the potency and volume of the sclerosant, as well as making it echogenic.

> ✔✔ For the treatment of truncal veins (such as GSV or SSV), foam sclerosant is superior to liquid sclerosant.

Setting and anaesthesia

UGFS can easily be performed in an outpatient treatment room. Access to a duplex machine and a treatment trolley are the only requirements. As the only injection involves the insertion of small cannulae or butterfly needles into the veins to be treated, the treatment is often possible with minimal or no local anaesthesia.

Technique

More than most other venous treatments, UGFS is associated with a significant learning curve. The ability to modify almost every component of the treatment (cannulation sites, volume and concentration of sclerosant) means that good training is imperative and techniques usually evolve and improve with increasing personal experience.

- Ultrasound-guided cannulation is performed as with other endovenous modalities. However, this may be more challenging with UGFS as multiple cannulae or needles may be required in tortuous varicosities.[37] It is worth noting that sclerosant activity is reduced in contact with blood, so multiple access sites are preferable to a single injection point.
- Foam sclerosant is created by combining liquid sclerosant with air in a 1:3 or 1:4 ratio using the 'Tessari' technique (**Fig. 17.9**).
- With the leg elevated (to empty the veins), foam should be injected and movement of the foam should be monitored using ultrasound (**Fig. 17.10**).
- The patient should be encouraged to move the ankle to promote deep venous flow.
- Although practice is variable, most practitioners would apply compression bandaging after the procedure, potentially using eccentric compression over the treated veins.

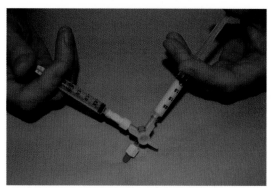

Figure 17.9 • Creation of foam by mixing liquid sclerosant with air (1:4 ratio) using 2 Luer-lock syringes and a three-way tap (Tessari technique).

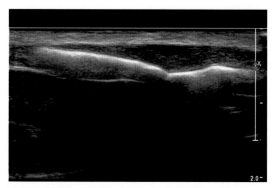

Figure 17.10 • Ultrasound image of highly visible echogenic foam sclerosant after injection within superficial vein.

Choice of sclerosant

Although several detergent sclerosants are available, the choice is usually driven by local availability. Most products are available in a range of concentrations. In general, the smaller and more superficial the vein to be treated, the lower the concentration of sclerosant should be. Pre-created foam sclerosant is now available as an alternative to physician-made foam, but cost and a lack of widespread regulatory approval have limited the use of proprietary foam.

Complications

Despite being the least invasive of endovenous treatment modalities, case reports of major neurological events after UGFS have raised safety concerns.[38] There is anecdotal evidence that adverse events may be more common with larger volumes of foam injection and neurological events may be more likely in patients with regular migraines. The volume injected will depend on the specific case, but most experts would suggest that 10–12 mL (of foam) should be considered a maximum for a single session.

1. Thrombophlebitis: Superficial thrombophlebitis is more common after UGFS than other modalities and presents with painful, hard lumpy areas and erythema. Inflammation may respond to topical anti-inflammatory creams, but may require early aspiration/expulsion of the thrombus, which usually results in a rapid improvement of symptoms.

2. Thromboembolic events: Although some foam inevitably enters the deep venous system during treatment, the risk of DVT remains low (approximately 1%). Encouraging ankle dorsiflexion after foam injection (to promote deep venous flow) may reduce the risk of DVT.

3. Skin pigmentation/staining: May occur (to varying degrees) in a significant proportion of patients. Pigmentation usually fades over 3–6 months, but may be permanent in some cases. Some experts suggest that aspiration of thrombophlebitis may reduce the severity of pigmentation.

4. Neurological symptoms/stroke: A review of neurological complications after UGFS demonstrated that transient neurological problems (usually visual disturbances) occur after around 1% of interventions and are more common in patients with a history of migraine.[38] Several case reports have described post-procedure strokes in patients treated with sclerotherapy, although this is extremely rare. These may be due to paradoxical emboli via a patent foramen ovale, although other scientific theories (such as the production of endothelins) have been proposed. Some experts have suggested that the use of carbon dioxide (rather than air) to produce foam may reduce the risk of neurological events, although robust evidence to support this assertion is lacking.[39]

> ✔ Neurological events after foam sclerotherapy have been described, but are rare. The incidence of adverse events is likely to be related to the volume of foam injected and may be higher in patients with migraines.

Non-thermal, non-tumescent endovenous modalities

The development of non-thermal, non-tumescent endovenous interventions has been the latest innovative advance for superficial venous interventions.[40] Although not currently in widespread use, many believe that these procedures are the future for varicose vein treatment.

Mechanochemical ablation (MOCA)

The MOCA catheter is positioned within the vein to be treated. A rapidly rotating fibre is activated and the catheter is slowly withdrawn while injecting liquid sclerosant. The combination of mechanical damage to the vein wall and chemical ablation deep into the damaged wall is purported to lead to fibrosis of the vein.

Cyanoacrylate glue closure

Cyanoacrylate glue has been used for a variety of medical indications for decades. In recent years, specific n-butyl cyanoacrylate preparations and customised catheters have been developed to permit endovenous use. Long-term evidence is awaited, but advocates believe that this offers enormous potential for virtually pain-free superficial venous treatments for the future.

Traditional surgery for varicose veins

Trendelenburg described ligation of the proximal GSV in 1890 and modifications of this technique have remained the mainstay of treatment for varicose veins for over a century. With the increasing popularity of minimally invasive, endovenous modalities, the proportion of patients treated with surgical stripping has declined in recent years.[41]

Setting and anaesthesia

Traditional varicose vein operations are usually performed in a sterile operating theatre, with virtually all varicose vein operations potentially performed as day case procedures. Although most procedures are performed using general anaesthesia, regional or local techniques may also be used. Epidural/spinal anaesthesia or femoral nerve blocks can facilitate surgery, but the motor block may persist for several hours, potentially hindering same-day discharge. Surgical stripping may also be performed using dilute local anaesthesia with adrenaline, injected in high volumes around the vein to be stripped ('tumescent' anaesthesia – see below). However, in a generally young and fit patient group, most surgeons (and anaesthetists) favour general anaesthesia for traditional varicose vein surgery. The routine use of prophylactic antibiotics has been shown to reduce the risk of wound complications in one randomised study.[42]

Technique

GSV stripping is performed with the patient in the supine position, with legs in a slightly abducted position, whereas SSV surgery is usually carried out with the patient prone. A 'head down' or Trendelenburg position can reduce venous bleeding during the procedure and while a detailed description of surgical technique is beyond the scope of this chapter, some important technical principles are listed below:

- In the modern era, all superficial venous interventions (including traditional surgery) should be guided by intraoperative ultrasound imaging to ensure appropriate location of incisions and technical success.
- Tributaries should be divided as distal as possible (ideally beyond the second branch).
- Stripping of the GSV after flush SFJ disconnection reduces varicose vein recurrence (compared to ligation alone).[43] Most surgeons would avoid stripping below the knee (to avoid the risk of nerve damage) and the use of tumescent anaesthesia is advisable.
- Ligation of the SSV should be performed at a safe level (not flush with the SPJ) and stripping of the SSV is controversial.
- Significant varicosities should be pre-marked in agreement with the patient and concomitant phlebectomies should be performed (with tumescent anaesthesia) with GSV or SSV surgery.

✔✔ Stripping of the GSV is an essential component of traditional varicose vein surgery.

Complications

Adverse events of specific relevance after traditional superficial venous surgery include:

1. Bruising/bleeding: Bruising is a very common early complication after surgery, particularly along the track where the truncal vein (GSV or SSV) has been stripped. Bleeding requiring a return to the operating theatre is usually due to persistent venous bleeding in the groin but is rare. Anecdotally, bruising may be reduced by using epinephrine-soaked swabs or tumescent anaesthesia with epinephrine infiltrated in the tract of the stripped vein.[44]

2. Thromboembolic events: The incidence of DVT after traditional varicose vein surgery ranges from 0.5% to 5.3% in the literature. The risk of pulmonary embolism has been estimated at 1 in 60.[45] Duplex studies have identified that many patients have small, below-knee DVTs of questionable clinical significance.

3. Nerve damage: A degree of sensory abnormality may be present in up to 40% of patients after traditional surgery, although this is rarely troublesome. True saphenous nerve injury after GSV stripping (to the knee) is likely to be <10%. The risk of sural nerve injury during SPJ disconnection is unknown, but is likely to be higher. Disabling motor nerve injury may occur, particularly involving the common peroneal nerve at the head of the fibula. This may be injured during stab phlebectomy in this area.

4. Recurrence: Poor results after traditional varicose vein surgery have often been attributed to poor surgical technique by inexperienced operators. While technical failure was certainly a problem, it has become clear that even with 'technically' successful surgery, performed by experienced operators, recurrence is common. Reported recurrence rates range from 20% to 80% at 5–20 years, although most patients remain satisfied with surgery.[45]

Treatment of recurrent varicose veins

Up to a quarter of patients presenting with varicose veins have had previous superficial venous surgery. These patients present a unique management challenge as the patterns of venous reflux may be significantly more complex than for patients with primary venous disease. Patients should undergo detailed clinical assessment and comprehensive colour duplex imaging to map the pattern of superficial and deep venous disease. Attention should be paid to sites and reasons for recurrent superficial reflux (such as neovascularisation, incompetent perforating veins or pelvic sources of reflux).[46] Redo groin surgery or popliteal fossa surgery is associated with an unacceptable risk of complications, including infection, seroma, DVT and nerve damage. Therefore, even for enthusiastic open vascular surgeons, endovenous interventions are widely considered the first line in the treatment of patients with recurrent varicose veins, particularly in the popliteal fossa.

> ✔ Endovenous interventions should be considered the first line for patients with recurrent varicose veins.

Areas of controversy

Treatment of incompetent perforating veins

Perforating veins connect the deep and superficial systems in the leg, with incompetent perforators (direction of flow from deep to superficial veins) seen in many patients with varicose veins. The optimal management of incompetent perforators remains an issue of controversy. Several studies have reported favourable outcomes when incompetent perforators are treated in combination with refluxing superficial veins. Conversely, there are numerous studies that have demonstrated that incompetent perforators may become competent after GSV or SSV treatment. Therefore, the additional value of perforator treatment over and above truncal vein ablation alone is unproven.[47] Although each case should be considered individually, a pragmatic approach adopted by many is to treat the refluxing truncal vein as an initial intervention and reserve perforator treatment for patients with residual/recurrent disease clearly attributable to an incompetent perforator. If perforator treatment is deemed necessary, options include endovenous thermal ablation (using a custom radiofrequency stylet or EVLA), open surgical ligation, cyanoacrylate glue closure or UGFS.[48]

> ✔ The routine treatment of incompetent perforating veins is not justified for patients with primary varicose veins.

Management of varicosities

Many patients with varicose veins have troublesome superficial varicosities. When traditional open surgery was the dominant treatment option, superficial varicose veins were usually treated (by stab phlebectomy) at the time of surgery, as the patient was already under general anaesthesia. However, the growing use of endovenous interventions, performed under local/tumescent anaesthesia in outpatient settings, has meant that treating the varicosities at the same time as truncal ablation may be less convenient or not feasible. This development has raised the question whether varicosities need to be treated at all (after saphenous ablation). Several authors have suggested that varicosities usually regress after truncal vein ablation and phlebectomy may be unnecessary, particularly if the refluxing superficial truncal vein is ablated to the lowest point of reflux. However, randomised studies suggest that synchronous treatment of varicosities may also have benefits, primarily by reducing the risk of further interventions.[49] The strategies for treating varicosities are:

1. Treat at the time of truncal vein intervention.
2. Do not treat varicosities at all.
3. Review the patient after truncal vein treatment and treat varicosities if required.

Local circumstances (type of treatment room, staff skill mix, reimbursement policies) are likely to influence the management approach to varicosities as much as clinician preference. Many clinicians prefer a selective policy for treating varicosities. Once a decision to treat varicosities has been made, options include:

- Stab phlebectomy: This is performed via a small incision using a specific hook (Oesch) to deliver the varicose vein through the incision. Care should be taken to avoid nerves and other structures,[50] particularly around the lateral knee (common peroneal nerve), the medial malleolus (posterior tibial vessels) and the regions of the saphenous and sural nerves. Ambulatory phlebectomy, performed under local anaesthesia in an outpatient setting, is gaining in popularity.
- UGFS: Sclerotherapy may be used to treat varicosities and can be performed in an outpatient setting. For more superficial veins, a lower concentration of sclerosant may be preferable to reduce the risk of phlebitis and skin pigmentation.
- Other options: Although powered phlebectomy has been available for many years, evidence demonstrating superiority over stab phlebectomy is lacking.

> ✔✔ When performing endovenous ablation procedures, concomitant phlebectomies should be considered.

Saphenous preserving interventions

CHIVA (French acronym for Ambulatory Conservative Haemodynamic management for Venous Insufficiency) and ASVAL (French acronym for Ambulatory Selective Ablation of Varicose veins under Local anaesthesia) are alternative techniques for the surgical management of superficial venous reflux.[51,52] Both popularised in parts of Europe, CHIVA aims to redistribute superficial venous flow into deep veins by strategically ligating tributaries and/or the saphenofemoral junction and ASVAL involves the selective ligation of specific incompetent tributaries, with the aim of restoring competence in the saphenous trunk. The aim of such 'saphenous-preserving' approaches is to maintain the venous drainage of GSV and to preserve the option of using the vein as a future vascular conduit. Prospective studies and randomised trials from enthusiastic units have reported favourable results in comparison to surgical stripping, but these techniques have not gained widespread acceptance.[53] This may be due to the excellent results that can be achieved using less esoteric and more reproducible ablation options.

Thromboprophylaxis after endovenous procedures

Although venous thromboembolism (VTE) is a recognised complication after superficial venous procedures, the approach to VTE prophylaxis varies dramatically between hospitals and clinicians. The thankfully rare occurrence of VTE events in this group makes it difficult to conduct trials to guide practice. However, high-profile fatal VTE events have occurred after varicose vein interventions, suggesting that there is a role for appropriate thromboprophylaxis in selected patients.[54] Although precise stratification models are yet to be defined, there is growing consensus that patients undergoing endovenous procedures should undergo some form of modified VTE risk assessment. High-risk patients should be prescribed pharmacological prophylaxis (such as low-molecular-weight heparins). The optimal duration of treatment is unknown, but as the VTE risk exists for several days after intervention, a course of 7–10 days may be reasonable for selected patients.

Compression after superficial venous interventions

There is considerable uncertainty regarding the use of compression therapy after superficial venous interventions. Compression bandages or stockings have been used commonly after open surgical procedures (stripping and/or phlebectomies), where there may be a role in reducing bruising and pain. However, the case for the routine use of compression after endovenous interventions alone is less clear.[55]

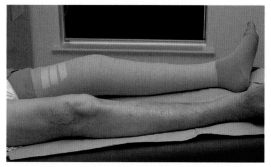

Figure 17.11 • Compression stocking and bandage applied after ultrasound-guided foam sclerotherapy procedure.

There are theoretical benefits after sclerotherapy treatments, as a compressed and empty vein may be less likely to develop thrombophlebitis (**Fig. 17.11**). However, evidence to support this assumption is lacking. In practice, many patients have advanced venous hypertension and therefore may be wearing compression long term. In the UK, most practitioners recommend compression after interventions. However, advocates of newer modalities such as cyanoacrylate glue closure, suggest that compression is usually not necessary. Results from ongoing studies will hopefully deliver some clarity on this issue.

Evidence for varicose vein interventions

The rapid expansion in available treatment modalities for superficial venous reflux has resulted in a confusing landscape for patients and clinicians. However, this expansion in treatments has been accompanied by a large volume of randomised and prospective clinical studies. Most comparative trials include two modalities, meaning that comparison between treatments often relies on inference.

Endovenous thermal ablation

Many studies have been conducted using EVLA and RFA interventions. A common criticism of these trials was that follow-up periods were short and outcome measures did not include patient-reported outcomes. However, there are now studies with reliable data to 5 years or longer, allowing clinicians to have greater confidence in the longer-term durability of these procedures. For thermal ablation procedures, early outcomes have proved to be an accurate surrogate marker for long-term treatment success. As a result, endovenous thermal interventions have largely superseded traditional surgery as the gold standard treatment for superficial venous reflux. Based on published studies,[56,57] the following broad conclusions can be drawn regarding the effectiveness of endovenous thermal ablation procedures:

- The early post-procedure outcomes (pain, bruising, time to mobilise, return to normal activity) are better after EVLA and RFA in comparison to traditional surgery.
- EVLA procedures performed using radial fibres using favourable laser wavelengths (such as 1470 nm) are probably less painful and associated with less bruising than previous generation forward-firing fibres.
- Target vein occlusion rates of >90% can be expected using RFA and EVLA procedures. Thermal ablation procedures are at least as effective as traditional surgery.
- It is difficult to distinguish between different types of RFA or EVLA devices in terms of technical success.

✓✓ Early outcomes (pain, bruising and return to normal activity) after endovenous procedures are superior to traditional varicose vein surgery.

Ultrasound-guided foam sclerotherapy

UGFS has unique advantages over other modalities, as it is probably the least invasive intervention and extremely versatile. In general, the efficacy and safety of foam sclerotherapy has been clearly demonstrated by studies published over many decades. However, most comparative studies have suggested lower GSV occlusion rates in comparison to traditional surgery and thermal ablation treatments.[57–59] The use of foam sclerosant has been shown to be superior to liquid sclerosant,[37] although comparative treatment success rates for different types or concentrations of sclerosants remain unclear. Although the reported incidence of visual disturbance is <1%, there have been reports of major neurological events after UGFS,[38] resulting in considerable unease, not least because the mechanism of neurological adverse events is unknown.

Mechanochemical ablation and cyanoacrylate glue closure

As non-thermal, non-tumescent ablation procedures have not been available for as long as other endovenous modalities, the evidence base is less extensive. However, recently published randomised studies have demonstrated that both MOCA and cyanoacrylate glue have comparable technical, clinical and patient-reported outcomes in comparison to RFA.[60,61]

Choosing between treatment modalities

The addition of this plethora of endovenous treatment options for varicose veins is welcomed by patients and doctors, but has led to significant confusion and heterogeneity in practice. The regular addition of new modalities, such as MOCA, cyanoacrylate glue and others, potentially compounds the confusion. Most of the available modalities are highly effective and choosing between interventions is likely to be driven by other factors such as cost, patient comfort, clinician preference and skill as well as unique advantages that specific modalities may have to suit individual circumstances. It is becoming clear that modern treatment of varicose veins may involve several different modalities, potentially performed at the same time.

There have been large randomised studies comparing multiple treatment modalities. In the CLASS trial, 798 patients were randomised to either traditional surgery, UGFS or EVLA. The authors concluded that UGFS was associated with lower ablation rates and slightly worse disease-specific quality of life.[57] In another randomised study of 500 patients comparing EVLA, RFA, UGFS and surgical stripping, 3-year results demonstrated that recanalisations and re-interventions were more likely after UGFS (in keeping with other studies).[59]

✓✓ Based on large randomised trials, technical success rates are likely to be best after EVLA/RFA and worst after UGFS.

To aid the decision-making of clinicians and commissioners, numerous guidelines (from the UK, Europe and the USA) have been published for the treatment of venous disease.[22,62–64] Some key messages are summarised below:

- Treatment of varicose veins is cost-effective for symptomatic patients and those with venous skin changes or venous ulceration (active or healed).
- For the treatment of GSV reflux, endovenous thermal ablation is recommended as the first-line treatment, in preference to traditional surgery or UGFS.
- When performing EVLA or RFA, concomitant phlebectomies should be considered.
- For the treatment of recurrent varicose veins, endovenous treatments should be considered in preference to open surgery.

> ✓✓ Traditional surgery and endovenous interventions are likely to be cost-effective in the treatment of patients with varicose veins.

Rationing of varicose vein treatments

At a time of global financial constraint and austerity, the cost and cost-effectiveness of venous treatments has come under great scrutiny. There is a widely held (and inaccurate) perception that varicose vein treatments are largely cosmetic and should be considered as low priority. In the UK NHS, commissioning guidance has become increasingly stringent, making it more difficult to treat superficial venous disease even in the presence of significant complications of chronic venous hypertension. This real-world commissioning landscape is in stark contrast to the published advice, including National Institute for Health and Care Excellence guidance for varicose veins, which recommends that patients with symptomatic varicose veins, skin changes, phlebitis, bleeding or ulcers should be offered treatment.[22]

The pragmatic view is that rationing is inevitable. The optimal approach to rationing is controversial. In many healthcare settings, the CEAP clinical grade is used to decide whether patients should be treated. However, this is a flawed strategy, as patients with severe, disabling symptoms may only be CEAP C2, whereas patients with a higher CEAP clinical grade may be totally asymptomatic. Vein diameter and patient-reported quality-of-life scores have also been proposed as rationing tools, without support. Accepting that rationing is inevitable, further work is needed to help define precisely which patients benefit most from varicose veins interventions.

Atypical varicose veins

Vulval and pelvic varices

In some cases, female patients may have varicose veins because of ovarian or internal iliac venous tributary incompetence. Varicose veins of pelvic origin may extend along the medial thigh and join the GSV, which may also be incompetent. Pelvic causes of venous disease should be considered in all patients, particularly those with recurrent varicose veins after GSV intervention. Duplex scanning can often identify an incompetent vein arising from the pelvis that is feeding the visible varicosities. Magnetic resonance venography or venography may be needed to identify the source of the pelvic reflux.

There remains considerable controversy over whether pelvic venous reflux needs to be treated aggressively. The treatment of choice is endovenous coil embolisation of the incompetent tributary, under fluoroscopic control. The use of foam sclerotherapy in addition to coils has also been described. Ovarian vein reflux may also be associated with the 'pelvic congestion syndrome', characterised by chronic pelvic pain and menstrual problems.[65]

Congenital causes of varicose veins

Patients commonly state that other family members have also suffered with varicose veins. The published evidence does suggest a hereditary or genetic contribution to the disease process in some cases, although specific genetic causes of varicose veins have not yet been identified. In one study, patients with varicose veins were over 20 times more likely to report a positive family history in comparison to controls. Varicose veins may also be part of some inherited disorders, such as Klippel–Trenauney syndrome.[66] Patients may present with a combination of cutaneous capillary malformations (port wine stains), limb hypertrophy/overgrowth and varicose veins. Most patients have varicose veins, which are commonly located on the lateral aspect of the leg. Although incompetent superficial veins may be treated, clinicians should be aware that there may be associated deep venous abnormalities, including atresia. Detailed venous mapping with colour duplex, with supplementary venous imaging in selected cases, is essential before considering intervention.

Conclusions

With a dramatic expansion in available treatment modalities, the management of patients with varicose veins has evolved rapidly in recent years. Endovenous thermal ablation procedures such as endovenous laser and radiofrequency ablation are considered the gold standard and have largely replaced traditional surgery. Non-thermal endovenous procedures such as ultrasound-guided foam sclerotherapy, mechanochemical ablation and cyanoacrylate glue closure may also have a role. After a century of open surgery and vein stripping, the modern management of varicose veins involves the routine use of colour duplex imaging and delivery of a range of minimally invasive, effective and well-tolerated treatments, under local anaesthesia in an office-based setting.

Key points

- Varicose veins are part of a wide spectrum of disorders caused by underlying chronic venous hypertension and are associated with significant quality-of-life impairment.
- Interventions for symptomatic varicose veins result in significant clinical, quality-of-life and health-economic benefits.
- All patients should undergo venous duplex imaging prior to planning intervention.
- Careful discussion of the risks and documented informed consent are essential in view of the risk of medicolegal consequences of adverse outcomes.
- Endovenous treatment modalities including endovenous thermal ablation (using laser or radiofrequency) and ultrasound-guided foam sclerotherapy (UGFS) have become the treatment modalities of choice, ahead of traditional surgery.
- Endovenous modalities are associated with lower early morbidity in comparison to surgical stripping.
- In a rapidly evolving area, non-thermal, non-tumescent options such as mechanochemical ablation or cyanoacrylate glue closure are the latest advances.
- Each of the endovenous treatments has advantages and disadvantages, but the technical success rates are likely to be greatest after EVLA or RFA.
- For patients with venous ulceration, superficial venous surgery has been shown to reduce the risk of recurrent ulceration.
- For the treatment of recurrence varicose veins, open surgery has been superseded by endovenous interventions.

Recommended videos:

- RF ablation – https://tinyurl.com/y8efytyr
- 'Clarivein' – https://tinyurl.com/yb9k2wba
- 'Venaseal' – https://www.youtube.com/watch?v=c2JEWfn-XQM

Full references available at **http://expertconsult.inkling.com**

Key references

6. Gohel MS, Barwell JR, Taylor M, et al. Long term results of compression therapy alone versus compression plus surgery in chronic venous ulceration (ESCHAR): randomised controlled trial. BMJ 2007;335:83. PMID: 17545185.

14. Bradbury A, Evans CJ, Allan P, et al. The relationship between lower limb symptoms and superficial and deep venous reflux on duplex ultrasonography: The Edinburgh Vein Study. J Vasc Surg 2000;32:921–31. PMID: 11054224.

16. Eklöf B, Rutherford RB, Bergan JJ, et al. Revision of the CEAP classification for chronic venous disorders: consensus statement. J Vasc Surg 2004;1248–52. PMID: 15622385.

22. Marsden G, Perry M, Kelley K, et al. Guideline Development Group. Diagnosis and management of varicose veins in the legs: summary of NICE guidance. BMJ 2013;347:f4279. PMID: 23884969.

28. Shingler S, Robertson L, Boghossian S, et al. Compression stockings for the initial treatment of varicose veins in patients without venous ulceration. Cochrane Database Syst Rev 2013;5:CD008819. PMID: 24323411.

42. Mekako AI, Chetter IC, Coughlin PA, et al. Antibiotic pRophylaxis in varicose Vein Surgery Trialists (HARVEST). Randomized clinical trial of co-amoxiclav versus no antibiotic prophylaxis in varicose vein surgery. Br J Surg 2010;97:29–36. PMID: 20013927.

43. Winterborn RJ, Foy C, Earnshaw JJ. Causes of varicose vein recurrence: late results of a randomized controlled trial of stripping the long saphenous vein. J Vasc Surg 2004;40:634–9. PMID: 15472588.

47. Nelzén O, Fransson I, Swedish SEPS Study Group. Early results from a randomized trial of saphenous surgery with or without subfascial endoscopic perforator surgery in patients with a venous ulcer. Br J Surg 2011;98:495–500. PMID: 21656715.

49. Lane TRA, Onida S, Gohel MS, et al. A systematic review and meta-analysis on the role of varicosity treatment in the context of truncal vein ablation. Phlebology 2015;30:516–24. PMID: 25135826.

56. Nesbitt C, Bedenis R, Bhattacharya V, et al. Endovenous ablation (radiofrequency and laser) and foam sclerotherapy versus open surgery for great saphenous vein varices. Cochrane Database Syst Rev 2014;95: CD005624. PMID: 25075589.

57. Brittenden J, Cotton SC, Elders A, et al. A randomized trial comparing treatments for varicose

veins. N Engl J Med 2014;371:1218–27. PMID: 25251616.

59. Lawaetz M, Serup J, Lawaetz B, et al. Comparison of endovenous ablation techniques, foam sclerotherapy and surgical stripping for great saphenous varicose veins. Extended 5-year follow-up of a RCT. Int Angiol 2017;36:281–8. PMID: 28217989.

60. Lane T, Bootun R, Dharmarajah B, et al. A multi-centre randomised controlled trial comparing radiofrequency and mechanical occlusion chemically assisted ablation of varicose veins – final results of the Venefit versus Clarivein for varicose veins trial. Phlebology 2017;32:89–98. PMID: 27221810.

61. Morrison N, Gibson K, McEnroe S, et al. Randomized trial comparing cyanoacrylate embolization and radiofrequency ablation for incompetent great saphenous veins (VeClose). J Vasc Surg 2015;61:985–94. PMID: 25650040.

62. Gloviczki P, Comerota AJ, Dalsing MC, et al. The care of patients with varicose veins and associated chronic venous diseases: clinical practice guidelines of the Society for Vascular Surgery and the American Venous Forum. J Vasc Surg 2011;53(5 Suppl):2S–48S. PMID: 21536172.

63. Wittens C, Davies AH, Bækgaard N, et al. Editor's Choice – Management of chronic venous disease: clinical practice guidelines of the European Society for Vascular Surgery (ESVS). Eur J Vasc Endovasc Surg 2015;49(6):678–737. PMID: 25920631.

64. Nicolaides A, Kakkos S, Eklof B, et al. Management of chronic venous disorders of the lower limbs – guidelines according to scientific evidence. Int Angiol 2014;33(2):87–208. PMID: 24780922.

18

Chronic leg swelling

Prakash Saha
Stephen Black

There are various conditions that can cause chronic lower limb swelling (Box 18.1). The three most common are chronic venous insufficiency, lymphoedema and dependent oedema, which may be associated with inactivity and obesity. This chapter explores these three conditions further.

Chronic venous insufficiency (CVI)

CVI encompasses disease of the lower limb veins in which venous return is impaired over a number of years, by reflux, obstruction or calf muscle pump failure. This leads to sustained venous hypertension and ultimately clinical complications including oedema, eczema, lipodermatosclerosis and, when severe, ulceration.

Clinical features

The clinical features of CVI include skin changes, varicose veins, swelling, ulceration and pain.

Skin changes

Varicose eczema presents as dry, scaly and itchy skin. The skin becomes friable and may become infected following scratching. Pigmentation, due to the deposition of haemosiderin in the tissues, produces a brown discolouration characteristic of CVI, which together with fibrosis leads to the clinical picture of lipodermatosclerosis around the ankle (**Fig. 18.1**). There may also be loss of pigmentation resulting in pale skin changes called atrophie blanche.

Varicose veins

Varicose veins may be present and a history of previous varicose vein treatment should be sought. The absence of visible varicose veins does not exclude the presence of significant superficial reflux. Varicose veins on the lower anterior abdominal wall are a sign of inferior vena cava or iliac vein obstruction and the patient should be examined standing in order to identify these.

Pain

The patient may complain of a general ache and heaviness in the leg after long periods of standing. This is worse towards the end of the day but improves with elevation or bed rest.

A history of deep vein thrombosis (DVT) should be sought. Venous claudication is an uncommon symptom that is usually due to iliofemoral vein occlusion or a significant stenosis. The symptoms differ from arterial claudication because the increase in arterial inflow during exercise combined with decreased outflow results in distension of the limb, giving rise to generalised pain and a severe bursting sensation in the leg. The pain often requires elevation for 10–20 minutes for relief after cessation of exercise.

Swelling

Swelling is due to an accumulation of oedematous fluid, which is initially pitting, but as the disease progresses subcutaneous fibrosis and induration occur. If there is any break in the skin, this can lead to copious exudation of fluid.

Venous disease
Primary varicose veins
Primary deep venous incompetence
Post-thrombotic syndrome
Arteriovenous malformations

Lymphoedema
Primary
Secondary

General disease
Lipoedema
Congestive cardiac failure
Pretibial myxoedema
Nephrotic syndrome
Hepatic failure

Tumours
Pelvic tumours causing extrinsic compression

Drugs
Dependency

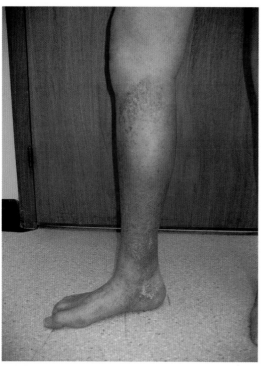

Figure 18.1 • Chronic venous insufficiency with pigmentation and severe lipodermatosclerosis resulting in the typical 'inverted champagne bottle' shape.

Ulceration

Ulceration is often precipitated by minor trauma and venous ulcers occur predominantly on the lower leg, more commonly around the medial aspect of the ankle. There may be surrounding eczema or pigmentation and frequently exudation of fluid can cause maceration of the surrounding skin. In patients presenting with lower limb ulceration, approximately 80%[1,2] will have evidence of venous disease and 10–25%[3] of limbs will have Doppler-verified arterial disease. Approximately 12% will have coexisting diabetes or rheumatoid arthritis.[4] Immobility is often a contributory cause, and can also cause stasis ulceration in isolation.

Epidemiology

The prevalence of CVI in the adult population lies between 2% and 9%, and may be higher in males than females.[5,6] The most serious feature of CVI is ulceration, which is a distressing and debilitating condition. Leg ulcers affect approximately 1% of the adult population in developed countries, with 50% of ulcers having been present for more than 12 months, and 72% are recurrent.[7] Within the UK, Australia, Sweden and Italy, overall rates for active ulceration range from 0.15% to 0.5%, and increase with age.[8–12] In the UK, the current total cost to the NHS is estimated to be around £1 billion a year.[13]

Aetiology

To understand CVI, the changes that occur in both the larger veins (macrocirculation) and the capillary bed (microcirculation) must be considered.

Macrocirculation

During exercise in the normal individual, effective contraction of the calf muscles combined with vein patency and valvular competence aids venous return and reduces venous pressure in the lower leg from about 90 mmHg to 30 mmHg. Failure of any of these mechanisms can result in postambulatory venous hypertension, which is accepted as the underlying haemodynamic abnormality in CVI. The recognised causes are outlined in Box 18.2.

Deep and superficial reflux

Most venous ulcers were thought to be secondary to a previous DVT but duplex scanning has demonstrated that some patients have primary deep venous reflux. Isolated superficial venous incompetence without deep venous incompetence occurs in between 31%[14] and 57%[15] of patients with venous ulceration.

Perforating vein reflux

The contribution of incompetent perforators to the development of CVI remains controversial. Isolated perforator incompetence occurs in only

Box 18.2 • Causes of venous hypertension

Superficial venous reflux
Long saphenous vein reflux
Short saphenous vein reflux

Deep venous reflux and occlusion
Primary (idiopathic)
Secondary to deep venous thrombosis or injury

Perforating vein reflux
Abnormal calf pump
Neurological
Musculoskeletal

Combination of the above

2–4% of limbs with skin changes, and perforator incompetence is usually associated with reflux in the superficial or deep systems. However, the prevalence of incompetent perforators increases linearly with the clinical severity of CVI.[16] There has been a recent trend towards treatment of incompetent perforating veins with laser or radiofrequency ablation, but the indications for this remain uncertain. In those cases where superficial and perforator reflux coincide, treating only the former results in healing rates of 95%.[17]

Microcirculation

The pathophysiology is still not fully understood but the following two hypotheses exist:

1. **White cell trapping hypothesis.** Increased venous pressures lead to white blood cell plugging of capillaries, adherence of white cells to the endothelium and release of proteolytic enzymes. This leads to increased capillary permeability and tissue damage causing ulceration.[18–21]

2. **Fibrin cuff hypothesis.** A rise in venous pressure causes widening of the pores between endothelial cells.[22] This results in leakage of fibrinogen out of the intravascular compartment into the tissues, which polymerises to form fibrin. A defective interstitial fibrinolytic system may also contribute to the build-up of fibrin.[23] Fibrin 'cuffs' form around the capillaries, which acts as a barrier to oxygen, resulting in local tissue ischaemia and cell death, producing ulceration.[24]

Matrix metalloproteinases help remodel the extracellular matrix by protein degradation, and enhanced matrix metalloproteinase activity has been demonstrated in lipodermatosclerosis.[25] This may also contribute to the development of ulceration.

Classification

CVI involves a variety of anatomical and physiological abnormalities and therefore a standardised system is required to allow uniformity of reporting.

✓✓ A classification was developed in 1994 by an international consensus conference under the auspices of the American Venous Forum and recommendations for change were made in 2004.[26]

The classification includes clinical signs (C), aetiology (E), anatomical distribution (A) and pathophysiological condition (P), and is therefore known by the acronym CEAP. This system is helpful in comparing limbs for the purposes of research, although it is rather unwieldy for everyday use (Box 18.3).

Investigation

Patients often present with mixed arterial and venous disease and so ankle–brachial pressure indices must be recorded if foot pulses are weak or absent and when compression therapy is being considered. The investigation of the venous disease is discussed below.

Box 18.3 • CEAP classification

Clinical signs (C_{0-6})
Limbs are placed into one of seven clinical classes according to objective signs as follows:
- Class 0: no visible or palpable signs of venous disease
- Class 1: telangiectases, reticular veins, malleolar flare
- Class 2: varicose veins
- Class 3: oedema without skin changes
- Class 4a: pigmentation or eczema class 4b, lipodermatosclerosis or atrophie blanche
- Class 5: skin changes as above with healed ulceration
- Class 6: skin changes as above with active ulceration
  Each limb is further classified as asymptomatic (A) or symptomatic (S)

Aetiology ($E_{C,P,S,N}$)
This classification refers to congenital (C), primary (P; unknown cause but not congenital), secondary (S; acquired) and no aetiology identified (N). These groups are mutually exclusive

Anatomical distribution ($A_{S,D,P,N}$)
This refers to superficial (S), deep (D), perforating (P) veins and no venous location identified (N). More than one system may be involved

Pathophysiological condition ($P_{R,O,N}$)
This refers to reflux (R) or obstruction (O), or both may be present. P_N implies no venous pathophysiology identified

Hand-held Doppler

Continuous-wave hand-held Doppler using an 8-MHz probe is a useful outpatient tool in screening for arterial and venous disease. Its limitations are that the exact vein being insonated is unknown, it is operator-dependent and the significance of reflux of short duration may be uncertain.

Duplex scanning

Duplex is an important investigation of lower limb venous disease and is now first line. Modern equipment allows easy identification of normal and abnormal venous anatomy, along with the presence of venous reflux. It is also extensively used for the diagnosis of DVT.

> ✅ An international consensus document recommends duplex scanning as an essential investigation for patients with CVI.[27]

Venography

Venography is invasive and to a large extent has been superseded by duplex scanning for the investigation of venous disease of the lower limb. Venography still has a place in the diagnosis of upper limb DVT when ultrasound is inconclusive and clinical suspicion persists and in patients with post-thrombotic limb syndrome where an obstruction in the iliac veins and inferior vena cava is not readily visualised by ultrasound. With the increased use of deep endovenous therapy, however, to treat such lesions, axial imaging with either computed tomography (CT) or magnetic resonance (MR) venography is often used for preoperative planning.

Computed tomography venography

Computed tomography venography (CTV) can be used to image thrombosis affecting the abdominal and pelvic veins. A contrast agent injected either directly into the dorsal veins (direct) or in the antecubital veins (indirect) is required. Extravascular anatomical structures can be visualised and the lungs can be imaged at the same time for the detection of pulmonary embolism. The main disadvantages of this technique are the use of ionising radiation, risk of contrast nephropathy and cost. CTV is mainly therefore used only when interventions are being considered.

Magnetic resonance imaging

Magnetic resonance imaging (MRI) techniques can be used for the assessment of the deep veins, particularly when intervention is being considered. MRI utilises non-ionising radiation, which is beneficial to the younger patient cohort, and by applying a number of different sequences both anatomical and functional information can be obtained. There are a number of limitations to the use of magnetic resonance,

however, including cost. Nevertheless, it is likely that this imaging technique will become first line for the assessment of patients with iliofemoral venous pathology before intervention is considered.

Intravascular ultrasound

Intravascular ultrasound (IVUS) is an invasive technique that can be used to visualise the vessel lumen and surrounding wall in real time. It complements venography and is a useful aid in measuring and deploying venous stents precisely. It is also more reliable than venography when assessing stent characteristics intraoperatively and is a vital adjunct to deep endovenous procedures.

Functional measurements

Various investigations may be used to examine the function of the venous system in the lower limb.

Ambulatory venous pressure measurement

This provides direct measurement of the superficial venous pressure at the ankle. This is achieved by cannulation of a vein on the dorsum of the foot connected to a pressure transducer, amplifier and a recorder. The pressure changes recorded in the long saphenous vein in the foot during and after 10 tiptoe exercises are shown in **Fig. 18.2**. This investigation is an indicator of overall lower limb venous function, including calf muscle pump function.

Plethysmography

There are many different types of plethysmography, which measure either alterations in calf volume directly or parameters that indirectly reflect volume change. These include photoplethysmography, strain gauge plethysmography and air plethysmography.

Treatment

The management of patients with CVI may be divided into either the prevention of or the treatment of clinical complications such as lipodermatosclerosis and ulceration. Correcting the underlying cause can help to stop or reverse these complications. In addition, vigorous treatment of conditions known to lead to CVI, particularly acute DVT, may reduce the incidence of this problem in the long term. Management of patients with ulcers of mixed aetiology will require treatment aimed at each specific cause but this section deals predominantly with the treatment of isolated venous disease.

General measures

These should include elevation of the legs at rest above the level of the heart. This helps to reduce oedema, decrease exudate from ulcers and accelerate regression of skin changes.[4] Immobility, occupation, obesity and

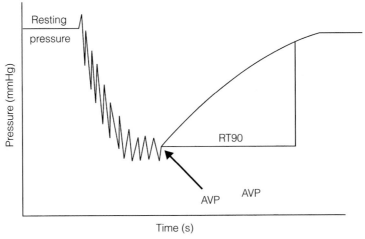

Figure 18.2 • Venous pressure trace recorded from a superficial vein on the dorsum of the foot during 10 tiptoe exercises and return to the resting value after exercise. AVP, ambulatory venous pressure; RT90, time for 90% refilling.

coexisting disease may also influence the development of skin complications and should be addressed. Placing the patient in bed reduces the venous pressure at the ankle to about 12–15mmHg and can help lead to ulcer healing. However, this is not a treatment enjoyed by most patients and may increase the risk of DVT. It is therefore generally reserved for ulcers that have failed to heal by all other methods.

Graduated elastic compression

Compression therapy remains the primary treatment for the majority of patients with CVI. It provides symptomatic relief, promotes ulcer healing and helps in preventing ulcer recurrence. Applying a sustained graduated compressive force that is highest at the ankle and decreases proximally has been shown to reduce venous pressure at the ankle, increase femoral vein blood flow and increase venous refilling time. This improves venous function and can heal up to 93% of venous ulcers.[28] Graduated elastic compression may be applied using either bandages or stockings but this is dependent on factors such as levels of exudate, amount of oedema and leg shape. It is important that these are applied by experienced staff as inexpertly applied compression can cause skin damage. Compression can also be used to treat mixed arterial and venous ulcers but this requires specialist assessment.

✔✔ In the healing of leg ulcers: (i) compression is more effective than no compression; (ii) elastic compression is more effective than non-elastic compression; (iii) multilayered high compression is more effective than single-layer compression; and (iv) there is no significant difference between four-layer bandaging and other high-compression multilayered systems.[29]

In the prevention of ulcer recurrence, there are no randomised trials comparing recurrence rates with and without compression.

✔✔ A review of trials comparing different grades of compression stocking concluded that higher grades of compression are associated with lower recurrence rates, but at a cost of lower patient compliance.[30] Approximately one-third of patients do not comply with the long-term use of compression hosiery.[31]

Stockings are classed according to the pressure they exert at the ankle and are designed to provide a linear graduated decrease in pressure above this, although in practice this may not always be the case. Pressures of up to 60mmHg may be produced by elastic stockings, and conventional pressure classes and indications are given in Table 18.1.

Table 18.1 • Conventional pressure classes of compression stockings

Class	Pressure at ankle (mmHg)	Indications
I	<25	Mild varicosis, venous thrombosis prophylaxis
II	25–35	Marked varicose veins, oedema, chronic venous insufficiency
III	35–45	Chronic venous insufficiency, lymphoedema, following venous ulceration to prevent recurrence
IV	45–60	Severe lymphoedema and chronic venous insufficiency

For the majority of patients with CVI or mild lymphoedema, a knee-length compression stocking designed to apply compression of 25–35 mmHg is ideal, but this will be influenced by how well they tolerate the stockings and their ability to apply them. Thigh-length stockings seem to confer little benefit over knee-length ones and as shorter stockings are easier to put on, compliance with these tends to be better. Stocking applicators may also aid patient compliance.

Intermittent pneumatic compression

✔✔ There is some evidence that intermittent pneumatic compression may provide accelerated ulcer healing when used either alone or in combination with elastic compression, although there is a need for further trials in this area.[32]

Laser and electromagnetic therapy

✔✔ A review of low-level laser therapy for venous leg ulcers has not found any benefit in healing rates.[33] Similarly, there is no high-quality evidence that electromagnetic therapy increases the rate of healing of venous leg ulcers.[34]

Pharmacotherapy

Dressings

For those patients with venous ulceration, there are a wide variety of topical dressings available.

✔✔ The type of dressing applied beneath compression has not been shown to affect ulcer healing, although dressing choice has an impact on pain, frequency of dressing change, maceration and odour. Decisions regarding which dressing to use should be based on local costs and practitioner or patient preference.[35]

Additional factors to consider in choosing a dressing are exudate, odour and patient comfort. Whatever dressing is chosen should be used in conjunction with treatment of the underlying venous insufficiency, usually by adequate graduated elastic compression. Simple non-adherent dressings are all that is required for many ulcers. Vacuum-assisted closure dressing systems are sometimes useful for deep ulceration and can be used under compression. There is recent evidence that they reduce time to healing at a lower cost when compared to conventional dressings.[36] The Vulcan trial suggested that silver dressings made no impact on ulcer healing when compared to any other dressing, although this has been questioned as many of the ulcers treated with silver within the trial would not have had silver applied in clinical practice.[37]

Emollients

These soothe, smooth and hydrate the skin and are indicated for all dry or scaling disorders, such as varicose eczema. Their effects are short-lived and frequent application is necessary. Preparations containing an antibacterial should be avoided unless infection is present.

Oxpentifylline (pentoxifylline)

✔✔ There have been several randomised controlled trials of oxpentifylline compared with placebo, with or without compression, in the healing of venous leg ulcers.[38] These have demonstrated that this drug is more effective than placebo in ulcer healing.

Nutrition

Adequate nutrition is important for ulcer healing; protein, vitamins A and C, zinc and other trace elements are all important. It may be appropriate to consider dietary supplements if these are deficient.

Superficial venous intervention

Superficial venous surgery

Superficial surgery may be of benefit in healing ulcers in situations of isolated superficial venous incompetence or combined superficial and deep venous incompetence. Surgery for isolated superficial venous incompetence may also reduce long-term recurrence rates. With the advent of minimally invasive techniques it may be possible to treat some patients who previously were not fit for conventional varicose vein surgery. These techniques include radiofrequency ablation (RFA), endovenous laser ablation (EVLA) and foam sclerotherapy, and are discussed in Chapter 17.

✔✔ A randomised controlled trial comparing superficial venous surgery plus elastic compression with compression alone for venous ulceration has demonstrated no difference in initial healing rates but a reduction in recurrence rates at 12 months in the surgical group (12% vs 28%). The authors concluded that most patients with chronic venous ulceration will benefit from addition of simple venous surgery.[39]

Perforating vein surgery

There has been renewed interest in medial calf-perforating vein incompetence with the advent of subfascial endoscopic perforating vein surgery, and more recently with minimally invasive techniques such as EVLA and RFA. The evidence for the benefit of treatment of incompetent perforating veins by any of these methods is weak and the precise indications and benefit of perforator treatment remain unclear.

Deep venous valvular reconstruction

Worldwide experience of deep venous valvular reconstruction is limited as most patients with CVI can be managed adequately with superficial venous surgery and the conservative measures described above. Therefore it is usually reserved for those patients with severe symptoms that prove resistant to conservative treatment.

The benefit of deep venous valvular reconstructive surgery is unclear as many of the published series have included ancillary procedures such as high saphenous ligation and stripping, and in the few series where the influence of these procedures has been excluded the numbers involved tend to be small or the follow-up short. A number of different procedures have been described and these are shown in Box 18.4.

> ✔✔ A Cochrane review[40] has found no evidence for benefit (or harm) of valvuloplasty in the treatment of patients with CVI secondary to primary valvular incompetence. The individual trials included in the review were small and of poor quality and the benefit of valvuloplasty remains uncertain.

Skin grafting

Large ulcers may be treated with a split-skin graft or pinch grafts which, if successful, may reduce the healing time. Before this is undertaken, it is important that the ulcer bed is clean and free from infection (particularly β-haemolytic streptococci, *Pseudomonas* and *Staphylococcus aureus*). However, unless the underlying venous abnormality is also treated, failure of the graft and subsequent recurrence is inevitable.

Endovascular management of venous outflow obstruction

Following DVT, a degree of recanalisation can occur in affected venous segments, usually by 90 days.[41] Many patients are, however, left with functional outflow obstruction and deep venous reflux. When the iliofemoral vein is affected and there is persistent venous outflow obstruction, symptoms tend to be severe, resulting in a persistent swollen leg, skin changes and venous claudication, which leads to a poor quality of life. Until recently, the majority of these patients were treated conservatively with compression hosiery; however, the development of endovascular treatments in recent years has led to the use of endoluminal stenting to treat iliac venous occlusions. These interventions have been shown to be of benefit in selected patients and Raju et al.[42] have reported treating long iliac venous occlusions, with primary and secondary patency rates at 2 years of 49% and 76%, respectively. Further studies have reported patency rates in the region of 90% at 1 year for stenting of iliac venous stenoses (May–Thurner syndrome).[43,44] This refers to the chronic pulsatile compression of the proximal left common iliac vein by the overlying right common iliac artery or aortic bifurcation, resulting in an intraluminal venous spur, web or membrane. This common lesion (20% of the adult population) is an increasingly well-recognised cause of left iliac vein thrombo-occlusive disease, particularly in young patients. The clinical picture is of left leg venous hypertension or DVT and is likely to explain the preponderance of left-sided DVT. The development of dedicated nitinol venous stents is likely to increase the use of these interventions, which show promise in the short term, and long-term data are awaited.

Venous bypass

Surgical bypass of an obstructed vein may be possible, but this should be reserved for those patients in whom there is measured evidence of outflow obstruction, endoluminal interventions have been exhausted and there are severe symptoms. Two principal surgical procedures have been described:

1. The femorofemoral crossover graft for iliac obstruction (Palma operation; **Fig. 18.3**).[45] Only a small number of patients are suitable for this procedure, but in these patients long-term patency and relief of symptoms may be achieved in up to 70% of cases.[46] The long saphenous vein on the unaffected side is used as a crossover graft.

2. Limbs with functional outflow obstruction due to stenosed or occluded deep thigh veins may be suitable for saphenopopliteal bypass, which uses the long saphenous vein as a bypass channel. The theoretical difficulty with this procedure is that the long saphenous vein may already be acting as a collateral channel and to interfere with this may make matters worse should thrombosis occur.

Box 18.4 • Procedures for correction of deep venous valvular incompetence

Valvular repair
Valvuloplasty
Valve transposition
Valve transplantation

External support of vein wall
Dacron cuff
Vein wall plication

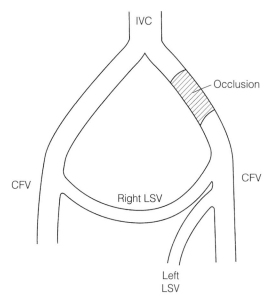

Labels in figure: IVC, Occlusion, CFV, CFV, Right LSV, Left LSV

Figure 18.3 • Femorofemoral crossover graft using the long saphenous vein (LSV) to bypass unilateral iliac obstruction. CFV, common femoral vein; IVC, inferior vena cava.

Preventing the post-thrombotic limb

CVI developing secondary to previous DVT is commonly referred to as post-thrombotic syndrome (PTS) or postphlebitic syndrome. The management of DVT has historically been directed at preventing thrombus extension and pulmonary embolus in the acute phase. There has been little focus on long-term treatment in order to prevent the development of PTS. However, 30% or more will develop features of mild or moderate PTS.[47–49] This risk increases with more proximal DVT and recurrent episodes of thrombosis. Even with isolated calf vein thrombosis there is a risk of development of PTS.

✓✓ The risk of developing severe CVI with ulceration following DVT is of the order of 2–10% at 10 years.[47,50]

The causes of PTS related to previous DVT are either valvular incompetence or residual outflow obstruction with eventual calf muscle pump failure. Treatment of the primary DVT should be aimed not only at preventing thrombus propagation and pulmonary embolism, but also at preventing venous damage and preserving or restoring venous function. This may include anticoagulation, limb elevation and elastic compression therapy. Increasingly, thrombolysis and catheter thrombectomy are being used in the management of acute iliofemoral DVT and should be considered first-line therapy in young patients without contraindications. Patients who have had a DVT should be encouraged to wear lifelong elastic compression hosiery, in particular those patients with residual reflux and who are on their feet all day or travel long journeys.[44] They should be encouraged to take regular exercise to stimulate the calf muscle pump and maintain ankle mobility. These simple measures are often recommended for life but there is controversy as to their success in preventing PTS.

Summary

Investigation and treatment must be tailored to the individual patient but a simplified everyday management plan is shown in **Fig. 18.4**.

Dependency and inactivity

Patients who sit for long periods are exposed to a raised venous pressure at the ankle for longer periods of time. Normal daily activity includes activation of the calf muscle pump by walking, thereby decreasing the venous pressure, but without this pressure reduction the effects on the lower limb are similar to those seen in venous reflux due to prolonged venous 'hypertension'. As a result inactive patients, for example those confined to a wheelchair, can develop venous-type leg swelling in the absence of any true venous pathology. Those with a stiff or fused ankle may also be affected. The use of prophylactic compression therapy should therefore be considered in these patients. Morbid obesity adds to this problem and is becoming a major aetiological factor in lower limb ulceration. The management of obesity is an important component of treatment in these patients and whilst this may be done in primary care in the majority of cases, some may require referral for gastric banding or bypass.

Lymphoedema

Lymphoedema is a progressive, chronic and debilitating swelling that can affect any part of the body, most commonly the limbs, leading to distortion in shape, size, reduction of mobility and impaired function.

Aetiology

Lymphoedema can be caused by intrinsic factors (primary) or extrinsic factors (secondary).

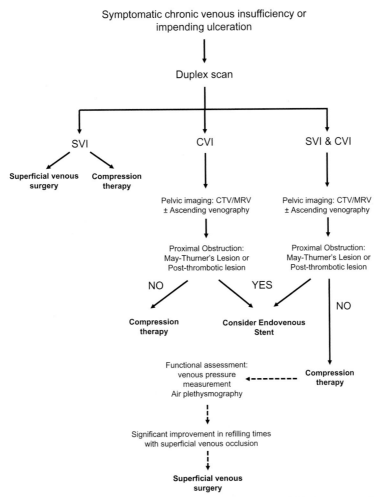

Figure 18.4 • Flow diagram for the management of chronic venous insufficiency. DVI, deep venous incompetence; SVI, superficial venous incompetence.

Primary

The traditional classification of primary lymph-oedema is shown in Box 18.5. Congenital lymphoedema occurs at or soon after birth and in some rare cases it is autosomally inherited (Milroy's disease). Lymphoedema praecox presents up to the age of 35 years and is more prevalent in females. Typically this is not familial, although lymphoedema–distichiasis syndrome, which develops at puberty, is familial and is linked to the *FOXC2* gene mutation.[51] Lymphoedema tarda presents over the age of 35 years. It is likely that these three groups represent different parts of the same spectrum of disease, which has been attributed to aplasia, hypoplasia or hyperplasia of the lymph vessels during development. A fibrotic obstruction in the lymph nodes has also been described.[52]

In addition to this, a functional classification more orientated to the treatment of these conditions may be used. This type of classification was first described by Browse.[53]

- Obliterative (80%): the distal lymphatics undergo progressive obliteration. This occurs predominantly in females and is often bilateral.
- Proximal obstruction (10%): proximal occlusion occurs in the abdominal, pelvic or inguinal lymph nodes. This is predominantly unilateral.
- Lymphatic valvular incompetence and hyperplasia (10%): development of the valve system is incomplete and lymphatic dilatation and hyperplasia occur. This is usually bilateral.

Box 18.5 • Causes of lymphoedema

Primary
Congenital (age <1 year)
- Familial (Milroy's disease)
- Non-familial

Praecox (age <35 years)
- Familial
- Non-familial

Tarda (age >35 years)

Secondary
Malignant disease
Surgery
- Radical mastectomy
- Radical groin dissection

Radiotherapy
Infection
- Parasitic (filariasis)
- Pyogenic (β-haemolytic streptococci, *Staphylococcus aureus*)
- Tuberculosis

Impairment
- Arterial surgery
- Venous disease and venous surgery

Secondary

Secondary lymphoedema develops following extrinsic damage to part of the lymphatic system. The lymphatic channels distal to the obstruction become dilated and the valves secondarily incompetent. The commonest cause worldwide is filarial infestation but in Europe the commonest cause is neoplasia and its treatment, for example post-mastectomy lymphoedema. The causes of secondary lymphoedema are also listed in Box 18.5.

Presentation

Initial presentation is with peripheral oedema. History and examination will usually differentiate lymphoedema from other causes of limb swelling and may distinguish between primary and secondary causes.

History

The patient complains of a slowly progressive swelling of the whole or part of the limb, which typically does not reduce overnight with elevation. Limb swelling usually commences distally and may progress during the day, particularly on standing for long periods. The patient may describe the limb as heavy and up to 50% will complain of pain requiring analgesia.[54] There may be a history of recurrent lymphangitis.

The age of onset and a history of previous surgery, malignancy or radiotherapy should be sought.

Lymphoedema can also occur secondary to lipoedema. Lipoedema is abnormal symmetrical swelling due to excess deposit and expansion of fat cells. It is always bilateral, occurs from the waist down and spares the ankles. It cannot be lost through diet and exercise, and often causes pain, particularly surrounding the tibial area. It occurs almost exclusively in women, and can occur in women of all sizes and can be inherited. The expanding fat cells interfere with the lymphatics so many lipoedema patients develop lymphoedema, which is difficult to treat due to the inability to tolerate compression because of pain.

Examination

Examination reveals swelling of the limb, which may be unilateral or bilateral. Initially it will pit like other types of oedema, but with time the swelling becomes non-pitting due to hypertrophy of adipose tissue and increasing subcutaneous fibrosis. The swelling is uniform and as it progresses the leg becomes like a tree-trunk (**Fig. 18.5**). The skin develops a 'peau d'orange' appearance with hyperkeratosis of the toes and skin fissuring with secondary fungal

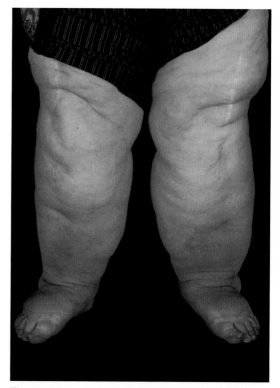

Figure 18.5 • Chronic lymphoedema of the leg with tree-trunk appearance and 'buffalo hump' of the foot.

infection. The skin gradually thickens, becoming less elastic until it is not possible to pick up a fold in the lower leg. This inelasticity produces a positive Stemmer sign (the inability to pinch the skin of the dorsum of the second toe between the thumb and forefinger). The dorsum of the foot is usually involved, producing the characteristic 'buffalo hump' appearance, and chylous vesicles may occur on the pretibial area.

Ankle ulceration is unusual with lymphoedema as the skin remains more elastic than in venous disease, allowing expansion to occur without increased tension.[55] The presence of surgical scars or skin telangiectasia following radiotherapy may indicate a cause of secondary lymphoedema.

Clinical staging

There is no consensus on a universal clinical staging system for all forms of lymphoedema, but the consensus document of the International Society of Lymphology suggests the staging system in Table 18.2.[56,57] Within each stage, severity based on volume difference can be assessed as minimal (<20% increase) in limb volume, moderate (20–40% increase) or severe (>40% increase).

Investigation

The diagnosis of lymphoedema can usually be made clinically. Investigation is needed when the diagnosis is uncertain, to exclude sinister underlying causes or, if surgery is being considered, to confirm the diagnosis and plan treatment.

Duplex ultrasonography

This is useful to exclude CVI. The B-mode image will also detect the changes in the dermis and subcutaneous layers and can therefore be used as a means of monitoring the disease.

Table 18.2 • Clinical staging of lymphoedema

Stage 0	Latent or subclinical condition where swelling is not evident despite impaired lymph transport
Stage I	Early accumulation of fluid that subsides with limb elevation. Pitting may occur
Stage II	Limb elevation alone rarely reduces tissue swelling and pitting is manifest. Late in stage II, the limb may or may not pit as tissue fibrosis supervenes
Stage III	Lymphostatic elephantiasis where pitting is absent and trophic skin changes such as acanthosis, fat deposits and warty overgrowths develop

Lymphangioscintigraphy (isotope lymphography)

This is now one of the most frequently performed investigations as it provides an overall assessment of lymphatic drainage by demonstrating isotope flow up the lymphatics, and in the majority of cases avoids the need for conventional lymphangiography (**Fig. 18.6**). Radiolabelled (usually technetium) colloid is injected into the interdigital space between the second and third toes on both sides and gamma-camera pictures are taken at 5-minute intervals to assess transit through the lymph channels. Scintigraphy has been demonstrated to have a sensitivity of 92% and a specificity of 100% for the diagnosis of lymphoedema.[58] A negative scintigram effectively excludes the diagnosis.[59]

Computed tomography

Computed tomography may show the presence of dilated lymphatic channels, thereby aiding the diagnosis of obstructive lymphoedema and lymphatic valvular incompetence.[60] It will also provide evidence of lymphoedema by the presence of a honeycomb appearance of fluid in the subcutaneous tissues, and has been used to monitor the response to compression therapy by measuring the cross-sectional area of limb compartments. Patients with a previous history of pelvic or abdominal malignancy should be scanned for recurrent disease in order to diagnose enlarged lymph nodes or pelvic masses that may be compressing the lymphatic channels.

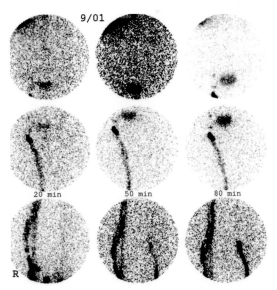

Figure 18.6 • Lymphoscintigram confirming left-sided lymphoedema. On the right, the isotope is travelling up the lymphatics of the leg with concentration in the ilioinguinal nodes (normal). On the left the isotope has remained in the leg.

Magnetic resonance imaging

In patients with chronic lymphoedema, MRI has been shown to demonstrate circumferential subcutaneous oedema, thickening of dermis and a honeycomb pattern of fibrosis between the muscle and subcutis, increased subcutaneous fat and variability in lymph node size and appearance.[61,62]

Interstitial magnetic resonance lymphangiography

Interstitial magnetic resonance lymphography involves intracutaneous injection of a paramagnetic contrast agent for the visualisation of lymphatic vessels.[63] Dilated lymphatic channels are a common finding and collateral vessels along with dermal backflow indicate proximal obstruction.[64,65] Dynamic MR lymphangiography is more sensitive and accurate than lymphoscintigraphy in the detection of anatomical and functional abnormalities in the lymphatic system.[66]

Fluorescence microlymphangiography

Fluorescence microlymphangiography (FML) involves visualisation of the superficial network of lymphatics with a fluorescence microscope following intracutaneous injection of fluorescein isothiocyanate–dextran. It can confirm the clinical diagnosis of lymphoedema and can distinguish various forms of oedema.[56,67] Emanating from the fluorescent spot, the surrounding network of microvessels is filled and becomes easily visible and is recorded by photography or video. In Milroy's disease, a lack of microlymphatics (aplasia) is typical, while in other primary and secondary lymphoedema the network remains intact but the depicted area is enlarged. In lipoedema, lymphatic microaneurysms are seen.

Contrast lymphangiography

This investigation is now used only rarely in the diagnosis of lymphoedema and has been largely replaced by scintigraphy. It is for patients being considered for microvascular lymphatic reconstruction.

Treatment

The aim of treatment is to reduce limb swelling, reduce the risk of infection and improve function. If management begins early in the disease process when pitting oedema is present, conservative measures should be successful. Once achieved, the improvement must be maintained. Surgical options are available in a few centres for resistant and severely symptomatic cases.

General measures

Once the diagnosis is made, a clear explanation of the condition and its non-life-threatening nature should be given to the patient, along with referral to a specialist service.[51] The treatment is improved by empowering the patient to manage their own condition, and the earlier education and treatment are instituted the better the outcome, hence information leaflets can be helpful. In the early stages elevation of a lymphoedematous limb while resting and at night can reduce oedema by increasing venous return and reducing the production of interstitial fluid. Exercise, such as on an exercise bicycle, encourages movement of lymph along non-contractile vessels and increased contractility of collecting lymph vessels. Managing obesity is also important.

Manual lymphatic drainage

This involves manipulating the leg by squeezing just above the most proximal area of oedema and then working from proximal to distal. This enhances lymphatic flow.

Graduated elastic compression

Compression stockings need to exert a pressure of approximately 50 mmHg or higher. The stockings can be used for maintenance of the limb after oedema reduction but compliance is low in the summer months, and the elderly and frail find them difficult to apply. Multilayer bandaging is an essential stage of the intensive phase of management. Inelastic bandages are applied to the limb, providing a low resting pressure but high exercise pressure. This is used to reduce severe swelling, and improve limb shape and skin condition prior to fitting compression hosiery.

> ✔✔ If graduated elastic compression is used initially followed by a stocking for maintenance, a greater and more sustained limb volume reduction is achieved than if stockings alone are used throughout.[68]

Intermittent pneumatic compression

Intermittent pneumatic compression (IPC) involves placement of the limb in a multicompartmental sleeve. Each compartment consists of air cells that are sequentially inflated to a pressure of about 80 mmHg and deflated from distal to proximal, thus massaging the lymph centrally. Patients use this for 4 hours a day and it can be done at home. If the lymphatic system is obliterated or obstructed more proximally, massaging the lymph centrally can precipitate collections elsewhere, such as the genitals, and high pressures may injure peripheral lymphatics. Reports combining IPC with stockings quote figures of 90% for immediate benefit and long-term maintenance.[69] The poor responders have usually had oedema for more than 10 years. In these chronic patients, compression using the hydrostatic pressure of mercury has had some effect.[70] The leg is placed in a cylinder and is covered by two membranes, which are filled and emptied with mercury in cycles. Pressures of up to 80 mmHg are generated at the foot and this linearly decreases towards normal atmospheric pressure at the surface. This is well tolerated and improvement is even seen in those with fibrosclerotic oedema. Despite its theoretical simplicity, the application and safety precautions are complex.

Thermal treatment

Hyperthermia of the leg is produced by microwave heating or immersion in hot water. There is no change to the flow of lymph but it does reduce the local inflammatory infiltrate and extracellular protein matrix.[71] A reduction in limb volume follows, along with a decrease in the rate of recurrent infections.

Complex decongestive physiotherapy (complex physical therapy)

Complex decongestive physiotherapy generally involves a two-stage treatment programme over 2–4 weeks. The first phase consists of skin care, light manual massage, range of motion exercise and compression, typically applied with multilayered bandage wrapping. Phase 2 aims to conserve and optimise the results obtained in phase 1. It consists of compression by a low-stretch elastic stocking or sleeve, skin care, continued 'remedial' exercise and repeated light massage as needed. With good compliance a 65–67% reduction in limb volume can be achieved, with 90% of the reduction being maintained at 9 months.[72] As an added benefit the incidence of infection almost halves and quality of life is improved.[73]

Prevention of infection

The lymphatic system transports lymphocytes, enabling rapid response to foreign antigens. Stagnation of lymph prevents this and so increases the risk and severity of infection. The common pathogens are β-haemolytic streptococci and *Staphylococcus aureus*. With each attack of cellulitis or erysipelas the organisms further obliterate the lymph channels, making the oedema worse. Well-fitting comfortable shoes prevent small cracks in the skin that may act as a portal of entry. Meticulous skin care is essential and the patient should develop a routine that includes washing followed by thorough drying of the limb, application of an emollient and monitoring the skin for any problems that develop into cellulitis. Any early signs of infection should be treated aggressively with antibiotics. Recurrent infection can be managed by long-term low-dose prophylactic antibiotics such as amoxicillin, flucloxacillin or a cephalosporin.

✔ Current guidelines recommend that antibiotics be taken for at least 14 days after signs of clinical improvement are observed.[74]

Drugs

Benzopyrones are thought to reduce oedema by reducing vascular permeability and thus the amount of fluid forming in the subcutaneous tissues. Advocates for this treatment method believe that the drugs have some beneficial effect on pain and discomfort in the swollen areas. Proponents also claim that these drugs increase macrophage activity, encouraging the lysis of protein, which in turn reduces the formation of fibrotic tissue in the lymphoedematous limb. A Cochrane review concluded that it is not possible to draw conclusions about the effectiveness of benzopyrones in the management of lymphoedema from the available trials.[75] Diuretics are not recommended in the management of lymphoedema as there is no evidence that they improve lymphatic drainage.[51]

Surgical treatments

Surgical options are available in some specialist centres. They should be reserved for severely symptomatic patients (e.g. lymphorrhagia or recurrent lymphangitis) in whom all conservative methods have failed. The patient must have realistic expectations of the likely outcome and will need long-term compression therapy after treatment. Surgical procedures can be divided into debulking operations (for obliterative causes) and bypass procedures (for lymphatic obstruction).

Debulking operations

These procedures aim to excise variable amounts of the excess skin and subcutaneous tissue from the affected limb. The techniques range from removal of ellipses of tissue and primary closure (Homan's operation; **Fig. 18.7**) to the radical Charles operation, which excises all the skin and subcutaneous tissues of the calf down to and sometimes including the deep fascia. Primary skin grafting is then required. Good functional results have been obtained with this method but cosmesis is poor and it may be complicated by warts, resistant

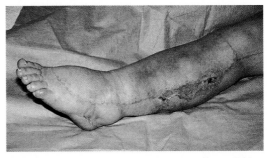

Figure 18.7 • Homan's operation. A long ellipse of skin and subcutaneous tissue has been excised from the lateral side of the leg after a previous procedure on the medial side. Poor wound healing is common.

ulceration, lymph weeping and pantalooning of the thigh. Suction lipectomy, which has good results in the postmastectomy arm,[76] has been advocated in order to overcome these problems but only in the less severe situation because there is a tendency for greater fibrosis in the lower limb. Modern liposuction devices along with the use of tumescent solution and power-assisted cannulae are thought to improve efficacy.[77]

Bypass procedures

These are very rarely performed and are reserved for regional blockage of the lymphatics, due to either primary obstructive or secondary causes. If an iatrogenic secondary cause is suspected, a period of 6 months should elapse to allow any procedural swelling to subside before embarking on a lymphatic bypass. The bypass procedures are listed in Box 18.6.

Skin, muscle and omentum have been used to bypass regional obstructions but these tissues tend to have a paucity of lymphatics and, as the technique relies

Box 18.6 • Bypass procedures for lymphoedema

Skin and muscle flaps
Omental bridges
Enteromesenteric bridges
Lymphatico-lymphatic anastomosis
Lymphatico-venous anastomosis

on the development of new channels, high levels of success have not been reported. The technique of enteromesenteric bridging was designed to overcome this problem. A 10-cm segment of ileum is resected on its mesentery and opened along its antimesenteric border. The mucosa is dissected off, leaving a submucosal area rich in lymphatics and blood vessels. The uppermost normal nodes are identified and bisected. The submucosal patch is then stitched in place over the top. Investigation has shown the early development of a lymphatic bridge and follow-up for 6 years has demonstrated a maintained improvement in 75% of legs, but the numbers are very small.[78]

Autologous lymphatic vessels harvested from the contralateral normal limb are used to perform lymphatico-lymphatic anastomoses and bypass obstruction. A suitable conduit is identified after the injection of patent blue dye into the interdigital spaces. The anastomoses are technically demanding. Limb volumetry reveals initial improvements in 66% of cases but this falls to about 50% at 1 year. Recent studies show that lower limb bypasses maintain improvement for up to 10 years.[79]

Lymphatico-venous anastomosis is physiological if one considers the termination of the thoracic duct at the subclavian vein. Excellent long-term results have been published, with volume reductions on average of 67% lasting more than 7 years in the 85% of patients followed up, along with an 87% reduction in the incidence of cellulitis.[80]

Key points

- CVI is the commonest cause of chronic leg swelling.
- The risk of mild to moderate chronic venous insufficiency after DVT is 30% at 10 years.
- The risk of severe CVI after DVT is 2–10% at 10 years.
- Superficial venous reflux alone may cause CVI.
- Graduated elastic compression is effective in healing ulcers and preventing recurrence.
- Superficial venous surgery may be of benefit in isolated superficial venous incompetence and combined superficial and deep venous incompetence.
- Deep venous reconstructive surgery with endovascular stents is playing an increasingly important role in the treatment of patients with post-thrombotic syndrome; though long-term data are awaited. In young patients with an iliofemoral DVT, thrombolysis should be considered as first-line therapy.
- Lymphoedema may be classified as primary or secondary.
- A further functional classification of obliterative, proximal obstruction, and valvular incompetence and hyperplasia may be used.
- The commonest cause of lymphoedema worldwide is filariasis but in Europe the commonest cause is malignancy and its treatment.
- Oedema is initially pitting, but becomes non-pitting due to subcutaneous fat deposition and fibrosis.
- Ulceration is rare in lymphoedema.
- Diagnosis is usually confirmed by isotope lymphangioscintigraphy.
- Satisfactory treatment can usually be achieved by conservative measures, including manual drainage, elastic compression, complex decongestive therapy and prevention of infection.

● Full references available at **http://expertconsult. inkling.com**

Key references

4. The Alexander House Group. Consensus paper venous leg ulcers. J Dermatol Surg Oncol 1992;18:592–602. PMID: 1624633.
A condensed consensus report summarising the status of various aspects of epidemiology, diagnosis and treatment of venous ulcers. Various investigational and treatment approaches are summarised and recommendations given. Level II evidence.

26. Eklof B, Rutherford RB, Bergan JJ, et al. Revision of CEAP classification for chronic venous disorders: consensus statement. J Vasc Surg 2004;40:1248–52. PMID: 15622385.
This is an international consensus document produced under the auspice of the American Venous Forum that provides a classification for CVI.

29. O'Meara S, Cullum NA, Nelson EA. Compression for venous leg ulcers. Cochrane Database Syst Rev 2009;1:CD000265. PMID: 19160178.
This is a meta-analysis of 39 randomised controlled trials reporting 47 comparisons of compression versus no compression or versus other types of compression in the healing of venous leg ulcers.

30. Nelson EA, Bell-Syer SEM, Cullum NA, et al. Compression for preventing recurrence of venous ulcers. Cochrane Database Syst Rev 2000;4: CD002303. PMID: 11034749.
This is a review of two randomised controlled trials, one of which compared class III stockings with class II stockings and the other compared two different makes of class II stocking in the prevention of ulcer recurrence. Higher grades of compression are associated with lower recurrence rates. Also, not wearing stockings is strongly associated with ulcer recurrence.

32. Nelson EA, Mani R, Thomas K, et al. Intermittent pneumatic compression for treating venous leg ulcers. Cochrane Database Syst Rev 2011;2: CD001899. PMID: 21328252.
This is a review of seven randomised controlled trials; four compared IPC plus compression with compression alone. One of these found increased ulcer healing with IPC, while three found no evidence of benefit. One trial compared IPC without additional compression with compression alone and found no difference, and in one trial more ulcers healed with IPC than with dressings. One trial found that rapid IPC healed more ulcers than slow IPC.

33. Flemming K, Cullum NA. Laser therapy for venous leg ulcers. Cochrane Database Syst Rev 2000;1:CD001182. PMID: 10796615.
Four trials were available, two randomised controlled trials compared laser therapy with sham, one with ultraviolet light and one with red light. Neither of the two randomised controlled trials found a difference in healing rates and there was no significant benefit for laser when the trials were pooled.

34. Aziz Z, Cullum NA, Flemming K. Electromagnetic therapy for treating venous leg ulcers. Cochrane Database Syst Rev 2011;3:CD002933. PMID: 21412880.
This is a review of three randomised controlled trials comparing electromagnetic therapy (EMT) with sham treatment. One small trial of 44 patients reported significantly more ulcers healed in the EMT group, one reported no difference and one reported a greater reduction in ulcer size in the EMT group.

35. Palfreyman SSJ, Nelson EA, Lochiel R, et al. Dressings for healing venous leg ulcers. Cochrane Database Syst Rev 2006;3:CD001103. PMID: 16855958.
This is a meta-analysis of 42 randomised controlled trials evaluating various types of dressings in the treatment of venous leg ulcers. In none of the comparisons was there evidence that any one type of dressing was better than others in terms of the numbers of ulcers healed.

38. Jull AB, Arroll B, Parag V, et al. Pentoxifylline for treating venous leg ulcers. Cochrane Database Syst Rev 2007;3:CD001733. PMID: 17636683.
This is a meta-analysis of 12 trials, 11 of which compared pentoxifylline (oxpentifylline) with placebo or no treatment. Pentoxifylline is more effective than placebo in terms of complete ulcer healing or significant improvement. The relative risk of ulcer healing with oxpentifylline compared with placebo is 1.70.

39. Barwell J, Davies C, Deacon J, et al. Comparison of surgery and compression with compression alone in chronic venous ulceration (ESCHAR study): randomized controlled trial. Lancet 2004;363:1854. PMID: 15183623.
This is a randomised controlled trial of 500 consecutive patients with chronic venous ulcers randomly assigned to compression alone or in combination with surgery to assess the role of superficial venous surgery in the healing and prevention of recurrence of leg ulcers. There was no difference in initial healing rates but a reduction in recurrence at 12 months in the surgical group (12% vs 28%).

47. Janssen MC, Haenen JH, van Asten WN, et al. Clinical and haemodynamic sequelae of deep venous thrombosis: retrospective evaluation after 7–13 years. Clin Sci 1997;93:7–12. PMID: 9279197.
In this study, 81 patients with venographically confirmed lower-extremity DVT were clinically and haemodynamically re-examined 7–13 years after DVT (mean 10 years) to assess PTS; 7–13 years after DVT 31% of the patients had moderate and 2% had severe clinical PTS, while 57% of the patients had abnormal haemodynamic findings. Level II evidence.

68. Badger CM, Peacock JL, Mortimer PS. A randomised, controlled, parallel-group trial comparing multilayer bandaging followed by hosiery versus hosiery alone in the treatment of patients with lymphedema of the limb. Cancer 2000;88:2832–7. PMID: 10870068.

This is a randomised, controlled, parallel-group trial in which 90 women with unilateral lymphoedema (of the upper or lower limbs) underwent 18 days of multilayer bandaging followed by elastic hosiery or hosiery alone, each for a total period of 24 weeks. The reduction in limb volume due to multilayer bandaging followed by hosiery was approximately double that from hosiery alone and was sustained over the 24-week period. The mean overall percentage reduction at 24 weeks was 31% ($n = 32$) for multilayer bandaging versus 15.8% ($n = 46$) for hosiery alone, with a mean difference of 15.2% (95% CI 6.2–24.2, $P = 0.001$). Level I evidence.

19

The acutely swollen leg

Cees H.A. Wittens
Rob H.W. Strijkers

Introduction

The acutely swollen leg is a common presenting complaint in the emergency room. It may represent a sudden presentation of an underlying chronic disease or it may be the manifestation of a new acute problem, in particular deep vein thrombosis (DVT). A number of diseases can be associated with swelling of the lower extremity. It is important to identify the cause of the swelling, as treatment differs greatly depending on the underlying pathology. The underlying diagnosis may be life-threatening and make immediate action necessary, and will also influence long-term prognosis and follow-up.

This chapter will help in the evaluation of the acutely swollen leg and will present up-to-date information on the treatment of DVT.

Pathophysiology of oedema

Acute swelling of the leg is caused by tissue oedema. Oedema formation is caused by excess water accumulation in the interstitial space of the tissue. Reasons for accumulation of water in the interstitial space are increased hydrostatic pressure, decreased colloid osmotic pressure, increased capillary permeability and lymphatic obstruction. These factors cause rapid fluid shifts in the body. There are also chronic states that cause oedema, but these are beyond the scope of this chapter. The mechanisms causing the shift in fluids are described below.

Increased hydrostatic pressure forces fluid out of the intravascular space. This is usually seen with any process that increases venous pressure. Central causes for increase of hydrostatic pressure include congestive heart failure, right heart failure and tricuspid insufficiency. Focal or unilateral oedema is often the result of DVT causing venous outflow obstruction.

Decreased colloid osmotic pressure allows passive transfer of intravascular fluid to the interstitial compartment. This is generally the result of reduction of intravascular protein content (i.e. hypoalbuminaemia). This mechanism causes generalised oedema and is rarely acute.

Increased capillary permeability removes the barrier to water moving from the intravascular space to the interstitial space. This is observed with focal trauma, burns, infection, ischaemia and immunological injury. This can cause rapid oedema forming in a single leg or it can present as a generalised oedema.

Lymphatic obstruction (lymphoedema) may be the result of hereditary hypoplasia, acute infection, or a consequence of lymphatic ablation following surgery, trauma or radiation. The trigger is usually identifiable and presentation is rarely acute.

Medical history

A good medical history from the patient will often raise suspicion regarding the underlying pathology. A previous history of operations on the leg, trauma or a history of DVT may be useful, along with an overview of the patient's general health. There are often several differential diagnoses despite an accurate history. The correct diagnosis, or exclusion of DVT, is essential to prevent potentially life-threatening complications. Consequently, several decision tools have been developed, including the Wells score.[1] It is important to ascertain the precise time point when symptoms began, as this can influence both treatment and prognosis.

Physical examination

Upon examination of the leg, specific features should be identified. The swollen leg may be accompanied by redness, tenderness in the calf and increased temperature. An entry point may be found in cases of erysipelas. Swelling around a specific muscle or muscle compartment may increase suspicion of muscle rupture. Despite a good medical history and thorough physical examination, additional investigations are usually required to confirm a diagnosis. If DVT is suspected, additional imaging may be necessary. Severe pain and loss of sensory and motor function may point towards a compartment syndrome. Skin changes, varicose veins and ulceration of the leg may point towards a chronic venous insufficiency.

Differential diagnosis

There are a few differential diagnoses for the acutely swollen leg. The most frequent cause is a DVT. If DVT is suspected it should be ruled out before any other diagnosis is considered. Other possible causes for acute leg swelling include a ruptured Baker's cyst, erysipelas, cellulitis, fasciitis, muscle rupture or lymphoedema. These causes are mostly limited to one leg. If the patient has swelling of both legs, then alternative causes should be considered, in particular systemic causes such as chronic heart failure, renal failure or sepsis.

Musculotendinous rupture

Sudden intense pain of the calf usually suggests a musculoskeletal aetiology. If associated with sudden dorsiflexion of the foot, rupture of the musculotendinous portion of the medial head of the gastrocnemius muscle or the plantaris muscle (tendon) should be suspected. Localised pain in the medial or mid-calf area and swelling at the ankle level is common. Ecchymotic discolouration at the ankle level often follows 2–5 days later due to blood tracking down the fascial planes when the leg is dependent. Excluding DVT with a venous duplex examination is appropriate.

Treatment consists of symptomatic and supportive care until symptoms resolve. Leg elevation, ice early followed by heat, analgesics and reduced weight bearing may be necessary until symptoms resolve, usually within a month.

Baker's cyst

Patients presenting with sudden, instantaneously severe calf pain and swelling of the leg may suffer from a ruptured Baker's cyst. A Baker's cyst forms as a result of overproduction of synovial fluid secondary to an underlying cause such as degenerative arthritis, meniscal tears, gout or rheumatoid arthritis. It is common among adults, but can occur in children.[2] A Baker's cyst is usually located on the dorsolateral side of the knee. If the cyst bursts, immediate pain occurs, with swelling of the leg and redness, often mimicking a DVT.[3] The Baker's cyst is usually easily identified with duplex ultrasound.[4] Treatment consists of anti-inflammatory medication, leg elevation and application of cold packs.[5]

Cellulitis and erysipelas

Sudden swelling of the leg, combined with redness, pain and increased warmth, is seen in patients with erysipelas or cellulitis. Accompanying complaints can be nausea, vomiting, headaches and fever. The terms erysipelas and cellulitis are both used. There is, however, a small distinction between the two diagnoses. They differ in that erysipelas involves the upper dermis and superficial lymphatics, whereas cellulitis involves the deeper dermis and subcutaneous fat. This manifests in a different presentation in erysipelas, where there is a clear line of demarcation of the redness and the skin involved. In cellulitis there is no clear demarcation visible. Upon physical examination it is important to look for a break in the skin as a portal for entry of bacteria. Common skin barrier breaks are abrasions, insect bites, or tinea pedis. Any fluid coming from the wound should be cultured. The most likely causative bacteria are *Staphylococcus aureus* and Group A streptococci.[6] Treatment comprises antibiotics targeted towards Gram-positive bacteria, rest and elevation. Duplex ultrasound should be considered to exclude DVT. Patients treated for erysipelas or cellulitis should experience symptom improvement within 24–48 hours.

Necrotising fasciitis

Fasciitis is a very serious condition with a high morbidity and mortality. While this may present as excruciating pain,[7] other clinical signs may be absent. Possible clinical signs include erythema, crepitations due to gas formed by subcutaneous bacteria, fever, nausea, vomiting, local oedema, blisters, and necrosis of the skin and underlying structures. The underlying mechanism is a bacterial colonisation of *S. aureus* or Group A streptococci. The micro-organisms produce endotoxins, which cause a severe inflammatory reaction, with destruction of the deep fascia and surrounding structures. Patients with a compromised immune system are more susceptible to infection with opportunistic bacteria. If this situation is left untreated the destruction of the fascia will spread and eventually lead to the death of the patient. Treatment of necrotising fasciitis consists of aggressive surgical debridement of the infected tissues. Broad-spectrum antibiotics should be given to include coverage for Gram-positive, Gram-negative and anaerobic organisms.[8] Additional intensive care support is vital to improve the chance of survival. Even with optimal treatment, the mortality rate is over 30%.[9]

Lymphoedema

Although lymphoedema usually presents as a chronically swollen leg, it can occasionally present acutely. Lymphoedema is the result of impaired lymphatic drainage due to obstruction or destruction of lymphatic tissue. The major causes of lymphoedema can be classified as primary (hereditary) or secondary (acquired). Causes of primary lymphoedema are congenital lymphoedema, lymphoedema praecox and lymphoedema tarda. These causes manifest themselves in childhood (congenital lymphoedema), puberty (lymphoedema praecox) or early adulthood (lymphoedema tarda). Secondary lymphoedema can be caused by malignancy, surgery with lymph dissection, radiation therapy, infection of lymph nodes, recurrent cellulitis or a connective tissue disease. The management of lymphoedema is discussed in Chapter 18.

Bilateral swelling

Swelling of both legs is usually a sign of a systemic problem, such as heart failure, renal failure, liver failure, sepsis, pulmonary hypertension or drugs (non-steroidal anti-inflammatory drugs (NSAIDs) and calcium channel blockers), but it is essential to rule out bilateral DVT or vena caval obstruction. History and examination will usually guide further investigation.[10] If the patient has a bilateral swelling caused by a systemic disease, treatment should focus on the primary cause. If the patient uses calcium channel blockers or NSAIDs, alternatives for these medications can be considered.

Deep venous thrombosis

DVT is very common in the Western world, with an incidence of 1.6 per 1000 persons per year.[11] The incidence of DVT increases exponentially over the age of 70. In people under 18 years of age, DVT is very

uncommon, with an incidence of 0.07 per 10 000 per year.[12] In the 19th century, Virchow postulated the mechanisms for clot formation. The three main mechanisms are stasis of blood, vessel wall damage and hypercoagulability. Once the clot has formed it has the tendency to extend. Thrombosis in calf veins does not usually elicit much in the way of symptoms. Once the clot has propagated in the popliteal vein, symptoms may become more apparent. If the clot further propagates to the femoral vein and common femoral vein, obstructing venous outflow from the leg, more severe symptoms are likely. At the most severe end of the spectrum is phlegmasia cerulea alba or phlegmasia cerulea dolens (see **Fig. 19.1**). These conditions require immediate attention from the physician, because of possible limb ischaemia and loss of the leg.

Pathophysiology of DVT

DVT should be viewed as a dynamic condition, and often results from a combination of risk factors that shift the balance of coagulation to a hypercoagulable state. A number of risk factors have been identified, which can be categorised relating to Virchow's triad (Table 19.1).[13] Thrombus usually forms around valves on the endothelium. In 80% of cases one or more risk factors can be determined in the patient.

Clinical decision rules

Because clinical signs are not very specific for DVT, clinical decision tools have been developed to aid patient management. The Wells score is the most widely used and validated clinical decision tool.[14,15] The patient's risk for having a DVT is assessed by the criteria shown in Table 19.2. The patient is then categorised into either a high- or low-risk group. A Wells score of 2 or more indicates that the patient has a high risk of DVT.[1] A Wells score of 0 or 1 puts the patient in the low-risk group. The Wells

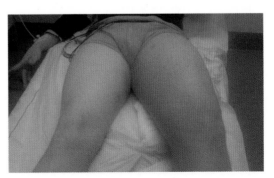

Figure 19.1 • Leg with phlegmasia cerulea dolens.

Table 19.1 • Risk factors for DVT

Risk factor	Hypercoagulability	Stasis	Venous injury
Age	X	X	
Immobilisation		X	
Surgery	X	X	
Trauma	X	X	X
Malignancy	X		
Primary hypercoagulable states	X		
History of DVT	X		
Family history	X		
Oral contraceptives	X		
Oestrogen replacement	X		
Pregnancy and puerperium	X	X	
Entiphospholipid and anticardiolipin antibody	X		
Central venous catheters			X
Inflammatory bowel disease	X		
Obesity		X	
Myocardial infarction/congestive heart failure		X	
Varicose veins		X	

Table 19.2 • Wells score for DVT

Score	Clinical factor
1 point	Active cancer <6 months or palliation
1 point	Paralysis, paresis or recent plaster immobilisation of the lower extremities
1 point	Recently bedridden for more than 3 days or major surgery within 4 weeks
1 point	Entire leg swollen
1 point	Calf swelling by more than 3 cm when compared with the asymptomatic leg
1 point	Pitting oedema
1 point	Collateral superficial veins (non-varicose)
1 point	Previously documented DVT
−2 points	Alternative diagnosis more likely or greater than that of deep vein thrombosis
Total score	
<2	Low risk of DVT
≥2	High risk of DVT

excluding DVT.[16] The clinical decision flow chart is shown in **Fig. 19.2**.

> ✔✔ If the patient has a low Wells score combined with a negative D-dimer, DVT can safely be ruled out without the need for a duplex scan.

Imaging techniques

The current standard for diagnosing a DVT is a two-point duplex scan.[17] The non-invasive two-point ultrasound examination looks at the popliteal vein and the common femoral vein. The physician will compress the vein at these two points. If the vein is non-compressible, the presence of thrombus is proven. Thrombus may also be visible on sonography and venous flow may be absent. Alternative diagnoses, such as a Baker's cyst, may also be identified on ultrasound. If the duplex scan is inconclusive, but the suspicion of DVT is still high, a conventional venogram or other imaging may be considered. Conventional venography is still the gold standard, but duplex ultrasound is much more accessible, less invasive and easier to perform. In cases of recurrent DVT it may prove difficult to differentiate between newly formed thrombus and old residual thrombus. Standardised documentation of the previous thrombus location may be helpful. The size of the vein and the identification of scarring may help guide the clinician, with small scarred veins most likely to represent chronic changes. In experienced hands it is also possible to estimate thrombus age based on homogeneity. A thrombus with a homogenous aspect

score combined with a D-dimer test can guide the clinician with regard to the need for a duplex scan. A patient with either a Wells score of 2 or more and/or positive D-dimer test will need a duplex scan to look for a possible DVT. Conversely, a Wells score of 0 or 1 with a negative D-dimer almost entirely rules out DVT and the patient does not require a duplex scan. Studies show the negative predictive value for this combination of findings to be 99% for

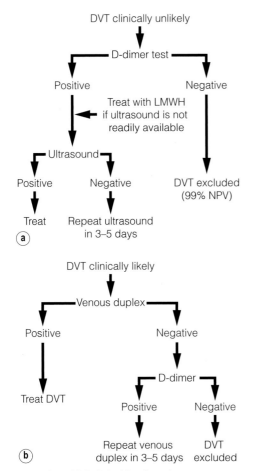

Figure 19.2 • Clinical decision flow chart.

New techniques are becoming more readily available for imaging of the venous system, including computed tomography and magnetic resonance venography. These techniques can be used to identify DVT but are especially useful in determining the precise extent of the thrombus and any underlying stenosis. In particular, the iliac vein segment and the inferior vena cava can be assessed in a simpler manner than with duplex ultrasound.[18,19] These techniques will become very important in identifying patients suitable for more aggressive intervention than standard anticoagulation therapy. New reporting standards have been developed to standardise the scoring of venous disease with different imaging techniques (LOVE score). With these standardised reports it is possible to identify and report DVT systematically and stratify patients into different treatment groups (LET score).[20,21] This will become more important as treatment options advance further. **Figure 19.4** shows a magnetic resonance venograph with a DVT present in the popliteal vein and femoral vein of the left leg.

Treatment of DVT

DVT needs to be treated immediately to prevent potentially lethal pulmonary emboli and to stop thrombus propagation. Standard treatment of DVT as formulated by the American College of Chest Physicians (ACCP) guidelines consists of three aspects, namely oral anticoagulation, compression therapy and mobilisation.[22]

Anticoagulation treatment prevents extension of thrombus and pulmonary embolism. Treatment should be started as soon as the diagnosis has been confirmed or in a patient with a Wells score of 2 or more and/or a positive D-dimer test while awaiting duplex scan confirmation. Anticoagulation is achieved

is more likely to be fresh. It should also be recognised that fresh thrombus may form within a recanalised area of old thrombus. **Figure 19.3** shows a duplex scan of the common femoral vein with intraluminal thrombus.

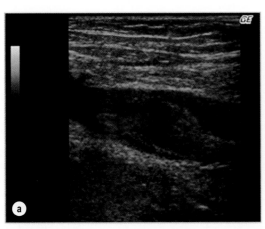

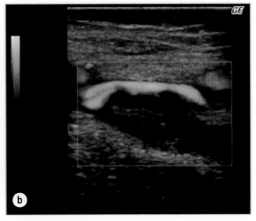

Figure 19.3 • Duplex scan of the common femoral vein with intraluminal thrombus.

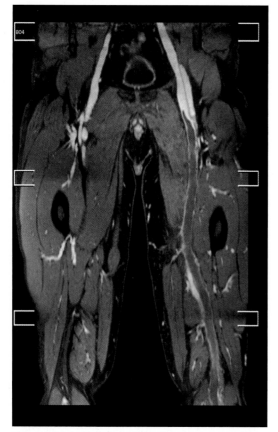

Figure 19.4 • Magnetic resonance venography with a DVT present in the popliteal vein and femoral vein of the left leg.

Hospitalisation for anticoagulation therapy is not necessary and treatment can be performed safely in the community.[28] Anticoagulation has no effect on the existing thrombus, resolution of which depends on the patient's own lytic system.[22,27]

> ✔✔ Patients with DVT should be treated with anticoagulation therapy for at least 3 months.

Compression therapy should be started as soon as possible. In the acute phase with leg oedema, compression therapy can be achieved with short stretch bandages. Once this has reduced the acute swelling, the patient can be switched to therapeutic elastic compressive stockings. The stockings should be to the knee, and effect a minimum pressure of between 30 and 40 mmHg. Current guidelines still advise to wear compression stockings for 2 years based on trials, which show a 50% reduction in post-thrombotic morbidity.[29] However, more recently a randomised controlled trial by Kahn et al. showed no reduction at all in post-thrombotic syndrome (PTS) in the group of patients with compression stockings compared to patients wearing sham stockings.[30] Despite encouragement, patient compliance for compression hosiery is low.

> ✔✔ Patients should wear compressive stockings for 2 years although their effect on preventing post-thrombotic syndrome is currently uncertain.

by immediate subcutaneous administration of therapeutic levels of low-molecular-weight heparins (LMWHs). Oral anticoagulation with vitamin K antagonists (VKAs) can be started simultaneously. Treatment with the LMWHs can be stopped after the international normalised ratio (INR) has reached the therapeutic range for 2 consecutive days. The INR range for a first-time DVT should be between 2 and 3.[22] Since 2012 new oral anticoagulants (NOACs) are available as alternatives for treatment with VKAs. Drugs like rivaroxaban, dabigatran, apixaban and edoxaban have been tested extensively on their effectiveness and safety. The NOACs have shown to reduce the risk of recurrent venous thromboembolic complications (VTE) equal to that of VKAs and are equally safe in regard to bleeding risk.[23–26] Anticoagulation should be given for at least 3 months. Depending on the balance of risk of bleeding and further DVT, the physician can choose to prolong the anticoagulation to 6 or 12 months.[27] Patients with malignancy should be treated with LMWHs for 3–6 months. Patients with a recurrent episode of DVT should be treated with lifelong anticoagulation.

Finally, immediate mobilisation is proven to be safe and does not increase the risk of pulmonary embolism.[31,32]

Thromboprophylaxis is discussed in Chapter 2 of *Core Topics in General and Emergency Surgery* in this Companion to Specialist Surgical Practice series.

Prognosis

If patients are treated according to the ACCP guidelines, the risk of recurrent DVT is 30% within 5 years of the initial DVT.[33] More worrisome is the high incidence of PTS, affecting between 20% and 50% of patients with DVT within 2 years,[34,35] because the variability in reported incidence relates to the use of different scales to assess PTS.[36] Patients with iliofemoral DVT have a twofold increased risk of developing PTS compared with patients with a below-knee DVT.[37] The CaVenT study showed that 56% of patients after iliofemoral DVT develop PTS within 2 years.[38]

Iliofemoral deep vein thrombosis

In iliofemoral DVT the thrombus is located proximally, having extended from the common femoral vein segment or commenced within the iliac veins or inferior vena cava. Thrombus in the common femoral vein obstructs outflow of the superficial and deep femoral vein, usually resulting in marked leg swelling and pain. Severe venous obstruction can result in phlegmasia cerulea dolens. This is a dangerous condition, where the circulation is compromised and may lead to amputation. Current ACCP guidelines suggest that immediate clot removal may be considered in specific patients with low bleeding risks. In all other cases of iliofemoral DVT, anticoagulation is still considered the gold standard,[22] though recent studies have challenged this.[39]

Post-thrombotic syndrome

PTS is a chronic disease following DVT, with significant impacts on patient quality of life and healthcare burden.[3] PTS incorporates a range of patient complaints and physical signs of venous disease. The severity of PTS can be recorded using the validated Villalta–Prandoni scale[40] (Table 19.3). The precise aetiology is unknown, though there are identified risk factors that increase the risk of developing PTS. Obstruction of the venous outflow tract together with

insufficiency, residual thrombus and recurrent DVT are significant risk factors correlating with the development of PTS.[35,41] In particular, poor recanalisation of iliofemoral DVT causes outflow obstruction and a state of venous hypertension, which in turn causes inflammation and vein wall damage.[42–44] The recanalisation process and inflammation also cause valves to be destroyed, resulting in venous insufficiency. Successful early thrombus removal or lysis should avoid these complications and thus lower post-thrombotic morbidity.[45] The concept of lysis is not new. Reports and case series from the 1980s stimulated interest in systemic thrombolytic therapy. While results of clinical trials showed that systemic thrombolysis slightly improved complete clot lysis, the high incidence of major bleeding complications has rendered the technique obsolete.[46,47]

> ✔✔ Systemic thrombolysis should not be given to patients with DVT, because of high major bleeding risk.

However, the severity and chronicity of symptoms is still well recognised,[48] stimulating interest in lysis delivered locally. Catheter-directed lysis has been shown to improve patient quality of life without the high rate of bleeding complications associated with systemic treatment.[49]

Table 19.3 • Villalta–Prandoni scale for post-thrombotic syndrome (also incorporates the presence or absence of venous ulceration)

Symptoms and clinical signs	None	Mild	Moderate	Severe
Symptoms				
Pain	0	1	2	3
Cramps	0	1	2	3
Heaviness	0	1	2	3
Paraesthesia	0	1	2	3
Pruritis	0	1	2	3
Clinical signs				
Pretibial oedema	0	1	2	3
Skin induration	0	1	2	3
Hyperpigmentation	0	1	2	3
Redness	0	1	2	3
Venous ectasia	0	1	2	3
Pain on calf compression	0	1	2	3
Venous ulcer	Absent	Present		
Total score	<5	5–9	10–14	≥15 or venous ulcer
PTS classification	No PTS	Mild PTS	Moderate PTS	Severe PTS

Catheter-directed thrombolysis

Catheter-directed thrombolysis (CDT) involves the placement of a catheter directly into the thrombus and local administration of the thrombolytic agent. The drug activates tissue plasminogen, which is converted into plasmin, which in turn can dissolve the fibrin strands of the clot.[50] Local administration in the thrombus enhances the thrombolytic effects but reduces the bleeding complications, because of the lower dosages needed. Retrospective studies have shown that successful lysis directly correlated with improved health-related quality of life.[51] Recently the randomised controlled CaVenT study showed that patients with iliofemoral DVT treated with catheter-directed thrombolysis had an absolute risk reduction of 14% in developing PTS compared to patients treated with standard therapy after 2 years. After 5 years of follow-up the absolute risk reduction increased to 28%, but quality of life did not differ between the intervention and conservative treatment group.[52]

There was a 3% incidence of major haemorrhage. This is the first randomised controlled trial showing the benefits of early clot removal in iliofemoral DVT with an acceptable bleeding risk.[38] Two other similar trials, ATTRACT and CAVA, are ongoing.[53,54]

The Society for Vascular Surgery (SVS) and American Venous Forum have developed guidelines for the use of CDT and other clot removal techniques (see below).[55] They recommend early thrombus removal in ambulatory patients with good functional capacity and a first episode of iliofemoral DVT of <14 days' duration (level 2c evidence). They strongly recommend such a strategy in patients with limb-threatening ischaemia secondary to iliofemoral DVT (level 1a). The guidelines suggest a role for pharmaco-mechanical strategies over CDT alone if resources are available, and that surgical thrombectomy be considered only if CDT is contraindicated (level 2c).[55]

A meta-analysis has suggested that the evidence for surgical thrombectomy is of low quality, reinforcing the recommendation of the SVS. It does, however, confirm the reduced incidence of PTS and venous obstruction following CDT.[56]

A number of CDT studies have demonstrated underlying iliac vein stenosis as a potential contributing factor for further DVT.[57,58] May–Thurner syndrome is the most prevalent of the stenotic lesions in the left common iliac vein. This syndrome is a condition where the left common iliac vein is compressed by the overlying right iliac artery, as demonstrated in **Fig. 19.5**.[59] Treatment of the underlying stenosis with balloon venoplasty, stenting, or both, can be performed

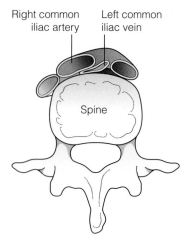

Right common iliac artery   Left common iliac vein

Spine

Figure 19.5 • Schematic overview of the May–Thurner syndrome.

to relieve venous outflow obstruction, though the role of these interventions remains ill-defined.[60,61] As more data become available regarding CDT for iliofemoral DVT, we will obtain greater understanding of the role and appropriate management of underlying iliac vein stenoses.

✔ Patients with iliofemoral DVT should be considered for catheter-directed thrombolysis to reduce the incidence of post-thrombotic syndrome.

New treatment modalities

Although the results of lysis in the CaVenT study are good, the mean treatment time of 2.4 days is considered long. Future techniques will focus on shortening the treatment time, lowering bleeding risk and avoiding the need for expensive intensive care hospitalisation. Therefore, the addition of a mechanical component has been suggested to speed up clot removal. This technique is called pharmaco-mechanical thrombolysis (PMT). Different PMT catheters are commercially available. A number of them are discussed in the next section.

EKOS endowave

The EKOS endowave catheter combines the standard CDT with ultrasound elements. These elements emit high-frequency, low-energy ultrasound waves that enhance the penetration of the thrombolytic drug into the thrombus, enhancing the lytic effect. In vitro studies have shown better permeability of the agent in the thrombus and reduced treatment time. Retrospective

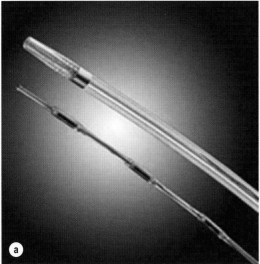
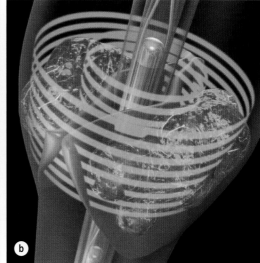

Figure 19.6 • EKOS device.

case series have shown that thrombolysis with the EKOS catheter is feasible and safe. The ongoing randomised controlled Dutch CAVA trial is further investigating the role of the EKOS endowave system in patients with iliofemoral DVT (**Fig. 19.6**).[54]

Angiojet

The Angiojet Power Pulse system (**Fig. 19.7**) uses a complex mixture of rapid fluid streaming and hydrodynamic forces to fracture the thrombus, allowing extraction at the catheter tip as a result of negative pressure (the Bernoulli effect). The catheter infuses normal saline through an infusion port while simultaneously suctioning through the effluent port. If the effluent port is clamped, the infusion port acts as a mechanical 'pulse spray' that delivers the preloaded thrombolytic drug to the thrombus. This is the only device that can be solely used as

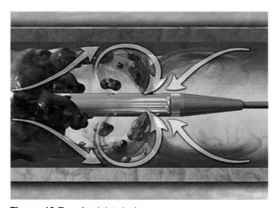

Figure 19.7 • Angiojet device.

a mechanical thrombectomy device. Safety and feasibility of the Angiojet have been demonstrated in retrospective case series only.[62]

Other PMT devices

The AngioVac Cannula (AngioDynamics, Latham, New York) (**Fig. 19.8**) is a mechanical suction device that is designed for removal of intravascular material such as thrombus, tumour, foreign bodies and vegetation, while maintaining flow during extracorporeal circulation. The suction cannula is a 22-Fr device that can be advanced over a wire using an internal dilator. The device has an expandable tip that opens up to 48-Fr. This tip serves as the suction end of a veno-venous non-oxygenating bypass circuit that filters removed blood and returns it to the venous system via a separate reinfusion cannula or sheath. The patient requires general anaesthesia to perform this procedure. Maximum anticoagulation is given to keep the bypass circuit open and a perfusionist monitors it. Evidence for this procedure is limited.

The Aspirex®S 10 F system (Straub medical AG, Wangs, Switzerland) is a new PMT device. The device has a corkscrew-shaped wire on the tip of the catheter, which fragments and aspirates fresh thrombus out of the veins. A close-up view of the tip of catheter is shown in **Figure 19.9**. Data on this device are limited to case reports,

The future

A more aggressive approach to the treatment of iliofemoral DVT will reveal underlying venous anomalies in approximately 50% of patients.[63]

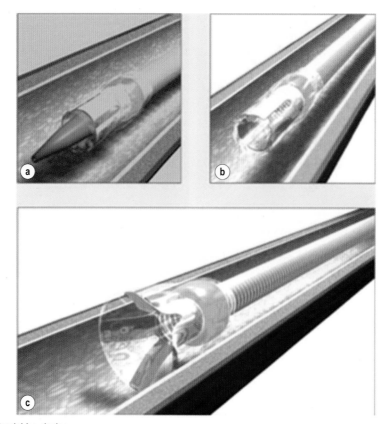

Figure 19.8 • AngioVac device.

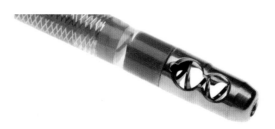

Figure 19.9 • Aspirex device.

Additional treatment of the underlying stenosis may enhance patency and improve the prevention of PTS. The ongoing randomised controlled trials ATTRACT and CAVA will provide us with more data on this subject. Dedicated thrombus removal devices and venous stents may further enhance clot lysis and long-term patency, but randomised clinical trials are essential to define their precise role in clinical practice.

Key points

- Acute leg swelling can indicate a number of diseases. An important differential diagnosis is DVT, which needs to be treated immediately to prevent potentially lethal pulmonary emboli.
- A low Wells score combined with low D-dimer levels is safe for ruling out DVT.
- Duplex sonography is the standard modality to confirm DVT.
- Standard treatment for DVT is oral anticoagulation, compressive stockings and mobilisation.
- Patients with iliofemoral DVT are associated with severe post-thrombotic morbidity and should be considered for additional CDT therapy.

Key references

16. Wells PS, Anderson DR, Rodger M, et al. Evaluation of D-dimer in the diagnosis of suspected deep-vein thrombosis. N Engl J Med 2003;349(13): 1227–35. PMID: 14507948.

    This randomised controlled trial evaluates the value of D-dimer testing in combination with the Wells score in evaluating the chance of the patient having DVT and the ability to safely exclude DVT.

22. Kearon C, Kahn SR, Agnelli G, et al. Antithrombotic therapy for venous thromboembolic disease: American College of Chest Physicians evidence-based clinical practice guidelines. 8th edition. Chest 2008;133(Suppl. 6):445S–54S. PMID: 18574272.

    These guidelines extend a level 1a recommendation for treating DVT with anticoagulation for at least 3 months. These guidelines have been composed after an exhaustive search of multiple studies carefully selected by authorities in the field.

29. Prandoni P, Lensing AWA, Prins MH, et al. Below-knee elastic compression stockings to prevent the post-thrombotic syndrome: a randomized, controlled trial. Ann Intern Med 2004;141(4):249–56. PMID: 15313740.

    This randomised controlled trial compares treatment of DVT with and without compression therapy and the impact on incidence of PTS on both groups.

38. Enden T, Haig Y, Kløw N-E, et al. Long-term outcome after additional catheter-directed thrombolysis versus standard treatment for acute iliofemoral deep vein thrombosis (the CaVenT study): a randomised controlled trial. Lancet 2012;379(9810):31–8. PMID: 22172244.

    The first randomised controlled trial to study the effects of additional CDT on the incidence of PTS in patients with acute iliofemoral DVT.

46. Watson LI, Armon MP. Thrombolysis for acute deep vein thrombosis. Cochrane Database Syst Rev 2004;4:CD002783. PMID: 15495034.

    Systematic review reporting on the effects of systemic thrombolysis for acute DVT. The results show an increase in clot lysis and a decrease in PTS incidence, and also a high rate of major bleeding. Systemic thrombolysis is therefore considered obsolete.

20

Vascular anomalies

Ian McCafferty

Introduction

Vascular anomalies are a complex broad group of developmental abnormalities that present significant challenges in diagnosis and management. The rarity and diverse presentation of vascular anomalies often means patients are seen by multiple specialists, before a correct diagnosis and treatment can be instigated. Accurate and timely diagnosis is crucial, and a multidisciplinary team approach is essential for their appropriate evaluation and management. The exact make-up of the multidisciplinary team varies but vascular surgery, interventional radiology and plastic surgery typically play a central role, along with other specialities, e.g. maxillofacial surgeons, dermatologists and laser specialists.

Mulliken and Glowacki[1] originally proposed a new way of classifying vascular anomalies in 1982, based on the biological and pathological differences of lesions. The classification broadly separates vascular anomalies into two groups: proliferative vascular tumours and vascular malformations. In 1992 Mulliken and Young founded the International Society for the Study of Vascular Anomalies (ISSVA) and the classification was adopted by the society. The classification has been modified over the years as the understanding of vascular anomalies developed. Vascular malformations are due to errors in development at various stages of vasculogenesis or angiogenesis and are further classified on the basis of the main vessel involved: capillary, lymphatic, venous, arterial or combined.

Classification

One of the original aims of ISSVA was to achieve a uniform classification for the understanding and management of vascular anomalies. Following the proposed biological classification by Mulliken and Glowacki in 1982, and adoption by ISSVA in 1992, the system has become widely accepted, helping to resolve the confusing terminology in the field of vascular anomalies. In 2013 a group of experts within ISSVA met to update the classification to include new understanding, and elements of other classification systems, e.g. the Hamburg classification system. This system, described in 1988, separates malformations based on the timing of arrested development of the vascular system. Extratruncal lesions are defects at an early stage of angiogenesis, with immature amorphous vascular tissue and truncal lesions arising from pre-existing mature vascular structures. The updated ISSVA vascular anomalies classification was published in 2014 at the 20th ISSVA workshop. The new classification has updated the proliferative vascular tumour section into benign, locally aggressive or malignant, and the vascular malformation section into simple, combined, named vessel and association with defined syndromes (Table 20.1).

Vascular tumours

Infantile haemangioma

These are the most common benign tumours in children, occurring in 2.5% of all neonates and having a distinct life cycle. Infantile haemangiomata (IH) are not present on the day of birth but usually appear within days to weeks after birth. They are characterised in early infancy (<10 months) by an initial proliferative phase, which can be rapid, followed by an involutional phase leading to spontaneous complete regression in most patients.

Table 20.1 • Vascular malformations associated with other anomalies/syndromes:

Syndrome	Associated vascular malformation
Klippel–Trenaunay syndrome (KTS)	CM + VM ± LM + limb overgrowth
Parkes–Weber syndrome	CN + AVM + limb overgrowth
Servelle–Martorell syndrome	Limb VM + bone overgrowth
Sturge–Weber syndrome	Facial + leptomeningeal CM + eye ± bone and soft tissue
Maffucci syndrome	VM ± spindle cell haemangiomata + enchondroma
Proteus syndrome	CM + VM ± LM + asymmetrical somatic overgrowth
Macrocephaly and microcephaly	CM
CLOVES syndrome	LM + VM + CM ± AVM + lipomatous overgrowth
Bannayan–Riley–Ruvalcaba syndrome	AVM + VM + macrocephaly + limb overgrowth
Rendu–Osler–Weber syndrome	CM
Blue rubber bleb naevus syndrome	VM
Gorham–Stout syndrome	LM

Malformations: CM, capillary; VM, venous; LM, lymphatic; AVM, arteriovenous.

IH occur in 5–10% of Caucasian infants and are three times more common in females. Some 10% have a history of an affected family member and they are more common in prematurity, multiple births and low birth-weights. In 30–50% of individuals a premonitory mark 'herald spot', i.e. focal area of pallor, is present. The precise pathogenesis is unknown; however, IH have a unique phenotype which closely resembles placental vasculature rather than mature cutaneous vasculature, and as such is glucose transporter-1 (GLUT-1)-positive. Cellular markers of angiogenesis, e.g. vascular endothelial growth factor (VEGF), are also increased, especially during the proliferative phase.

The diagnosis is clinical, with lesions having a typical natural history and being warm to palpation, due to the fact that they are high-flow lesions. IH involving the superficial dermis produce lobulated, bright red lesions that are commonly referred to as 'strawberry birthmarks' (**Fig. 20.1**), whereas deep dermal involvement produces a swelling with either no discolouration or a blueness of the skin. Anatomical location plays a critical role in determining whether complications may occur. IH can occur anywhere, although 60% occur in the head and neck region, with their distribution typically along facial developmental subunits.

The proliferative phase of an IH varies in its duration, but rapid growth will usually occur during the first 6–10 months of life, followed by gradually involution of the IH. This process is complete in 50% of individuals by 5 years, in 70% by 7 years, 90% by 9 years and virtually all by 12 years. Residual skin changes following

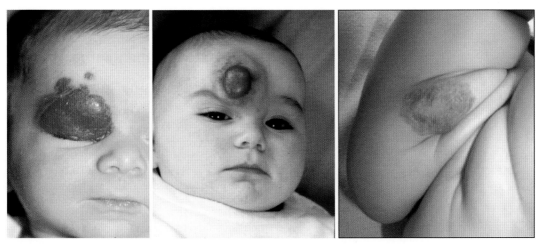

Figure 20.1 • Typical infantile haemangioma with a 'strawberry-like' appearance, a rapidly growing infantile haemangioma and a non-involuting congenital haemangioma.

complete involution are common; in the majority they are mild and inconspicuous, but 20–50% have significant changes of skin distortion and a fibro-fatty remnant.

Diagnosis and imaging

The diagnosis of IH is straightforward based upon the clinical history and examination; imaging is often unnecessary unless there is a concern about associated underlying structural anomalies. It may occasionally be difficult to differentiate deep haemangiomata from other vascular anomalies or tumours; in such instances further investigation, and occasionally biopsy, may be necessary. GLUT-1 positivity on the pathological specimen is pathognomonic.

The imaging features during the proliferative phase are usually characteristic; ultrasound demonstrates a well-defined, reflective lesion that is highly vascular, with central feeding vessels. Magnetic resonance imaging (MRI) will demonstrate a well-defined lobulated tumour that is isointense or hypointense when compared with normal muscle on T1-weighted images and hyperintense on T2-weighted images. If intravenous contrast is given the tumour will enhance avidly and homogeneously.

Complications and structural associations

The majority of complications of IH occur when growth is most rapid in the first 6 months. These include ulceration, bleeding, infection, compromise to vital organs and in rare instances cardiac failure. Cutaneous ulceration is the most common complication, occurring in 10%, and is often when the lesions become painful. Significant bleeding is very uncommon.

- **Amblyopia:** Is a complication of periocular haemangioma. Closure of the eye can lead to occlusion of the visual axis which will prevent light stimulation and result in loss of vision. Close ophthalmic review and early intervention is essential in these cases.
- **Subglottic haemangioma:** Infants with large segmental haemangiomata of the neck and 'beard area' require careful follow-up during the first 12–16 weeks of life as they have a 60% risk of associated airway haemangiomata. These tumours may be life-threatening.
- **PHACE syndrome:** PHACE syndrome[2] (an acronym for: Posterior fossa; Haemangioma; Arterial anomalies; Coarctation of the aorta and other cardiac defects; Eye abnormalities) describes the association between large segmental facial haemangiomata and several structural abnormalities. Affected individuals are nearly always female and the haemangioma most commonly involves the upper face and forehead, but this is not invariable. A child with such a lesion should be carefully examined for signs and symptoms of the syndrome and appropriate investigations should be performed to exclude associated anomalies, especially heart and aorta.

Management

Haemangiomata are extremely heterogeneous in location, size and growth characteristics. The majority of the smaller lesions can be treated conservatively with parent information and clinic visits to wait for resolution after the involuntary phase. Intervention is indicated when a lesion causes significant mass effect or disfigurement, when it involves the airway and when it obstructs the visual axis or in the presence of secondary complications. The mainstay of management is medical, with treatment with beta-blockers the preferred first-line therapy.[3] Bleomycin injections have also been used to treat complications of ulceration and vision as first-or second-line therapy.[4] Occasionally, in visceral haemangioma particulate embolisation techniques are required to treat severe bleeding or cardiac failure.

The surgical management of haemangioma can be divided into two main areas. Early surgery, during the proliferative phase, is generally reserved for lesions obstructing the visual axis when more conservative measures have failed, following partial or complete involution, between the ages of 3 and 5 years, and may be considered for persistent cosmetic deformity or when a large haemangioma persists and is having a detrimental effect on the child's social development because of its appearance. The surgical scar that is likely to result from such an operation should, however, be weighed against the likely outcome if the haemangioma were allowed to involute completely.

Congenital haemangioma

These haemangiomata differ in their natural history and prognosis when compared with infantile haemangiomata.[5] They are rare, with an estimated incidence of 0.3%. They are present and fully grown at birth and often regress rapidly before 1 year of age, remain stable or partially involute. On this basis, they have been divided into two main distinct groups: rapidly involuting congenital haemangiomata (RICH) and non-involuting congenital haemangiomata, (NICH) (**Fig. 20.2**). Both types are histologically and immunophenotypically distinct from infantile haemangiomata; they are high-flow lesions composed of capillary lobules where endothelial cells do not

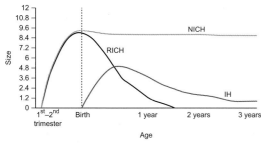

Figure 20.2 • Evolution scheme of natural history of untreated infantile haemangioma and congenital haemangioma (NICH and RICH). IH appears after birth and grows rapidly before stabilising. CHs are fully-grown at birth, with RICH involuting rapidly and NICH persisting. (For abbreviations, see text.)

express GLUT-1 positivity and are associated with large extralobular veins, arteries and lymphatics. RICH may be associated with transient thrombocytopenia and consumptive coagulopathy.

Tufted angioma

Tufted angiomas (TA) appear as brown or erythematous plaques in children and young adults. Occasionally they are present at birth and can be associated with hyperhidrosis or hypertrichosis. Tufted angiomas are composed of small tufts of capillaries characteristically surrounded by a crescentric slit-like vessel dispersed throughout the dermis in a cannonball pattern.

Kaposiform haemangioendothelioma (KHE)

Kaposiform haemangioendotheliomas (KHE) are rare lesions that may affect the skin but often affect deeper tissues and organs, e.g. liver. They are high-flow lesions and can occur as a focal abnormality or as diffuse organ involvement. The majority present in early infancy. Histologically, KHE resembles a tufted angioma with larger and tumour lobules in a more infiltrative pattern.

Both TA and KHE tumours express lymphatic endothelial markers and are GLUT-1 negative. Many authors consider the two tumours to be part of a spectrum rather than distinct entities. Both may be associated with the life-threatening Kasabach–Merritt phenomenon (KMP), which is characterised by profound thrombocytopenia and a severe consumption coagulopathy and is associated with a high mortality. KMP is not a complication of the common infantile haemangioma[6] and should not be confused with the less profound coagulopathy that may be associated with large venous malformations.

Vascular malformations

Vascular malformations are believed to be present at birth, but they may not become evident clinically for many years. They are sporadic and persist for life, never spontaneously regress and commonly may undergo periods when they increase in size and become painful.[7] This is most common during puberty or pregnancy, or following trauma or spontaneous thrombosis (a triggering event is not always recognised). They can be localised or diffuse lesions, which do not respect anatomical boundaries, and their clinical presentation, and prognosis is often dependent on degree of anatomical involvement. They are most conveniently divided into low-flow and high-flow subsets, a differentiation that is usually evident on clinical examination (see in subsections below). Low-flow malformations are further subdivided into capillary, venous and lymphatic subtypes, which may exist as a single entity, combined or associated with other anomalies in syndromes as described in updated 2014 ISSVA classification. High-flow malformations are termed arteriovenous malformations (AVMs) and are further subdivided on the basis of the predominant level of fistulous communication.

Capillary malformations

Capillary malformations come in a variety of forms.

Salmon patch (naevus simplex; erythema nuchae)

A salmon patch is a red macule present at birth, which most commonly involves the skin of the nape of the neck, the upper eyelids or glabella. It is usually central, does not follow a dermatomal distribution and will usually fade by 2 years of age, especially if it involves the skin of the face; the nuchal lesion is more likely to persist into adult life.

Port-wine stains (naevus flameus)

Port-wine stains are well-demarcated vascular stains that are present at birth and increase in size commensurately with the child's growth. They are relatively uncommon and have an equal sex distribution. They tend to follow a dermatomal distribution and are usually unilateral, although they may occasionally cross the midline. Those involving the face are usually flat in early childhood but have a tendency to become thickened and nodular over time and may be associated with bony and soft-tissue hypertrophy. Most of these facial lesions occur as an isolated abnormality but some are part of a syndrome complex, e.g. Sturge–Weber syndrome,[8] which describes the triad of a facial port-wine stain in a V1 distribution, an ipsilateral leptomeningeal vascular malformation and a choroidal vascular malformation of the eye that can cause glaucoma. MRI is helpful to document an intracranial abnormality, although only 10% of children with a port-wine stain in the V1 distribution will have the syndrome.

Low-flow vascular malformations

These have a varied clinical presentation depending on whether the lesions are focal or diffuse and which anatomical compartments are involved. They are present at birth, although they may not be apparent until adolescence or adulthood, and can fluctuate at certain times e.g pregnancy. Venous malformations are the commonest low-flow entity, with a prevalence of 1% in the general population. These lesions are often described as having the 'iceberg phenomenon' as the portion clinically apparent is often the tip of the underlying abnormality.[9]

A detailed history and clinical examination commonly reveals the diagnosis and can help differentiate from other sinister pathology, e.g. sarcoma. Clinical features are typically related to the focal mass and patients present with pain and swelling, often intermittent and associated with acute flare-ups lasting 3–5 days. Clinical features that are atypical for low-flow vascular malformations, including a short clinical history with rapid increase in size or pain, a poor response to treatment or atypical imaging, should lead to a percutaneous biopsy to ensure the correct diagnosis and to exclude the rare mimics of these malformations, e.g. angiosarcoma, low-grade sarcoma, B-cell lymphoma, Ewing's tumour.

Vascular malformations tend not to respect anatomical boundaries and the prognosis, to some degree, depends on the tissues involved. The Birmingham classification[10] defined malformations dependent on the level of tissue involvement from skin to bone, eye and peritoneum and association with syndromes as identified on MRI imaging. The classification defined four types (1–4), which increased in complexity and difficulty in management (Table 20.2).

Low-flow venous malformations (LFVM)

Venous malformations consist of dilated venous spaces of varying size, within which blood flow is slow. They vary considerably in size and can be focal or diffuse. The morphology of venous malformations is dependent on the composition of degree and size of the vascular spaces to cellular matrix component. They can be subdivided into those with macrovascular spaces, matrix-rich (solid) or mixed lesions. This is an important distinction for treatment planning and prognosis. They occur anywhere in the body but are most common in the head and neck and limbs. Most commonly the LFVM causes a dull ache accentuated by activity, extremes of temperature, Valsalva manoeuvre or dependency. Frequently there are more severe bouts of pain, secondary to localised thrombophlebitis. There is frequently a localised coagulopathy with low fibrinogen levels and raised D-dimers.[11] The extent of symptoms depends on the size, location and proximity to adjacent structures. Superficial lesions often exhibit a bluish discolouration and can be associated with dilated veins. On examination, the lesions are characteristically soft, compressible, non-pulsatile and demonstrate filling on dependency (**Fig. 20.3**). Phleboliths are pathognomonic and 75% progress during adolescence.[12] Most venous malformations are single but they may rarely be multiple or combined with capillary, lymphatic and high-flow lesions or as part of syndromes like the blue rubber bleb naevus or Bean syndrome. Most of these cases are sporadic, although some are inherited in an autosomal dominant fashion.

Low-flow lymphatic malformations (LFLM)

Lymphatic malformations are best subclassified into macrocystic and microcystic lesions; although there is no agreed definition, most authors consider macrocystic lesions as those that can be easily accessed with a small needle to administer therapy.

Table 20.2 • The Birmingham classification of low-flow vascular malformations

	Limbs	Head and neck	Trunk
Type 1	Superficial (skin and subcutaneous tissue) (a) Localised (b) Diffuse		
Type 2	Fascia/muscle involvement	Fascia/muscle/mucosa involvement	Fascia/muscle involvement
Type 3	Bone/joint involvement	Bone/joint/airway involvement	Spinal/central nervous involvement
Type 4	Diffuse whole limb involvement ± hypertrophy (e.g. Klippel–Trenaunay)	Ocular/intracranial involvement	Intraperitoneal involvement

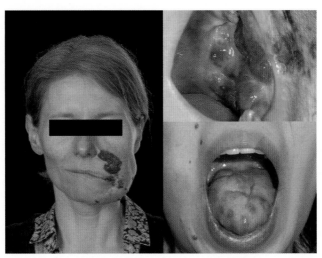

Figure 20.3 • Typical clinical features of a low-flow venous malformation that affects skin and mucosal surfaces; blue discolouration with mass effect that exhibits dependency.

Most are evident at birth but some may not become apparent until early childhood. Macrocystic LFLMs most commonly affect the head and neck, trunk and extremities (90%); lesions do not exhibit dependency, are not compressible but transilluminate. Microcystic LFLMs can infiltrate tissues, most commonly skin and mucous membranes but they can also affect bone and organs. They have a typical clinical appearance, with multiple vesicles overlying the affected area, which often bleed, leak lymph and are frequently complicated by infections, which cause acute expansion and pain. LFLM lesions are most likely to progress during adolescence.

Diagnosis and imaging

The vast majority of low-flow vascular malformations are diagnosed with a detailed history and examination. Usually one can differentiate them further into lymphatic and venous types based on anatomical position, features of dependency (LFVM) and transillumination (LFLM). Imaging is primarily required to identify the extent of tissue involvement, confirm the diagnosis and plan treatment options (conservative, percutaneous sclerotherapy or surgery).[13] The most useful imaging is ultrasound (US) and magnetic resonance imaging (MRI). Angiography has no role and direct stick venography will be discussed later.

Ultrasound is portable and can be performed in clinic at the time of outpatient attendance. A malformation typically appears as a low reflective or heterogeneous defined mass lesion, which can be unilocular, multilocular or solid (matrix-rich, or post haemorrhage). Duplex US can help differentiate LFVMs from LFLMs by demonstrating low-velocity flow within the lesion, although in up to 20% of LFVMs no flow is seen. It should be noted that US has limitations with depth penetration and assessment of associated structures such as nerves, bone and defining the extent of lesions not located in the extremities.

MRI is the imaging modality of choice as it has superior contrast resolution to identify soft-tissue involvement. The assessment with MRI can give prognostic information and should include a description of the extent – focal, multifocal or diffuse, tissues involved, including joint involvement, and evidence of prior haemorrhage. There are numerous MRI protocols described in the literature but a simple approach is to optimise imaging to identify slow-moving fluid – lymph or blood. T1-weighted imaging defines anatomy and the presence of previous haemorrhage and fat suppression techniques (either fast spin-echo T2-weighted or short inversion time inversion recovery, STIR) to increase lesion detection by suppressing the bright fat surrounding the bright LFVM (**Fig. 20.4**). The addition of contrast imaging is useful to aid differentiation of low-flow vascular malformations; LFLMs demonstrate peripheral enhancement whereas LFVMs enhance homogeneously throughout the lesion and help in identifying a differential diagnosis, e.g. vascular tumour.

Management

A multidisciplinary team approach is essential for the best patient outcomes, with the aim of treatment to improve symptoms and the cosmetic appearance.[13,14] The management of LFVMs and LFLMs can be considered together as there is much overlap in the techniques, although the agents used for treatment may differ slightly. The majority of patients only require assessment and advice of the diagnosis and natural history, along with made-to-measure compression garments

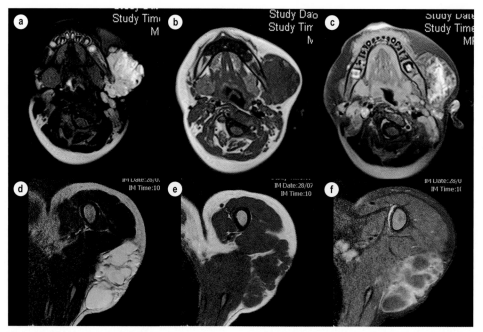

Figure 20.4 • MRI features of low-flow vascular malformations. Both show similar appearances on the T2-W **(a, d)** and T1-W **(b, e)** sequences. Venous malformations **(a–c)** demonstrate central homogeneous enhancement **(c)** whereas lymphatic malformations demonstrate peripheral edge enhancement post IV gadolinium **(f)**.

and treatment of complications, e.g. infection, thrombophlebitis. When patients are particularly symptomatic there are essentially two treatment options available: direct stick sclerotherapy or surgery.

Direct stick sclerotherapy (DSS) is a minimally invasive technique that uses ultrasound and fluoroscopy to guide needle access into the vascular malformation to allow the safe and controlled instillation of a sclerosant agent. Once the needle has been image-guided into the lesion, contrast can be instilled under fluoroscopy to confirm intralesional position and outline the malformation. In LFVMs this direct stick venography (DSV) classifies the malformation using the Puig system.[15] There are a variety of sclerosant agents used which aim to destroy the endothelial linings of venous and lymphatic malformations[16] (**Fig. 20.5**). Each agent has its own unique technique for use and safety profile, and it is essential that operators have a detailed knowledge of these agents in order to manage these patients.[13] Agents commonly used to treat these malformations are sodium tetradeycl sulphate (STS),[17] ethanol, bleomycin,[18] doxycycline and picibanil (OK432). These agents are injected into the malformations in either their liquid form or more commonly in LFVMs as a foam using a 1:2 or 1:3 mix with air/CO_2 using the Tessari method.[19] In matrix-rich LFVMs and microcystic LFLMs bleomycin treatment has become first-line;[4,17] furthermore, some authors are combining sclerosant

therapies when lesions are mixed or contain both cystic and solid components.

Surgery has traditionally been used to treat low-flow malformations and there are a number of surgical techniques employed.[20] There is, however, a high recurrence rate for these lesions and surgery can potentially be quite morbid. The use of surgery after sclerotherapy for cosmetic reasons has been suggested and in very large malformations there is some logic to debulking surgery to prevent secondary compression effects and then treat remaining areas with DSS.

High-flow vascular malformations

Arteriovenous malformations (AVMs) are defects of the circulatory system that can arise during fetal development or be acquired after birth. Many, however, do not become apparent until puberty or even adult life. Progression of AVMs may also occur in response to pregnancy or trauma; trauma may be accidental or iatrogenic (e.g. surgery).

AVMs typically present clinically with a pulsatile soft-tissue swelling associated with pain and discomfort or due to symptoms due to complications. Clinical examination with palpation demonstrates the high-flow nature of the lesion and the complications of AVMs, including thinning of the overlying skin, skin discolouration, frank ulceration, infection and bleeding, should be documented. AVMs are classified utilising

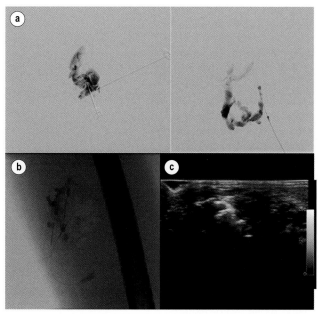

Figure 20.5 • Direct stick sclerotherapy with needle placement into the venous malformation. Venography confirms intralesional position **(a)**; post foam sclerotherapy air can be seen within the malformation on fluoroscopy **(b)** and ultrasound **(c)**.

a clinical classification developed by Schobinger (Table 20.3), which is a simple grading system (1–4) that aids decision-making in the timing of intervention. Biopsy should be performed only if there are any atypical history or clinical features to exclude differential diagnosis of a vascular soft-tissue tumour. An acquired post-traumatic arteriovenous fistula (AVF) may have an identical appearance on clinical examination to that of an AVM, except there is typically a history of previous blunt trauma or penetrating injury. A single fistulous communication is usually present and this will sometimes be the first indication of this diagnosis; appropriate embolisation often results in a cure.

Diagnosis and imaging:

The diagnosis of an AVM is typically clinical although deep-seated lesions may be less obviously pulsatile. US examination aids detection of an arteriovenous signal and reveals high flow with loss of normal venous damping on Doppler studies. MRI is the mainstay of diagnostic non-invasive imaging for AVMs for a number of reasons. AVM is a term that is commonly used (incorrectly) for all vascular malformations and cross-sectional imaging with

Table 20.3 • Schobinger clinical grading system for AVMs

Grade 1	Quiescent – stable
Grade 2	Enlargement – growth
Grade 3	Symptomatic – pain, bleeding
Grade 4	Decompensation – high-output cardiac failure

protocols similar to those used in low-flow vascular malformations will ensure the correct diagnosis, as well as identify combined complex malformations. AVMs typically demonstrate flow voids on both the T1- and T2-weighted sequences with lack of mass lesion; fatty hypertrophy and muscular atrophy are frequently associated. Gadolinium-enhanced magnetic resonance angiography (MRA) can be performed to identify the vascular anatomy, although the spatial resolution is poor when compared to formal angiography. New sequences are being developed and image quality is significantly improving, e.g. Siemens TWIST (Time-resolved angiography With Interleaved Stochastic Trajectories). TWIST is a time-resolved 3D MRA technique with very high temporal and spatial resolution, that can capture multiple vascular phases.

Catheter angiography is an invasive procedure that is essential to understand the morphology of an AVM and plan treatment, which may be endovascular or combined with surgery following embolisation. The procedure can be performed just prior to treatment but more commonly is a separate investigation to allow all interested parties to understand and plan the treatment in these most complex patients.

AVMs are abnormal communications between an artery and a vein and are classified based on the level of communication using the Houdart system[21] described in 1993:

Type I: Arteriovenous. AVMs with a 'nidus' (first venous component) that is supplied by three or fewer arterial pedicles.

Type II: Arteriolovenous. AVMs with a 'nidus' (first venous component) that is supplied by more than three (often very many) arterial pedicles.

Type III: Arteriolovenulous. AVMs with communications that are minute and numerous such that they cannot be separately identified from multiple 'nidi' at a distance.

Cho et al. modified this classification system in 2006 by developing a type IIIa and type IIIb and linked classification type to clinical outcome following embolisation. The type III lesions were the commonest (60%) and the most difficult to treat.[22]

Management

AVMs that are quiescent, not associated with significant symptoms and cause little in the way of cosmetic deformity are usually best left alone. Patients should be informed that a change in the malformation might warrant re-evaluation. Patients with symptomatic AVMs who require treatment are often best managed by embolisation, although surgical excision or debulking, often combined with embolisation, may be necessary in some individuals.

The general principle of embolisation is that occlusion is performed at the site of the abnormal arteriovenous shunts; this is defined as the first dilated segment of vein and is referred to as the 'nidus' and acts as a venous sump that drives the AVM. This entity is paramount to the successful treatment of an AVM with embolisation. If one considers the 'nidus' as a traffic roundabout, with multiple roads entering and exiting the roundabout as feeding arteries and draining veins, then one can understand that only blocking the roundabout itself will prevent travel; blocking a feeding artery or draining vein will not. There are a number of access routes that can successfully be used to treat AVMs: transarterial (TA), direct stick (DS) and transvenous (TV).[23,24] The best approach is to treat each AVM case by case, depending on site, Houdart classification and choice of embolic agent (**Fig. 20.6**). However, commonly DS or TV approaches best treat these lesions as they give the best access to the nidus (venous sump). When used with a liquid embolic agent such as sodium tetradecyl sulphate or absolute alcohol, then a long-term improvement in symptoms can be achieved with total obliteration. Type I and type II lesions are particularly suited to this form of treatment. New liquid embolic agents that are controllable and pushable are now on the market and have opened up opportunities to treat some of the most complex type III AVMs in the periphery and brain via a TA approach. Onyx (Medtronic) and PHIL (Microvention) are ethylene vinyl alcohol copolymers mixed with a radio-opaque agent for visualisation that are cohesive and can be pushed through very small arteries in the nidus segment to achieve success.

AVMs with a largely intraosseous component are especially well suited to treatment by this method of embolisation because they usually have a type II (arteriolovenous) anatomy and are usually best approached by a direct, transosseous, puncture of the dilated venous component of the malformation.

With developments in embolic materials and catheter equipment, primary treatment of AVMs should be endovascular and surgery has a secondary role either as a planned staged procedure to improve the aesthetics following embolisation or to treat skin complications. These surgical techniques often require complex plastic surgery with the use of tissue expansion and muscular flap transfer techniques. Surgery is performed as a primary procedure only if the AVM can be totally excised and even then preoperative embolisation may be very helpful by reducing the vascularity of the AVM. It is important not to embolise feeding vessels with coils or plugs even when distal embolisation has been performed with particles, as this will only hamper future angiographic assessment or treatment if the malformation recurs.

Follow-up and outcomes

The best results are achieved in dedicated specialist centres with multidisciplinary malformation teams able to provide all aspects of care in these complex patients. Treatment is mainly aimed at symptomatic improvement and prevention of progression/complications in this heterogeneous group of congenital anomalies. The outcomes of vascular tumours are highly dependent on early and accurate diagnosis and implementation of the appropriate treatment pathway. Within the vascular malformation group the outcome is determined predominately by patient education, managing patient expectations and treating the appropriate cohort of patients where the benefits of sclerotherapy or embolisation significantly outweigh potential serious complications, e.g. skin loss, neuropraxia and muscle loss.

Sclerotherapy procedures for low-flow malformations frequently require a course of treatment rather than a single session to obtain satisfactory patient symptom improvement. Outcomes are better for localised malformations involving superficial structures or focal intramuscular lesions. Those involving multiple compartments and that are multifocal fare worse, but treatment can still be focused on the symptomatic areas within. Microcystic LFLMs have always been a significant challenge, however, work by

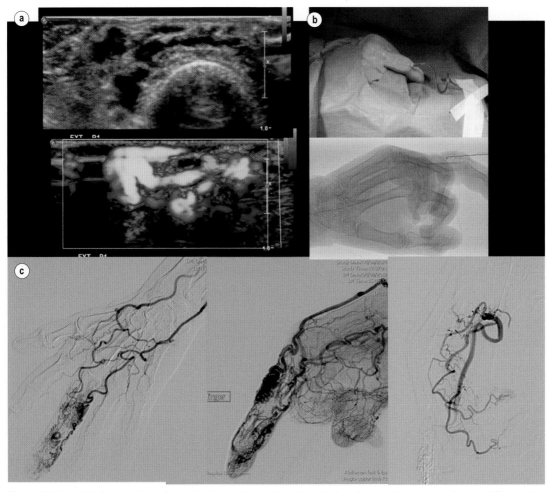

Figure 20.6 • High-flow malformation of the finger demonstrated on duplex ultrasound and colour Doppler **(a)** treated with direct stick 'nidus' puncture **(b)** following placement of a super-selective catheter to outline the AVM by angiography before and after Fibrovein (STS 3%) injection under orthopaedic tourniquet control **(c)**.

Muir et al. has demonstrated remarkable results using intralesional bleomycin injections.

AVMs represent a significant challenge and it is clear that the outcomes are worse for the higher-type lesions.[21] Outcomes significantly improve with a full understanding of the AVM morphology and appropriate access to achieve nidal ablation. Whilst a significant number of type I and II lesions have good long-term success rates, in the type IIIa and IIIb AVMs one can often only achieve a downgrading, in terms of Schobinger grade and angiographic complexity. This is very important for the patient but often means that repeat treatments are inevitable.

Conclusions

Vascular anomalies are simply classified into vascular tumours and vascular malformations. The common haemangioma of infancy makes up the vast majority of the former group and most of these will involute spontaneously without the need for active intervention.

Vascular malformations are difficult to treat successfully and a cure is unlikely. Patients with these anomalies are best treated in specialised units providing multidisciplinary expertise, including diagnostic and interventional radiology and surgery.

Key points

- Vascular anomalies are classified into vascular tumours and vascular malformations.
- The commonest vascular tumour is the infantile haemangioma.
- The majority of infantile haemangiomata require no treatment.
- Vascular malformations are inborn errors of vasculogenesis and persist throughout life.
- Vascular malformations are most conveniently classified into high- and low-flow lesions.
- A significant proportion of vascular malformations do not require treatment.
- Venous and lymphatic malformations may cause marked disfigurement.
- The main treatment of symptomatic venous and lymphatic malformations is direct stick sclerotherapy.
- Large venous malformations may have a localised coagulopathy with low fibrinogen and elevated D-dimers, which may result in severe bleeding during surgery.
- High-flow malformations are equally difficult to manage and may require multimodality treatment, including embolisation and surgery.
- An understanding of the angioarchitecture of a high-flow malformation is essential as this influences the approach to treatment and predicts the likely response to embolisation.

Full references available at **http://expertconsult. inkling.com**

Index

F

G

H